harness your hormones and
get your cycle working for you

period power.

maisie hill

GREEN TREE
LONDON · OXFORD · NEW YORK · NEW DELHI · S

GREENTREE
Bloomsbury Publishing Plc
50B edford Square, London, WC1B 3DP, UK
29 Earlsfort Terrace, Dublin 2, Ireland

BLOOMSBURY, GREEN TREE and the Green Tree logo are trademarks of
Bloomsbury Publishing Plc

First published in Great Britain 2019

Text copyright © Maisie Hill, 2019
Illustrations © Jasmine Parker, 2019

Maisie Hill has asserted her right under the Copyright, Designs and
Patents Act, 1988, to be identified as Author of this work

A catalogue record for this book is available from the British Library

Library of Congress Cataloguing-in-Publication data has been applied for

ISBN: TPB: 978-1-4729-6361-1; ePub: 978-1-4729-6358-1; ePDF: 978-1-4729-6359-8

20

Typeset in Minion Pro by Deanta Global Publishing Services, Chennai, India
Printed and bound in Great Britain by CPI Group (UK) Ltd, Croydon, CR0 4YY

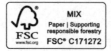

FSC
www.fsc.org

MIX
Paper | Supporting
responsible forestry
FSC® C171272

To find out more about our authors and books visit www.bloomsbury.com
and sign up for our newsletters

To Mum, for sowing the seeds of everything in this book.
And to Christine, for bringing them all to life.

HOW TO USE THIS BOOK

Section One is all about understanding your body and I've done my best to avoid it feeling like the biology lessons that you might have struggled with in school. That being said, if it feels a bit science-heavy for you at the moment, it's totally okay for you to skip ahead to The Cycle Strategy in Section Two so that you can start implementing it, and refer back to Section One when you want to. You'll also find a glossary on page 314, so if there's a term that you're unsure of, head there for a quick explanation.

CONTENTS

INTRODUCTION

In my profession as a women's health specialist I get asked a lot of questions; questions that my clients have had since they were 13 that they still don't have the answers to in their thirties. Questions that usually begin with why, such as:

- Why is my period so painful/short/light/long/heavy?
- Why are they so frequent/irregular/rare?
- Why have they stopped altogether?
- Why do I feel so great one week and so bloody awful the next?
- Why is my vagina so dry/wet/sensitive?
- Why does sex hurt sometimes/all the time?
- Why don't I want to have sex?
- Why am I so horny?
- Why am I so goddamn tired all the time?
- Why do I get so bloated that my dress size jumps up by two sizes?
- Why do I feel anxious/stressed/depressed?
- *Why am I so filled with rage?*

The answer to all those questions is – it's your hormones. Apart, that is, from the rage you feel; that rage is because women do the bulk of unpaid work and emotional labour in society, and that shit is exhausting, so it's your hormones that are trying to alert you to this gross imbalance.

Hormones rule the lives of all humans – not just women. They are the chemical messengers, secreted by the glands in your body, which travel through your bloodstream to their target organs and tissues, giving instruction on processes that need to be carried out in order to regulate your health and behaviour. When you feel hangry (hungry and angry) they tell you that you need to eat something, when you're stressed they get your blood pumping so that you can put up a fight or do a runner, and at the end of the day they let you know that it's time to go to bed. They also control your menstrual cycles and cause or contribute towards the variations in energy, mood, sexual desire, and changes to your body and behaviour that you experience as you transition through each menstrual cycle.

In the coming chapters, I'm going to give you all you need to make sense of your cycle. I'll offer accessible and practical suggestions through which you can improve your symptoms, and we'll focus on particular milestones that require an altered approach, such as the teen years, using hormonal birth control, infertility, pregnancy, motherhood and the perimenopausal years. This is The Cycle Strategy, which you'll come to know as your secret weapon when it comes to improving your relationships, career and health.

You'll discover how to attune your daily life with your cycle, *where possible*. I don't expect that you'll be able to make changes to your daily life in order to cater to every variation that you experience, because let's face it, who can? But I'm confident that you'll be able to make some adjustments here and there, and when you aren't able to, you'll make compensations that make the trickier days that bit easier. At the very least you'll simply be aware of what's going on and, instead of berating yourself, you'll talk to yourself with more kindness and love. It's The Cycle Strategy that I find to be truly transformational because it gives you a blueprint to work with your particular experience of your cycle – whatever that may be – so that you can get to grips with your cycle once and for all.

Before we get started, there's a few things that I'd like to make clear. This is a book about improving hormonal and menstrual health, and I am a huge believer in the health benefits of having a menstrual cycle as well as how it can benefit your life. There's no judgement from me though if you choose to use hormonal birth control like the pill which turns the menstrual cycle off. I do, however, find its prevalence in being prescribed to treat menstrual cycle issues disturbing, not least because although it may provide relief from some symptoms, it can't actually treat the issues. But anything that you choose to do for your mental or physical health, or situation in life, is up to you. It's your body, and your life, and I encourage you to tune in to your own wisdom.

Period Power is a no-nonsense guide to your hormones and your cycle. I'll give you the scientific basis for why each season of your cycle gifts you with a set of superpowers, and the pitfalls to watch out for. We are all different and science doesn't have all the answers, but your curious spirit might!

I'm not by any means including all the research that's out there. I've had to make judgements about what to include and what not to, and when you consider that someone might do a PhD thesis on just one of the topics in this book, you can imagine the scale and scope of what I've left out. You can, of course, use what I have included to go off and do your own research, and the Resources and References sections at the back will help you to do so.

In this book I'll give you a practical set of tools to do the in-depth internal work required to prepare you for all of life's challenges, including the demands of having a career and possibly juggling it with your relationships and potentially motherhood too. But I make no assumption in this book that you are someone who wants to be in a relationship, have children, or that you identify as female. Most reproductive and sex education resources still use cissexist language and frameworks, such as gendering hormones as 'male' or 'female' and referring to all people who have a womb as 'women', but this is problematic. When we talk about testosterone as a 'male' hormone, we attribute what it's associated with – ambition, sexual desire, and muscle mass – with men, and that does those of us with female reproductive systems a disservice because these factors are important in our lives too. Not everyone who is a woman has a menstrual cycle or womb, and not everyone who has a menstrual cycle and a womb is a woman. I want to acknowledge that people of all gender identities can have a menstrual cycle and have avoided the use of pronouns in order to keep language inclusive and reflective of this diversity. My use of the term 'menstruator' is not always ideal, because if you're not currently menstruating then you may not feel that it applies to you, and there will be people who feel that it reduces them to a bodily function. Using 'people with periods' goes some way to improve this, though it doesn't resolve the issue if you're not currently menstruating. In cases where I have used 'girls' and 'women', I am either reflecting the language used in the relevant research papers (and I feel to change this to the term 'menstruators' would be damaging in that there is virtually no research around menstruation and transgender issues) or using them to make a point about patriarchy. I hope that my choice of language comes across in the balanced and inclusive way that it is intended.

What I do assume is that you're someone who deserves to know just what the hell goes on inside you every month, and that you'd like to make your life easier and more pleasurable. Understanding how you move through your menstrual cycle gifts you with flow. I grew up believing that my biology would hold me back in life, that it would bring me trouble and couldn't be trusted. This book grew out of a desire to counter those beliefs, to show how our physiology can be used to great advantage, and that it needn't hold us back. The menstrual cycle is unappreciated, but I hope that by the end of this book you'll see that it is the most unused and underrated tool for improving our lives.

Yes, we are hormonal, and that's a very good thing.

My Story

I used to get hit hard by period pain. Really hard. I've had to lie down in public places because I couldn't stand up or face trying to get home, where I desperately wanted to be. I have regularly woken up in pain and run scorching hot baths at 2am whilst impatiently waiting for painkillers to kick in. I have felt like my coccyx and hips were about to snap open with pressure. I have burned my skin to the point of causing blisters, three months in a row, because the extreme heat of a water bottle was the only thing that helped to mitigate such bad period pain. There have been times when I have been close to calling 999 and begging for morphine.

I have spent years healing that pain – casually at first, and then with fierce commitment. Acupuncture, Chinese herbs, Western herbs, osteopathy, reflexology, massage, homeopathy, nutrition, menstrual cycle awareness, cognitive behavioural therapy, psychotherapy, hands on healing, yoga, divorce, masturbation … I have tried them all. I have begged for drugs, in my head and out loud. I have prayed. I have taken copious amounts of painkillers and let me tell you, all hail the power of painkillers, be they natural or pharmaceutical. I don't know what I would have done without them.

For the last five years, period pain hasn't bothered me at all, and my journey to healing was the reason why I got serious about helping other people to sort their menstrual and hormonal issues out. I was inspired by the wise women who treated me and intrigued by the therapies they used. I completed a BSc in Acupuncture, and gained diplomas in the Arvigo Techniques of Maya Abdominal Therapy® (ATMAT, a form of abdominal massage – see page 272), aromatherapy, and reflexology. Then, being the geek that I am, I apprenticed with several world leaders in the growing field of menstruality, learning about how nutrition and lifestyle can impact on our cycles, as well as the psychological impact of them.

Bit by bit, my personal and professional life became increasingly focused on menstrual health, and because I'd taken one for the team and tried so many different ways of improving my own menstrual health, I knew how to help my clients and what techniques would work well for their specific situation or condition. But the one approach that was consistently the easiest and most effective for my clients to implement was knowledge of what actually happens in a cycle and how to attune daily life to suit their rhythms and needs. My clients kept asking me to draw diagrams and write notes so that they could share them with their friends, which is why, in addition to working with women one on one, I started running menstrual health workshops. That's where things got really interesting and my work got a lot bigger, because there's something hugely powerful about sitting with a group of women and exploring our cycles together. Attendees cried. I cried. We got angry that nobody had told us this crucial information when we were fourteen, or thirty or forty. And in a couple of cases, fifty. There were women who grieved that they had gone through menopause and would not bleed again with this knowledge to guide them, but who felt great relief at finally understanding what had been happening to them during their menstruating years. We felt sad that nobody had told our mothers either, and so they didn't know how to tell us. We discovered the common themes that bind us together as menstruators – that *her* story is often *your* story too. More and more women started getting in contact with me, saying that they'd love to come to a workshop, but they lived on the other side of the country or in another country. Everybody was asking if there was another way to work with me and that's how I knew I had to write this book.

The Red Tide is Turning

The idea that your period can act as a report card of your overall health has been expressed by the American College of Obstetricians and Gynecologists. In 2015, the ACOG recommended that the menstrual cycle be used as a fifth vital sign when evaluating the health of menstruating teenagers, with some experts recommending that this consideration extend beyond adolescence and into the rest of a woman's reproductive years, something that I'm wholly on board with.

And media organisation NPR (National Public Radio) coined 2015 'the year of the period' after usage of the word 'menstruation' tripled in major news outlets between 2010 and 2015, thanks to prominent news items such as Instagram censoring Rupi Kaur's photo of herself lying on a bed with blood stains on her trousers and bed linen, Kiran Gandhi's freebleeding London marathon run, and the #PeriodsAreNotAnInsult response to Donald Trump's taunting of Megyn Kelly. Around the same time, menstrual activism gained ground as calls to abolish the tampon tax swelled. Why is it that tampons are taxed but Jaffa cakes and Viagra are not?

We are making headway. Following a successful pilot scheme, the Scottish government has spent over £500,000 on a larger plan in which people from low-income homes will receive free menstrual care products and they recently began distributing them to pupils in every school, college, and university. Frustratingly, the Tory government and the Department of Education in the UK have not followed suit.

The #freeperiods campaign led by teen menstrual activist Amika George received massive public support and after a demonstration outside parliament organised by The Pink Protest, the government pledged to spend £15 million on addressing period poverty in the UK, which we can all agree was an incredible result. But despite them promising to abolish the tampon tax, and the British Medical Association backing a motion to end period poverty, they still haven't axed the tax.

Thankfully there are some politicians who are using their voices to continue to drive the conversation. MP Danielle Rowley recently stood up in parliament to speak out about period poverty and announced that she was on her period *fist bump*. In the US, Representative Sean Maloney, Democrat of New York, was shocked when he was ordered to reimburse the Committee for House Administration for the $37.16 expense he had claimed to cover the tampons his office purchased for staff and visitors. Maloney stated that, 'we need to stop acting like women's daily needs are something we can't handle.' Men who want to be allies, take note.

An increasing amount of universities and businesses are providing free menstrual products for students, staff, employees, and visitors. Kenya and Uganda have eliminated their tax on menstrual products, and India has just abolished its 12 per cent tax on pads. Canada abolished their sales tax in 2015, six US states have also achieved this, and Australia look set to get rid of their tax later on this year.

This is progress, but it's not enough, because it's not just access to products that must be tackled. If we are to continue to diminish the shame and stigma that has long been associated with bleeding, then we must push on and improve access to education and change the language that we use when we discuss menstruating bodies. It's pregnancy and the absence of blood that's prized in our society, and as long as we are viewed as reproductive vessels our periods will remain disgusting and hidden, a sign of our failure to reproduce and live out our capacity as breeders. The stigma that dominates the language and behaviour surrounding periods is all about cleaning up the shame of a failed cycle. When menstrual products are described as *sanitary pads* and *feminine hygiene products* it infers that we're dirty and unhygienic. And then there's the new line of tampons from Tampax®, Pure and Clean – because you can be a good girl, remain a virgin like you're supposed to, and be sparkly and clean all whilst using a tampon.

Some companies *are* tackling taboos. Incredibly, an actual pad hadn't been included in an advert until Bodyform® did in 2016, so it's great that when they did feature one, they acknowledged that we don't bleed blue and featured red liquid, as well as showing blood trickling down a woman's leg while she showered. In India, girls and women are said to be able to rot pickles when they're bleeding, and the #touchthepickle campaign for Procter & Gamble menstrual pad brand Whisper® garnered a lot of attention and even won an award at Cannes. But we need to be wary of companies getting in on the act under the veil of activism. When Procter & Gamble brand Always® announced their (marketing) campaign to end period poverty, with a paltry donation of one pad per pack of Always Ultra pads purchased by customers in April 2018 (one month!), they were accused of trying to cash in on period poverty, and rightly so. Gabby Edlin, founder of Bloody Good Period, an organisation that distribute donated menstrual supplies to asylum seekers, refugees and those who can't afford them, responded to the campaign by stating that, 'They're not lending their voice. They are using period poverty as a marketing tool … This is the most minimal thing they could do.' Contrast that with companies like Hey Girls, Conscious Period, and Ruby Cup who have a buy one, give one business model. Also, The Cup Effect sell menstrual cups on a not-for-profit basis and for every cup sold two are donated to people experiencing period poverty.

So how do we continue to change the conversation? We need to share our stories because it's conversations that will keep moving the menstrual movement forward. The more we talk about our experiences and issues, the less they can be ignored. It is not acceptable that menstrual cycles are dismissed because they don't apply to half of the population. People with wombs are not a niche.

In her hilariously accurate 1978 essay, 'If Men Could Menstruate', author, activist, and feminist, Gloria Steinem, described how if men had periods, 'menstruation would become an enviable, boast-worthy, masculine event: Men would brag about how long and how much.' And they would certainly have an emoji to do so – something charity Plan UK are calling for to encourage conversation around periods. They make the valid point that; 'girls and women in the 21st century still can't use one of the fastest growing global languages to talk about their periods.' Surely a red drop – Plan UK's suggested emoji – would get more use than a levitating man in a suit?

A simple act of revolution is to learn about your body, to get to know the terrain of your cycle, and to take charge of your own health. Experts in hormonal and reproductive health, and the increasing number of medical tracking devices on offer can be hugely helpful, but you do not need them to get to know yourself in this way. All you need is the information that's in this book to help you understand what's going on, and a pen and some paper to keep track of how you feel. And if you want to track how your temperature changes over the course of a cycle so that you can identify when you ovulate, you'll need a digital thermometer too.

Our bodies have long been weaponised against us and used to keep us out of positions of influence and power, but the red tide is turning and it's time for us to take advantage of what our hormones can do for us.

SECTION ONE

GET TO KNOW YO'SELF

Knowing yourself is the beginning of all wisdom
– Aristotle

I want to give you all the tools you need to understand your body and your menstrual cycle, so let's start off with the things you should have been told in sex education at school but you probably weren't.

You have a right to know and understand your body, and being clued up on all things menstrual will make it a whole lot easier for you to identify when something isn't quite right. And understanding how everything works is a sure-fire way to eradicate the shame that many of us have been made to feel about our – usually very healthy and very normal – bodily functions.

Not to mention that your body is amazing and fascinating and worth getting to know, so let's take a peek under the hood …

Chapter 1

The notorious v.a.g.

Let's take a journey back in time to when you were a freshly fertilised egg inside your mum; an incredible bundle of developing cells. When your parents conceived you and their DNA met and mingled, your genetic sex was determined as either female or male, but in terms of sexual development, for another six weeks the early genital system in both sexes appears somewhat similar – something my clients are amazed by and you might be too, check out the illustration overleaf to see how the male and female genitals develop and differentiate throughout pregnancy.

By week seven of pregnancy, embryos that are destined to develop male genitals begin to develop testes and start releasing testicular hormones which masculinise the external genitals. This causes the various folds to fuse, leaving behind a telltale seam that runs all the way from the penis down the middle of the ball sack and around to the anus, which can be seen in adulthood. Another hormone that is produced prevents male embryos from developing female reproductive structures, whereas in female embryos the absence of these hormones allows for the development of the uterus, cervix and fallopian tubes. Externally the genital tubercle that became the glans (head) of the penis in male embryos, becomes the glans clitoris in female embryos. The genital folds don't fuse as they do in male embryos, and instead they form the labia minora (inner lips), and the labioscrotal swellings become the labia majora (outer lips). Essentially, male or female, we all have the same parts and start off looking the same, but in the early weeks of pregnancy a male embryo responds to hormones and develops male genitals. A female embryo simply continues as she was. Later in life, if a person has a gender identity which does not match the genitals they were born with, they can undergo gender confirmation surgery and the penis can become a clitoris, or the clitoris can become a penis. Isn't modern medicine wonderful?

Second month

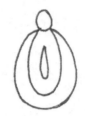

Female

Third month

Male

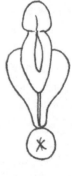

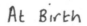

At Birth

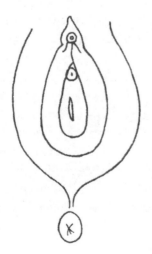

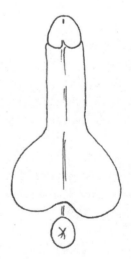

Head, Shoulders, Knees and Vagina

Now that you know where you came from, and how you ended up with your genital configuration, let's take a closer look at whatcha got. And if you want to take a peek at yourself, this is your cue to go and grab a mirror.

Vulva

Are you familiar with yours?

Do you know where it is? Research carried out by UK charity The Eve Appeal found that 60 per cent of the British women surveyed couldn't identify the vulva on a medical diagram, and it's no wonder given the concerning lack of sex education that we receive. So, let's make things easy: your vulva is all of your external genitalia, including your mons pubis (that's the mound of fatty tissue on top of your pubic bone that's populated with pubic hair), labia minora and majora, your clitoris and its beautiful hood, as well as your perineum and the external openings of your vagina and urethra (where you pee from).

What most of us commonly refer to as the *vagina*, is actually the *vulva*. Your vagina is the internal tube which connects your external genitalia – your vulva – with your womb, and it is only the opening to the vagina that can be seen once the labia are parted. Can you imagine men, or indeed women, confusing the different parts that make up the male genitals? I thought not, so let's all do what we can to take ownership of our bodies by using the proper terminology.

Now that you know what the vulva actually is, let's take a look at the individual parts in more detail, starting up top with my favourite; the clitoris.

Clitoris

Densely packed with an astounding 8,000 nerve endings (that's double the amount of the male equivalent; the glans or head of the penis), your clitoris is all about pleasure. *Your pleasure.* Whereas a penis has several functions – urination, ejaculation, penetration, and sensation – the clitoris is the only organ built solely for sexual stimulation and arousal. Because, newsflash – we are more than reproductive vessels.

The clitoris is only partially visible to the human eye, and not because it might be hidden behind its hood, but because the clitoris is less of a button and more of an iceberg. The clitoris is not 'pea-sized' as dictionaries and medical texts would have you believe (and that's if they include it at all – many don't). It is in fact 7 to 12 centimetres in length and the part that we're most familiar with is the 'head' or glans, which emerges at the top of the vulva.

So, where's the rest of it?

Thanks to Helen O'Connell, an Australian urologist who mapped the external *and internal* clitoris in its entirety, we now know that there's a lot more to the clit than meets the eye. Internally there's a bulb which extends deep into your vagina (some experts believe that this bulb is the infamous G-spot) and spreading like a wide wishbone are its legs (crura) which line the opening to your vagina. The legs and bulb are covered in muscular tissue which plays a crucial role when it comes to arousal and orgasm by creating the tension and involuntary contractions that you may have experienced.

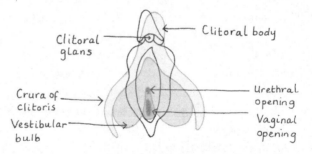

Wanna know when she discovered this? 1998.

Let that sink in for a moment, *1998*. We have only known about the full size of the clitoris for the last twenty years, and yet scientific texts and magazine articles still refer to it as a nub. They're also fond of describing it as *phallus-like* but given the fact that the clitoris in its entirety is larger than an average flaccid penis, I prefer to think of the penis as a small clitoris.

The glans varies in size from 0.5 to 3.5 centimetres long, it has a hood (the male equivalent being the foreskin) which, depending on your wonderful and unique configuration, will also vary in size. The hood can be pulled back by you or your lover, or it may retract by itself when you're feeling turned on. During arousal the clitoris becomes engorged and swells and the head may become more visible and easier to find. A small number of clitorises won't be fully visible, often due to the presence of clitoral adhesions. In such cases, the lining of the clitoral hood adheres to the clitoris and, depending on the severity of the adhesions, may hold the hood in place and cause irritation, pain, infection, and sexual dysfunction in the form of decreased sensation and muted orgasms, or none at all. If you experience these symptoms, please see a doctor who specialises in sexual health and who knows how to examine for clitoral adhesions, as one study found that 1 in 5 women attending a sexual health clinic had adhesions of varying degrees. When clitoral adhesions cause problems they can be removed surgically under a local anaesthetic.

The clitoris varies in size across the population, and also throughout your life. One small study found that the clitoris changes in volume over the course of a menstrual cycle, increasing in volume by 20 per cent around ovulation and decreasing premenstrually. Another study discovered that it can decrease in size when you use hormonal birth control, and research which followed 40 women who either used the birth control pill or the contraceptive vaginal ring, found that all forty women experienced a decrease in clitoral volume. Yep, clit shrinkage is a thing. But the clitoris also grows as you age, particularly after the hormonal shift that comes with menopause. Whatever yours looks like, your clitoris is beautiful and deserving of love and appreciation, just like the rest of you.

If you're someone who doesn't orgasm through penetration, you're not the only one; only 18 per cent of women orgasm through penetration alone, with the vast majority of us requiring clitoral stimulation, which is no surprise given that it's the clitoris, not the vagina, that's jam-packed with nerve endings. In fact, now that we know the full anatomy of the clitoris, some experts believe that 'vaginal orgasms' and 'G-spot orgasms' *are* clitoral orgasms – just ones that involve the internal parts of the clitoris.

Despite all of this, and the fact that when it comes to masturbation most of us solely focus on the clitoris, heterosexual sex largely focuses on vaginal penetration, which explains why there's such an orgasm gap between men and women. Imagine if the tables were turned and only a cursory minute or two of attention was bestowed upon the penis before sexual focus moved to their balls or thighs and that's how men were expected to orgasm; do you think they'd put up with it? No, so why should we?

During arousal we get wet, but did you know you get hard too? The clitoris has erections and they even occur throughout the night – you can have as many as eight erections per night, all whilst you're sleeping.

Labia

Despite what we see in medical diagrams and porn, labia are not symmetrical, and they vary in thickness, length, shape, hairiness, and colour. All variations are normal and magnificent.

Labia is the Latin plural for 'lip'. The outer labia (labia majora) are your set of outer lips. They're plumper than your inner labia, acting as protective cushioning that comes in handy when you ride a bike, and they have hair follicles, whereas your inner labia don't. Hair on your outer labia is also there as a form of protection, helping to prevent skin abrasions and acting as a first line of defence against foreign invaders; in the same way that you have nostril hairs to filter germs and pollutants as you breathe in air, pubic hair is there to help stop bacteria from heading internally. Whether you have dense or sparse hair growth on your outer labia depends on how many hair follicles you have.

Your inner labia (labia minora) are – yeah, you guessed it – the lips that are the inner set, and for some of you they may be tucked away, requiring you to part your outer lips to see them, or they may be clearly visible and extend beyond your outer lips. All normal, all wonderful.

Inner labia are thinner and more sensitive than your outer labia, and thanks to their rich blood supply, they swell when you're feeling turned on which can increase their sensitivity. They're covered in a mucus membrane, a layer of cells which is also found lining the other openings to your body; nostrils, mouth, eyes, ears, anus and urethra. It's there to prevent pathogens from invading and also keeps these tissues hydrated by secreting fluid. It's this function that can lessen when oestrogen declines during menopause and results in vaginal dryness.

Female porn models and actresses sometimes have labial surgery (labiaplasties) to 'perfect' their lips, and along with the use of editing to 'improve' the appearance of female genitals, this has led our visual reference for what vulvas look like to become exceedingly narrow, to the point where some teenage boys now think a hairless vulva is normal. Of course, what *you* choose to do with your body is up to you, but with labiaplasty rates increasing at a scary rate and children reportedly as young as nine years old seeking them out, something has gone awry. If you'd like to increase your visual reference for the tremendous variations of what vulvas look like, then I recommend checking out The Vulva Gallery on Instagram, where you can find drawings of vulvas along with the personal stories of those that they belong to.

Vulval Vestibule

If you were to spread your inner labia apart, your vulval vestibule would be revealed. It's the part of your vulva that lies between your labia and the opening to your vagina, a brief entrance court that has two holes; the urethral opening where you pee from which sits underneath the clitoris and above the second hole – the vaginal opening. On either side of the vaginal opening are two Bartholin's glands which are also referred to as Greater Vestibular glands, and although they *are* great – they secrete fluid when we're turned on – they are small and not usually visible to the human eye. When you get wet, this is where the fluid is coming from. The male equivalent is the Cowper's gland which sits beneath the prostate and releases pre-ejaculatory fluid (men get wet too).

Your Skene's glands (aka Lesser Vestibular glands) are located in your vaginal wall but come out into the open near your urethra. They produce around a third of the fluid you produce when aroused and if you've ever squirted, this is where your ejaculatory fluid came from.

Let's leave your pee hole alone (it's easily irritated) and head inside the vagina instead.

Vaginal Opening and Corona (Hymen)

At the entrance to the vagina is where the legendary hymen can be found (when it's there, that is), and it really is the stuff of legends, because most of what we are taught about the hymen is fictitious: the hymen is *not* a flat seal which is punctured during your first experience of vaginal penetration, leaving you forever broken and impure.

While a small number of hymens do cover the entirety of the vaginal opening (making the discharge of menstrual blood tricky and usually requiring surgery), most have either a hole in the middle, or lots of tiny holes

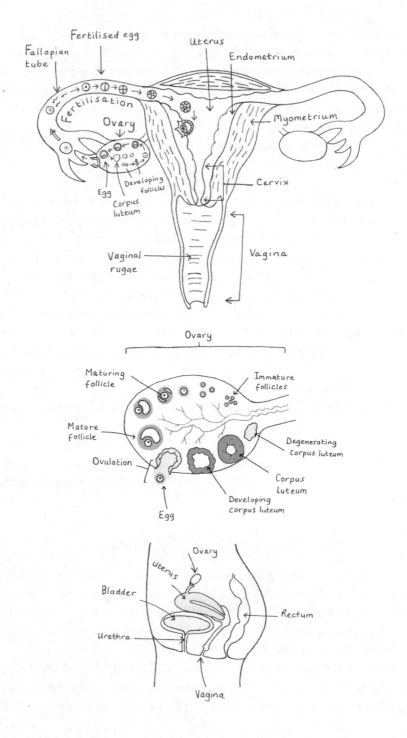

across its breadth (picture the rose at the end of a watering can that sprinkles fine sprays of water), and some look a bit like a fringe which partially covers your vaginal opening. Some hymens will atrophy (wither away) and disappear by adolescence, and some will tear easily as a result of movement and exercise or the use of tampons. Some will be more robust and stretch as they become accustomed to fingers, tampons, and penises being inserted into the vagina, and eventually atrophy. A small fraction will remain till later in life, and some of us are even born without them.

The hymen is simply a thin membrane along the edge of your vaginal opening, that for reasons which remain quite bizarre to me, many cultures place a great deal of emphasis on, to the point where hymenoplasty is sold to us so that we can restore our virginity. Because we're worth it.

Your hymen is not a treasured prize for your husband on your wedding night unless you want it to be. It's just a piece of tissue that's likely to be long gone by then.

Vagina

Your vagina is the internal tube that connects your vulva (external genitalia) with your womb (uterus). It cannot be seen externally. It runs at a 45-degree angle pointing backwards towards your bum, and the front of it (the anterior wall) is slightly shorter than the back of it (the posterior wall). Your bladder sits in front of your vagina and uterus, and your rectum (the last section of your large intestine) sits behind it.

The vagina is not a gaping hole just waiting to be filled, in fact the vaginal walls touch each other unless something – fingers, a tampon, penis, sex toy, or baby as it's being born – is inside it. The surface of the vagina is covered in ridges called rugae which you'll feel if you put a finger inside yourself. Rugae make the vagina highly elastic and capable of expanding, producing the so-called tenting effect that lifts your cervix higher when you're aroused and stimulated. At certain times in your menstrual cycle you may find that your vagina feels dry, and it can also feel dry during puberty, after giving birth, during breastfeeding and after menopause due to lowered levels of oestrogen. Vaginal dryness can also be caused by cigarette smoking, anti-oestrogen medications, and Sjogren's syndrome – an immune system disorder that often accompanies rheumatoid arthritis and lupus, which causes dry mucus membranes, including that of your eyes, mouth and vagina.

Your vagina doesn't have much of a nerve supply (imagine giving birth if it did), and one of its jobs is to act as a physical barrier to stop pathogenic microorganisms from entering your uterus. It does this by keeping its front and back walls pressed against each other, and by producing *Lactobacillus acidophilus* – the healthy bacteria used to make probiotic supplements and yoghurt – which secrete lactic acid and hydrogen peroxide, helping to maintain an acidic environment (pH 4.9–3.5) in order to reduce the chance of invading pathogens surviving and entering your uterus. In the same way that your gut has its own unique ecosystem of friendly bacteria, so does your vagina, and when they're out of balance you can end up with recurrent bouts of yeast infections and bacterial vaginosis. The vagina does not need to be cleaned or rinsed out and using vaginal cleaning products or douching can upset the balance of bacteria and cause harm. It's thought that a lack of a healthy vaginal microbiome can contribute to pelvic inflammatory disease, bacterial vaginosis, sexually transmitted diseases, miscarriage, ectopic pregnancy, premature birth, and cervical cancer.

Cervix

At the top of the vagina is the entrance to the womb; your cervix. Your cervix is a bit like a gate in that for most of your life its job is to stay closed, only opening around the time of ovulation to allow sperm in, at menstruation so that blood can come out, and during childbirth to allow a baby out.

Your cervix is actually the lowest and narrowest part of your uterus and is sometimes referred to as the neck of your womb. If you were to insert a finger into your vagina, you might be able to feel it (squatting makes this easier). It is circular and depending on where you are in your menstrual cycle, it can either feel a bit like a nose with a dimple in the middle of it or a set of puckered lips. If you've given birth or been in labour then the dimple in the middle will be more pronounced than if you haven't and you may be able to insert the tip of your finger into it.

Sometimes it's easy to feel, and at other times it'll be out of reach because as well as changes to how it feels, your cervix changes position throughout your menstrual cycle. Your cervix is lower before, during, and after your period, and as such you may find that penetrative sex in certain positions is uncomfortable during these times. Around the time of ovulation, the cervix retreats further up inside you in order to shorten the distance that sperm have to travel. Sperm are ejaculated at 28 mph, so they have no trouble reaching your cervix, but once they've been deposited, it's on them to complete the rest of their journey to your fallopian tubes which is where fertilisation takes place if it were to occur. And they've got a way to go, sure it's 'only' 15–20cm, but for a tiny cell swimming at 5 mm a minute, it takes them 2–7 hours to complete the journey, so your body assists by pulling your cervix upwards and lessening the distance for them.

Your cervix produces mucus, which acts as a barrier to help prevent infection. During the fertile window in the lead up to ovulation, rising oestrogen makes cervical mucus increase in volume and slipperiness, so much so that it resembles egg whites. This type of cervical fluid helps sperm travel and enter the uterus. You can read all about the changes it undergoes and how to use it to monitor your fertility in the next chapter.

During pregnancy, your cervix produces mucus that forms a plug over the entrance – yet another protective measure to keep germs out. We place great emphasis on how open and dilated the cervix is during labour, but the cervix has to undergo many other changes in order to dilate all the way to 10cm. It has to thin, soften, shorten, and move forward into a facing-forward (anterior) position. At 10cm dilatation, the cervix is fully open, and in fact has disappeared, whilst the upper part of the uterus – the fundus – has increased in size, resulting in more strength at the top of the uterus which helps to create the downward pressure required to birth a baby.

When you have a cervical screening test, cells are swabbed off the transformation zone of your cervix – the area of changing cells on the cervix which is the most common site for abnormal cells to develop – to analyse for abnormalities. If abnormal cells are found, then further investigation is suggested which takes the form of removing more cervical cells by cervical biopsy or a procedure called LLETZ (large loop excision of the transformation zone) which is also known as LEEP (loop electrosurgical excision procedure) and diathermy loop biopsy. Loop procedures such as these are carried out with a local anaesthetic and involve the use of a small wire loop with an electrical current running through it to remove the affected area of tissue whilst sealing the wound at the same time.

Cervical screening is incredibly important and saves lives, so it's crucial that you attend your screening appointments. There are downsides to some of the further investigations as they can increase your risk of having a preterm birth, a low-birthweight baby, and of giving birth by caesarean section. Most abnormalities usually go away by themselves without treatment but the increased awareness health screens bring of possible abnormalities can often lead to overtreatment, so later on this year the British Society for Colposcopy and Cervical Pathology will discuss its guidelines, and whether some women would benefit from 'watchful waiting' and repeating the PAP smear, instead of being referred for surgery.

Uterus (Womb)

Your uterus is an incredibly dynamic organ. Not only does it respond and change in a highly sensitive fashion to the hormonal signals it receives throughout the course of a menstrual cycle, but it also carries out hormonal signalling in its cells and to the cells that surround it – communicative functions which are vital when conception has taken place.

It resembles the shape and size of an upside-down pear. It's approximately 7.5cm long and 5cm wide, with walls which are 2.5cm thick. In front of it lies your bladder, and behind it sits your rectum.

When we look at diagrams of the female reproductive system, we're led to believe that the uterus is perfectly upright with its arms (fallopian tubes) outstretched, when in fact it's more like she's taking a modest bow with her arms extending slightly behind her. The uterus is hollow, but in the same way that your vaginal walls push up against each other, so do your uterine walls, with a thin layer of fluid separating them.

The uterus has three sections; the uppermost part which sits above the opening to the fallopian tubes is called the fundus, the middle section is the body, and down at the lowest and narrowest point of the uterus, connecting the uterus and vagina, is the cervix.

It also has three layers. The outermost layer is the thin perimetrium which is a bit like its skin. The middle layer is referred to as the myometrium and is composed of interlacing layers of smooth muscle. It's this muscular layer that comes into play during labour and birth, creating waves of contractions which pull the lower segment of your uterus upwards and cause the cervix to thin and open. The innermost layer is the endometrium, aka the lining of your womb. It's this layer that, thanks to its juicy blood supply, is able to fill and plump up in every menstrual cycle in preparation for possible implantation of a fertilised egg, and then degenerate if pregnancy hasn't occurred. It's the lining of your womb which is shed when you have your period.

Most uteruses tip slightly forwards and are referred to as anteverted, but around a quarter of us have a tilted womb, where the uterus tips backwards towards the bum and is referred to as retroverted. A retroverted uterus can sometimes occur as a result of endometriosis lesions or a pelvic infection, both of which can cause scarring and adhesions which can hold the uterus in this tilting backwards position, often causing or contributing towards pelvic pain, including painful periods and pain during sex. In some cases, a uterus can also flex itself, and no I don't mean it's in there pumping iron, but it can bend a little and even fold in on itself – either forwards or backwards – and can cause further problems. If a uterus is pointing backwards and it also bends backwards on itself, the top part of it can impinge on your rectum and cause pain whilst pooing. If it's tipped forwards and folds in, it can create pressure on the bladder and result in frequent urination. In fact, the bladder and the uterus are held closely next to each other by connective tissue, which means that when one moves, so does the other.

If you've been told, or you suspect that your uterus is in an interesting position, practitioners of the Arvigo Techniques of Maya Abdominal Therapy® (ATMAT – see page 272) and women's health physiotherapists can manually work on adjusting and releasing the ligaments and muscles which hold your uterus in place in order to help it back into an optimal position, though in some cases surgery is necessary.

Some people are born with a uterus that's formed in an unusual way. Instead of being shaped like an upside-down pear, the uterus can be heart-shaped and is referred to as a bicornuate uterus, or it can have a slight dip at the top (arcuate). It might have a wall of muscle coming down the centre of it which splits the internal space in two (septate), the womb can be split in two and each side has its own cavity (didelphic/double), and very rarely only one side of the uterus develops (unicornuate). You're unlikely to find out if your uterus has a variation like this unless you have an ultrasound to investigate a gynaecological condition or recurrent miscarriages. The more noticeable variations would be picked up during routine ultrasounds during pregnancy, at which point you would receive guidance and additional support as some variations are associated with preterm labour.

Fallopian Tubes (Uterine Tubes/Oviduct)

Extending from each side of the upper part of your womb is a fallopian tube, one on the right and one on the left. Each is approximately 10cm long and consists of two parts; the isthmus (the short, narrow, thick-walled portion nearest the uterus), and ampulla (the wider, longer portion of the tube nearer the ovaries). Think of each fallopian tube as a funnel; the narrow end is attached to your womb, and the wide end is next to your ovary. This wide end also has fronds extending from it – known as fimbriae – the largest of which is attached to your ovary, and their job is to catch the egg released from your ovary at ovulation, where it then journeys down the fallopian tube towards your womb.

If the egg is met by a lurking sperm cell, fertilisation usually occurs in the ampulla, and the fertilised egg travels towards your uterus, along the isthmus where its journey may be slowed in order for the lining of the womb to develop for implantation, and for communication between the fertilised egg and its mother to begin. In one in 80 pregnancies the fertilised egg implants somewhere other than the lining of the womb, resulting in an ectopic pregnancy that's non-viable and requires medical care. A fallopian tube is a common site for an ectopic pregnancy to occur and if a fertilised egg implants here it is usually removed using medication or during an operation and can result in the loss of the affected tube.

The fallopian tubes' main function is to facilitate transportation; to this end they are muscular and use a wave-like motion called peristalsis to create movement (your intestines do this too), and they are also lined with miniscule hairs called cilia which waft the egg along towards your womb. Your fallopian tubes also secrete mucus which aids the transport of both sperm and egg, in the same way flowing water carries and speeds your journey down a water slide. Smoking cigarettes and cannabis negatively impacts on the motility of your fallopian tubes and increases your risk of ectopic pregnancy.

Ovaries

The ovaries are two pearl-coloured glands the size of unshelled almonds which lie either side of the uterus just beneath the end of each fallopian tube. Ligaments which attach to the uterus and the pelvic wall hold them in place. They are the female sex glands and the male equivalent is the testicles.

They have two roles; producing a mature egg in each menstrual cycle which is released at ovulation and producing hormones such as oestradiol (the form of oestrogen we're most familiar with), testosterone, progesterone, and inhibin, all of which play a part in the hormonal dance of your menstrual cycle. We're going to delve into the role of these hormones in the next chapter, so hold tight and let's stick with the pool of ovarian eggs that they contain for now.

Unlike sperm which are produced regularly from puberty onwards, if you're born with a female reproductive system, then you're born with all the eggs you'll ever have. That means that the egg which produced you existed when your grandmother was pregnant with your mum. That means part of you was once inside your granny.

When you were growing in your mum's uterus in her twentieth week of pregnancy, you had the most egg cells (oocytes) you've ever had – an astounding 7 million – but from week 24 the number of egg cells rapidly declined so that by the time you were born, you were left with 1 million, and by the time puberty hit, that number further reduced to 400,000. The miniscule immature eggs that don't make it deteriorate and are reabsorbed by the body. From puberty, a few follicles commence growth every day and each houses an immature egg, so there's a continuous trickle of developing follicles which go through several phases of development before they reach the point of maturation which determines them as being contenders for ovulation, or not. Only around 400 of them end up being released as mature eggs at ovulation, accounting for the number of periods you're likely to have over your lifetime. The rest don't make the grade and undergo a process known as atresia, in which thousands of follicles in each cycle die off. You might find that only using 0.1 per cent of what you started out with depressing, but I find it incredible that our bodies do such a great job of selecting high quality eggs. Creating, growing and raising another human is a massive biological investment, so it makes sense that there's a highly selective process behind it all.

So that's your whistle-stop tour of the reproductive system. Now let's get stuck into what happens over the course of a menstrual cycle.

Chapter 2

What that wet patch in your knickers is all about

There are two pivotal moments in your menstrual cycle: menstruation, the discharge and movement of blood; and ovulation, the release and motion of an egg.

The poles of menstruation and ovulation determine the two main phases of your menstrual cycle. The follicular phase runs from day 1 of your cycle – the first day of your period – all the way through to ovulation. It's called the follicular phase because this is the stage of your cycle in which your hormones cause the rapid growth of ovarian follicles, and maturation of the egg each follicle contains. The follicular phase culminates when the egg bursts out of the follicle that has housed it – the moment of ovulation – so it can vary in length greatly depending on how long it takes for you to ovulate. For example, in a so-called 'textbook' 28-day cycle – which as little as 12.4 per cent of us actually have – you're likely to ovulate on day 14, but if your cycle is shorter at, say, 21 days then you'll ovulate earlier than day 14, and if your cycle is longer, at 36 days for example, then you probably don't ovulate until around day 22. In some people the variation can be even wider, and if you're someone who has a cycle that's shorter or longer then it's important that your doctor considers this when testing your progesterone level. Progesterone is usually tested on day 21 of your cycle, which would be appropriate if you have a 28-day cycle (as the ideal time is seven days after ovulation), but if your cycle is shorter or longer, then day 21 is not the ideal time for a progesterone blood test. If you have long cycles then be sure to tell your midwife and/ or obstetrician during pregnancy as many people are told towards the end of pregnancy that they're 'overdue' and are booked in for what could be an unnecessary induction. If you track your basal body temperature and are familiar with when you ovulate then you can ask your midwife to calculate your estimated due date (EDD) from ovulation rather than your last menstrual period.

Ovulation marks the start of the luteal phase, or second half of your cycle, and is so named because once an egg bursts out of its follicle, the follicle is left behind on the surface of your ovary and turns into a yellow body called the corpus luteum, a temporary gland which produces and releases progesterone, the hormone that runs the show in the second half of your cycle. The luteal phase tends to be fixed in length, ideally at around 14 days. It begins at ovulation and ends when your period begins again.

The incredible process of your menstrual cycle is orchestrated by the delicate dance of several hormones:

- **Gonadotropin-releasing hormone (GnRH)**
  GnRH is the boss of your cycle. The hypothalamus gland in your brain releases pulses of GnRH which are then carried to the hypothalamus' neighbour, the pituitary gland, which picks up on the messages GnRH is sending it and then releases follicle stimulating hormone and luteinising hormone (see below). These two hormones communicate with your ovaries and cause your follicles to mature and eventually release an egg at ovulation. Think of Meryl Streep in *The Devil Wears Prada*; her presence is felt everywhere, and nothing happens without her say so, though she gets her minions – FSH and LH – to do the actual work.
- **Follicle stimulating hormone (FSH)**
  Follicle stimulating hormone does exactly what it says on the tin – it *stimulates* your follicles to help the eggs they contain to mature. It arrives on the scene when hormone levels are low at the start of your cycle and stimulates your follicles to grow and glow (technically they don't glow, but I like to think of them all vying for attention – *pick me, pick me!*) then once the lead follicle has been selected and it starts to produce oestrogen, FSH stands down as its job is done, for now. But once the amount of oestrogen being pumped out by the maturing follicle reaches a threshold, FSH reappears and together with luteinising hormone (LH), they take turns nudging each other to do bigger and better, and their combined efforts result in the follicle releasing its egg. Imagine Tyra Banks in *America's Next Top Model*; at the beginning she's there pumping all the

contestants up, helping them to feel good and giving them all they need to mature, then she steps back to see who is going to truly blossom, and once a winner is declared, she comes back with lashings of praise and awards them their prize so that they can launch their career (or ovulate in this instance).

- **Oestrogen**
  Oestradiol is the form of oestrogen that is released by your developing follicles and reigns over the first half of your cycle. She is indeed queenly, and I like to think of oestrogen as the Beyoncé of hormones: confident, alluring, sensual, fertile, and able to learn complex dance routines because she's great at picking up new skills. She makes your features appear more symmetrical, clears your skin up, makes you feel good, changes your walk into a sassy strut, demands attention and is ready to conquer the world because she is oh so fabulous.

- **Luteinising hormone (LH)**
  LH is the power and strength behind the final moment of ovulation. In the 24 hours preceding ovulation and as oestrogen reaches its peak, it stimulates the secretion of LH, which in turn stimulates your follicle to produce more oestrogen and along with FSH results in ovulation. Whilst Beyoncé (oestrogen) may seem like the star of the show, it's Solange (LH) who has the power to make ovulation happen. Or kick the crap out of Jay-Z. LH is also responsible for instructing the corpus luteum on your ovary to produce progesterone after ovulation and is the guardian of the second half of your cycle.

- **Testosterone**
  Testosterone is *not* a male hormone, it is produced by all humans. It's active, ambitious, sexy and competitive, in other words, the Serena Williams of hormones. It helps you maintain and build muscle and bone density, not to mention give your libido a boost when it peaks in the lead up to ovulation.

- **Progesterone**
  Quiet, calm and introspective, progesterone dominates the second half of your cycle and it can be the culprit behind your anxiety, tears and mood swings. It slows you down and makes you want to stay in and eat comfort food. The Kristen Stewart of your reproductive hormones, she's edgy, doesn't want to be the centre of attention, prefers slouchy trousers and staying home to bake apple pie with female friends.

Hormones 101

The word hormone comes from the Greek verb *hormao*, which means to excite or arouse, and that's exactly what hormones do; they're powerful messenger molecules which travel around your bloodstream sending messages to specific sites in the body in order to create a response that would otherwise lie dormant. Some hormones cause quick, short-term responses, such as a faster heartbeat or sweaty palms, and others, such as those that control reproductive cycles or growth, take longer periods of time to complete their action.

Hormones are produced in glands, some of which are in your brain (hypothalamus, pituitary, and pineal gland), and others are found in the rest of your body (ovaries, adrenal glands, thyroid, parathyroid, and pancreas). There are hundreds of hormones circulating in your blood at any one time, though the concentration of many of them will fluctuate depending on the time of day, where you are in your menstrual cycle, and even with the seasons of the year. Their job is to maintain balance within the body and for every function under their control, the same general pattern is followed:

- A signal is received by a target cell which is designed to receive the specific signal that's been sent out;
- A chemical response takes place;
- And a reaction occurs.

The action of each hormone is very specific and in order for a hormone to have an effect it must be recognised by a target cell that's set up to receive its message. It achieves this by using a lock and key mechanism in which a hormone (the key) travels around the body looking for the receptor sites (the lock) that it can interact with, so if the key fits the lock, a reaction will take place and the door will open, but if it doesn't fit then nothing will happen.

Receptor sites can be found on particular glands and organs, and some are scattered around the body so that many areas are affected. This is essential when a large scale coordinated response is required, such as the fight or flight survival response that's designed to make you either fight or run away from a perceived threat.

There are different hormonal loops within the body in which instructions are sent to the other glands involved in a particular loop, and each of these loops is referred to as an axis:

- In the HPO axis (HPO = hypothalamic-pituitary-ovarian), your hypothalamus instructs your pituitary to tell your *ovaries* to make hormones. It's the HPO axis which controls uterine and ovarian cycles which occur concurrently. The ovarian cycle refers to the changes in the ovary over the course of a menstrual cycle in which the follicle matures, ovulation takes place, and the corpus luteum is formed. In the uterine cycle the lining of the uterus is prepared for the possible implantation of a fertilised egg, shed during menstruation if implantation doesn't take place or succeed, and then regenerated all over again.
- With the HPA axis (HPA = hypothalamic-pituitary-adrenal), your hypothalamus instructs the pituitary to tell the *adrenals* to make hormones such as adrenaline which is released during the fight or flight stress response. The HPA axis controls your stress response and it can inhibit your reproductive system and stop you from ovulating and menstruating if it perceives it to be an inappropriate time to conceive, such as a period of sustained stress, over-exercising, and/or inadequate food intake in relation to your energy expenditure.
- In the HPT axis (HPT = hypothalamic-pituitary-thyroid), the hypothalamus instructs the pituitary to tell your *thyroid* to make thyroid hormones. The HPT and HPO axes are intertwined and when thyroid function is underactive (hypothyroidism) or overactive (hyperthyroidism) it commonly results in menstrual disturbances (see page 290).

As well as making hormones, these axes also involve feedback loops in which the message can also be to stop producing a hormone – remember it's all about balance.

Now that you've got the gist of the main hormonal players of your menstrual cycle, let's take a look at what happens in each phase. It might seem like a lot of this chapter is about fertility, and it is, but fertility isn't just about conceiving, it's a marker of your overall health. Knowing where you are in your cycle goes beyond avoiding or achieving pregnancy because it improves body literacy (your ability to read yourself). The second half of your cycle is typically fixed in length at around 14 days, so knowing when you ovulate is going to be super helpful, especially if your cycle is erratic. It will allow you to calculate when your period is likely to start, which means instead of feeling in limbo, you'll feel more in control and able to plan for this time. Even if your cycle is regular, knowing where you are at any given time gives you a way to take your physical and emotional experiences of your cycle, and consider them within the context of what is happening hormonally.

When it comes to monitoring your cycle to aid conception or to use it as a contraceptive method, knowing when you're fertile is essential. Researcher Kerry Hampton found that only 13 per cent of women trying to conceive and who were seeking out fertility assistance at clinics could correctly identify when they were fertile, despite 68 per cent of them stating that they were timing sex to coincide with their fertile window.

Follicular Phase: Menstruation to Ovulation

Your period and your cycle are a reflection of your overall health and can be affected by little and large life events – the gallons of wine and platefuls of delicious stinky cheese you devoured over Christmas, the crazy-ass work project that nearly broke you, the relationship issues that kept you up at night, the death of a loved one, weight gain or loss, travelling, finally quitting smoking, the supplements you've been taking, the weekly yoga class you've been going to, the new job that you love, the great sex you've been having – they all have an impact on whether our periods are early or late, light or heavy, short or long, and painful or pleasurable.

While you may be aware that the events that have happened in your current cycle can have an influence on your upcoming period, it's important to look back even further, to what has transpired in previous cycles. Here's why: housed in your ovaries are dormant follicles, each of which contains an immature egg, and it takes them over a year to develop from their dormant state and reach the ovulatory phase. Around 190 days before ovulation takes place, they develop a blood supply and begin to respond to their environment, so we need to think beyond what's happened to us in the cycle we're in, the one before that, and go back even further to what has transpired in the last six months.

If your period takes a while to get going, you might be confused as to what counts as day 1. The first day of your cycle is one where you experience your period in full flow. Spotting a light amount of blood before your period starts is the tail end of a cycle, even if it continues for several days before your blood flow increases and your period actually begins. It can actually happen at any point in your premenstrual phase whenever progesterone drops and may be a sign that your body isn't producing enough progesterone, the hormone that supports the luteal phase and pregnancy, causing the lining of your womb to start shedding early. Spotting can happen around ovulation and it can also be a sign of implantation as an embryo embeds itself in the lining of your womb.

Now that you know how to identify day 1, let's backtrack a little to what initiates the bleeding process. Just before your period begins, and assuming you haven't conceived, progesterone and oestrogen levels fall, triggering the release of prostaglandins, which, in turn, cause the blood vessels in your endometrium (the lining of your womb) to constrict, thereby depriving your endometrial cells of oxygen and causing them to die. The dead cells are then carted off down and out of your vagina during your period. If you're blessed enough to experience cramps or period poos, you can thank prostaglandins for them. When prostaglandins are released they yell, 'Hey, get constricting over there!' to the smooth muscle that is your myometrium (the muscular middle layer of your womb) in order to stimulate contractions to help expel blood, but they can yell so loudly that your bowels get the message too, and hey presto, they also contract, leaving you running for the nearest bathroom.

The lining of your womb, aka your endometrium, generally begins its grand remodelling process within 48 hours of your period starting; by day 3 oestrogen and progesterone receptors (the lock that the key, or hormone, fits into) form, and by day 6 remodelling is complete. Your endometrium is now at its thinnest, measuring approximately 4–7mm thick.

Under My Tongue

An inexpensive, low-tech way of determining if and when you ovulate is to track your basal body temperature (BBT) by using a digital thermometer to take your temperature orally first thing in the morning. Your BBT is the lowest body temperature that your body reaches during sleep, which is why it must be taken after at least three hours of consecutive sleep, and before you eat, drink, or get out of bed in the morning. Prior to ovulation, your temperature is lower, around 36–36.5°C, and after ovulation it rises by 0.2°C or more due to the heating effect of progesterone, which is produced after ovulation. Some people will also find that their temperature dips slightly before they

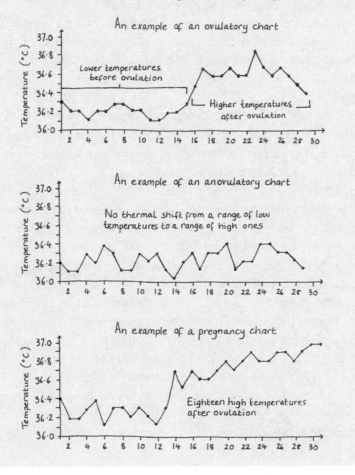

ovulate which can be a helpful heads up that it's about to happen. In the absence of pregnancy, progesterone falls towards the end of your menstrual cycle, causing your BBT to drop just before or as your period starts, whereas if conception has taken place, your temperature remains high and may climb even higher.

BBT tracking is an accurate way of assessing when ovulation takes place, and after a few months of charting your temperature to get to know your cycle in this way, you can establish when you're capable of conceiving (a period of time known as your *fertile window*). Then you can either get to it if you're hoping for a baby, or if you don't want to have one, avoid penis-in-vagina (PIV) sex or use a barrier method like a condom. The fertile window is generally considered to last for 6 days, because an egg is only viable for 12–16 hours after ovulation. Even if you were to ovulate twice in a cycle it would occur within 12 hours of the first egg being released, and once they're inside you, sperm can survive for up to five days in the presence of fertile quality cervical fluid.

When used correctly, taking your morning temperature and monitoring your cervical fluid and cervical position – collectively known as the sympto-thermal method – is a highly effective method of contraception, but tracking your BBT can provide other valuable information too which is why I often ask my clients to chart theirs. Temperatures that are below 36°C are suggestive of hypothyroidism, and post-ovulation temperatures that take a while to climb or which dip during the luteal phase can indicate progesterone deficiency (see page 159 for more on this), both of which would warrant investigation. Establishing when ovulation takes place can help to determine if someone is ovulating on the early side, or quite late, and if their luteal phase is sufficiently long, which is particularly relevant if they plan on having a baby. My clients find it to be fascinating homework, and for those that have irregular cycles, they love being able to predict when their period will start because once they know that ovulation has taken place, they can count forward the number of days that their luteal phase typically lasts for, and calculate when their period will start.

The Sympto-Thermal Method

If you want to use the sympto-thermal method as a form of contraception, I really recommend working with a fertility awareness practitioner to learn how to chart and how to interpret your charts – even if you plan on using an app or a device which monitors your fertility status – before you take the plunge and put your trust in it. Or in the very least read a dedicated book about it (*see* Resources). I've used it as my main method of contraception for 15 years, and I have to admit, after 10 years of it working perfectly, I started to wonder if it was just working well because I was infertile, but since then I have had two planned pregnancies, and both occurred very quickly, probably because I knew exactly when I was fertile. These days I use Daysy, a fertility tracker with a 99.4 per cent effectiveness rate that I use to take my temperature in the morning. Daysy uses my temperature to evaluate my fertility status for the next 24 hours based on the data it's previously collected and then displays either a red light if I'm in my fertile window, or a green one if I'm not. It also displays a yellow light whilst it's learning your cycle and doesn't have enough data to establish your fertility status, or if there's a fluctuation in your temperature (basal body temperatures can be thrown off by drinking alcohol, illness, and fevers), and a yellow light should always be interpreted as a red/fertile day. And of course, you and your partner should both be tested for STIs before embarking on condomless sex.

Interesting Facts About Periods

- You'll have around 400 in your lifetime.
- You can have a cycle in which you don't ovulate and still have a period.
- If you're taking hormonal birth control you're not having periods, you're having withdrawal bleeds which are caused by the lack of hormones when you take the dummy pills in your pack (placebo pills which don't contain hormones but help you to stay in the habit of taking them every day), whereas a period is the result of a full month of biological processes, the key one being ovulation.

- We don't sync up with each other. Research conducted by the menstrual app Clue found that rather than menstrual synchronicity occurring among menstruators who live together, their periods were more likely to diverge over time. If there are periods of time when you menstruate at the same time as someone you live with, it's likely because cycles vary in length for some individuals as well as varying between different individuals, so it makes sense that there will be periods of overlap when you're bleeding together.
- If you swim whilst you have your period, you won't get attacked by sharks.

A Selection is Made

Towards the end of your previous cycle, a group of immature follicles are chosen to continue the maturation process that will see them competing to be the egg that makes it to ovulation, under the influence of follicle stimulating hormone (FSH). It's a bit like all their CVs have been collected, reviewed, and then a group of candidates are selected for interviews. By day 6 the interviewing process is complete, and one candidate overshadows the others in maturity and size. This dominant follicle congratulates itself on getting the job by starting to produce oestrogen – your Beyoncé hormone that prevails over the first half of your cycle. The production and release of oestrogen (along with another hormone produced in your ovaries called inhibin) sends a signal to your pituitary – that pea sized gland in your head – to produce less FSH because now that the follicle for this month has been recruited, we don't want any others trying to compete for the job. FSH still has a role to play, but for now it can take a back seat.

As your dominant follicle continues to grow and ripen, oestrogen levels climb and cause the lining of your womb to thicken to around 10–11mm. Rising oestrogen also stimulates the glands in your cervix to start producing mucus, and you'll be relieved to know that *that's* what that wet patch in your knickers is all about. In fact, there can be a hell of a lot of fluid down there, enough to make you question if you have something weird going on. But what you're feeling and seeing is cervical fluid and it's a sign of good health. Thank flip for that.

Cervical fluid is produced in the lead up to ovulation and is massively important when it comes to fertility. It works in several wondrous ways by:

- Letting you know you're getting ready for ovulation. Cheaper and, in my opinion, more effective than so-called ovulation sticks, which by the way *do not* detect ovulation (see page 46).
- Making sex more comfortable due to its lubricating nature (though it is different from the fluid you produce when you're turned on).
- Creating a route for sperm to get from your vagina and into your womb via your cervix. Think of how salmon jump up waterfalls when they're returning to breed.
- Literally speeding sperm up on their epic journey to your egg.
- Producing a fern-like pattern to guide sperm on their merry way. Whereas the non-fertile cervical fluid during the rest of your cycle, which is drier and more sticky, stops them in their tracks.
- Nourishing sperm to keep them alive and in tip-top shape.
- Providing a more alkaline environment to protect sperm from the acidic nature of your vagina.

The Different Types of Cervical Fluid

Throughout your cycle (remembering that we're all different) you might find that after your period finishes you experience a few days of feeling dry or being slightly moist, but that the moisture evaporates within a few seconds of being exposed to air. This is then followed by the production of cervical fluid that tends to be quite sticky, a bit like rubber cement – rubbery, springy and relatively thick – a consistency that sperm would struggle to do their thing in (warning, if you're using fertility awareness (see page 33) as a method of contraception, you should still treat this fluid as fertile to be on the safe side). Next up comes cervical fluid that is increasing in its moisture content and fertile abilities: it's creamy, runny and milky or lotion-like, and it can also feel quite cool at the opening to your vagina. This fluid is typically white and opaque. You'll start to feel wet even when you're not turned on, which in itself can get you feeling really horny ... yup, Mother Nature's pretty clever when it comes to creating ways to get you to have sex when you're about to ovulate.

Finally, the most fertile mucus arrives. This magical stuff resembles raw egg white and is mega slippery and stretchy; it can stretch for several inches and may just fall out of you (don't worry, there's more inside, you haven't just flushed your fertility for this month down the toilet). Many people I've spoken to have been grossed out by this and assumed there was something dodgy going on. There isn't. This is a normal and an ideal occurrence; you want the egg white goo to be present, particularly if you're trying to conceive. Besides, if a man produced something that could stretch so much, don't you think he'd be boasting about it?

At this stage cervical mucus can be clear or a bit streaky, and at ovulation 4.8 per cent of menstruators will experience spotting and find that their mucus is tinged with pink or red blood. Ovulation spotting is thought to occur because of the relative balance between oestrogen and progesterone immediately after ovulation, when oestrogen drops suddenly but progesterone hasn't risen. Not all mid-cycle bleeding is due to this hormonal shift and it can be a sign of an underlying health issue, so it's important to discuss it with your GP.

You might be wondering how to tell the difference between cervical fluid and semen. Great question! If you're trying to conceive, you're going to have semen inside you pretty regularly, so how do you know what's what? Semen tends to be thinner, breaks apart easily and dries quickly on your finger. Egg white cervical fluid is slippery and stretchy, so doesn't break apart easily. Semen will be absorbed into toilet paper, whilst egg white cervical fluid will sit on top of it without being absorbed.

If you're trying to conceive, you really want to be having sex or directly inserting sperm inside you by the time the milky-lotiony fluid arrives, and certainly when you're producing the egg white mucus. The egg white mucus can keep sperm alive for up to 5 days, hence why it shows up in the days *preceding* ovulation. Some of the sperm that have made it to the cervix will be stored in the side channels called *crypts* that line it before being allowed to proceed any further, and, in rapidly dwindling numbers as the journey continues, those sperm that do make it through the cervix, the uterus, and all the way to the fallopian tube will be temporarily bound to the lining of the fallopian tube where they will wait for the egg. Then, when the egg drifts on by, some sperm will be released and allowed to approach the egg. So rather than it being the sperm racing to reach the egg, it's more of a case of them lurking around until she is ready for them and decides which ones may approach.

That means if you want to conceive YOU NEED TO BE HAVING SEX IN THE LEAD UP TO OVULATION. Don't just wait for day 14 to arrive – you may be leaving it too late as your egg only hangs around for up to 24 hours, plus, not everyone ovulates on day 14. Pay attention to your fluid!

If you're using the sympto-thermal method as contraception, then this is when you need to take other measures, e.g. abstaining (boring, particularly if your libido spikes around ovulation), using condoms (still a bit boring but highly effective), or 'pull and pray' (fun but it requires a lot of prayer, i.e. arguably not a safe method of contraception because it relies on your lover having an excellent level of control). One study found that sperm can be present in pre-ejaculate fluid which dribbles out prior to the main event – though other small studies found no sperm in some pre-ejaculate (and the failure rate of using the withdrawal method is 4–18.4 per cent which is similar to the 2–17.4 per cent achieved with condoms).

So now you're all ready to start keeping an eye out for your cervical fluid, you might be wondering exactly how you'll find it. Here's a radical idea: put your fingers inside your vagina. I know there are people who aren't into doing this and there are lots of reasons why that may be the case, all of which I respect. However, our hesitancy to put a finger or two inside ourselves is really no surprise: most of us have been silently but effectively raised by the powers that be (your parents/religion/school/mass media) to believe that vaginas are dirty and that we're sexual deviants if we touch ourselves – this is the real reason behind tampon applicators. Whatever your feelings about your body, I'm here to tell you that you are wonderful, all of your body parts included.

You may also notice your cervical fluid when wiping yourself after doing a poo (it's okay, we all do it). The slippery nature of the egg white mucus means that your hand may speed up and glide past your vulva as you wipe. As you poo it may also move out of you and go down the toilet. If you suspect that you're approaching ovulation and want to be super attentive, you may want to hold a piece of toilet paper underneath your vulva as you poo so that you can see if any fluid comes out. You may cringe at the idea of doing that now, but if you want to be a parent, you may as well get used to dealing with body fluids now.

Finally, the wet patch in your underwear is a clue to the quality of your fluid. The most fertile fluid has a high-water content and therefore tends to leave a symmetrical patch that stays damp in your undies, whereas the non-fertile stuff that you produce post-ovulation is more likely to leave streaky patches which dry quickly.

Something Fishy Going On?

Cervical fluid is very healthy, but vaginal discharge that smells, or which is different in colour or texture can indicate a vaginal infection such as a yeast (candida) infection, bacterial vaginosis, or trichomoniasis.

- **Thrush** is caused by an overgrowth of a yeast (usually Candida albicans), which lives on the lining of your gut, skin, and vagina without causing us any harm. It's usually kept in check by your immune system and by the naturally acidic environment of the vagina, but there are times when the pH of the vagina becomes more alkaline, such as during menstruation, pregnancy, having diabetes, undergoing chemotherapy, using birth control pills, and taking some antibiotics which kill off the healthy bacteria that usually compete with candida for food and space (ever had a urinary infection, taken antibiotics but gone on to develop thrush?). In this more alkaline environment, yeast-like organisms can proliferate and cause a thick white discharge that often resembles cottage-cheese and severe genital itching, though some people with thrush will experience vaginal itching without a discharge, or the discharge may be thin and watery. Other symptoms include a sore vulva, pain during sex, and a burning sensation whilst peeing. Thrush typically doesn't result in a discharge which smells, and if there is an odour it will smell yeasty, not fishy. An over the counter antifungal medicine such as fluconazole can be used to treat it which is taken orally and/or in the form of a vaginal pessary, and because candida loves yeast and sugar all forms of them should be cut out of the diet, including alcohol and fruit. Eating fermented foods, taking a probiotic which includes a strain called *Sacchararomyces boulardii*, and oregano oil (taken orally) can help to prevent and treat candida overgrowth.
- **Bacterial Vaginosis (BV)** is a bacterial infection that's caused by a disturbance of the ecology of the vagina. A decrease in the number of dominant beneficial bacteria such as Lactobacilli causes numbers of unfriendly bacteria such as Gardnerella to rapidly increase. It can result in a thin, watery, grey, yellow or green discharge that has a strong fishy smell to it but which doesn't usually cause itching or irritation. If your discharge smells fishy, it's important that you tell your doctor because

careful washing before your appointment may mean that they're not alerted to this key sign of BV, and untreated BV is linked to miscarriage and premature birth (pregnant women with untreated BV are five times as likely to have a late miscarriage or premature labour than a woman without BV), as well as periods that are heavy and painful, and breast abscesses. A study conducted by Dr. Anona Blackwell, a consultant in Genito-Urinary Medicine at the Singleton Hospital in Swansea, found that women with untreated BV undergoing terminations have an increased risk of developing a pelvic infection afterwards. As a result of the study, Dr. Blackwell recommended that doctors screen for BV before terminations and caesareans. Risk factors for BV include: vaginal douching, bubble baths, using a copper IUD (which doubles your risk of developing it), smoking, the presence of other sexually transmitted infections, and being sexually active (BV isn't thought to be directly transmitted through sex, though it's identified more frequently in people who are). Antibiotics are usually offered if you are pregnant, undergoing a termination of pregnancy, or have symptoms which bother you such as its characteristic smell, but BV often resolves by itself, particularly if you avoid douching, excessive washing of the vulva (i.e. more than once a day) and the use of products which can upset the balance of bacteria in your vagina and result in BV, such as bubble bath and bath oils, scented soaps and shower gels, strong laundry detergents, and 'intimate hygiene' products (which FYI nobody needs). You should also use condoms during penetrative sex and avoid non-vagina friendly lubricants which are full of additives, flavours and colours (stick to water-based ones instead).

- **Trichomoniasis**, or 'trich' is a sexually-transmitted parasite. This delightful disease produces a discharge which is heavier and/or thicker than usual, or one that's frothy, and that may be yellow, green, grey, or blood-tinged. It may smell fishy or of rotten meat. It also causes itching and burning when you pee, your labia may be red and swollen, and sex might be painful. Antibiotics are used to treat it and to avoid passing it back and forth, sex should be avoided for at least one week following treatment and sexual partners should be treated at the same time. But rather than risk contracting it, why don't you and your partner just get yourselves tested for STIs before opting not to use condoms?

Don't Have Much Fertile Fluid?

Here are the reasons for a low level of fertile fluid:

- You have less as you age – depressing but true. When I started using fertility awareness as contraception in my early twenties, I would consistently have four days of very slippery stretchy egg white fluid, whereas now that I'm 37 I have between one and three days, depending on how well I'm taking care of myself.
- You've recently come off birth control.
- Some common medications can dry your cervical fluid up. These include NSAIDs (e.g. ibuprofen and aspirin), antihistamines, cold and sinus medications that include a cough suppressant or dry up your mucus, clomid (a fertility drug), some sleep aids and antidepressants, propantheline (pro-banthine) and some epilepsy drugs.
- Dehydration.
- Poor circulation to the reproductive organs, which can be related to a sedentary lifestyle, e.g. sitting at a desk all day.
- Cervical cone biopsies, which tend to be performed after an abnormal cervical smear, can occasionally – apparently rarely – affect the ability of your cervix to produce and release cervical fluid as the crypts that produce the fluid can be removed during the biopsy.
- Oestrogen production is low.
- Tampons are hugely absorbent; just think about the blue water being sucked up by a tampon on a TV ad. If you experience vaginal dryness and have a lack of fertile fluid, you might want to experiment with using pads for a few cycles and seeing if there's a difference.

Along with producing and secreting cervical fluid, your cervix also starts showing off. As in, it gets Soft, High, Open and Wet (SHOW). When you feel your cervix internally – this is your cue to put a foot on the side of your bath or loo and assume the classic 'this-is-how-you-insert-a-tampon' pose, or, you know, just squat – you'll feel changes throughout your menstrual cycle. In the run up to ovulation your cervix feels:

- Soft, like your lips. During the rest of your cycle it will feel firm, like the tip of your nose.

- High. It rises up to the top of your vagina so that the distance between your vagina and womb is shorter, giving sperm more of a chance to make that momentous journey. At other points in your cycle it will be lower, which may mean that penetrative sex could feel painful.
- Open. As in, the door is open, come on in you guys!
- Wet, thanks to all that cervical fluid your body has done an amazing job of making.

You Might Get All Tingly, Down There

Thanks to rising oestrogen, blood flow to your genitals is increased, creating delicious sensations that'll have you fantasising when you're meant to be working. Annnnnd you're more likely to orgasm. Hands up if this is your favourite time of the month.

That extra blood flow can also make your clit get bigger around ovulation too, so combined with extra lubrication and an increase in libido thanks to oestrogen and testosterone, this makes for a great time to have some quality me time or grab your lover.

By now your dominant follicle has grown all the way from under 4mm at the start of your cycle up to 25mm in diameter, and ovulation – the moment when the mature egg contained in your follicle is released – is now on the cards.

As oestrogen levels secreted by the follicle peak prior to ovulation, a hormonal sequence is triggered, which instigates the final growth spurt that your follicle needs to mature the egg it contains. This surge of growth creates a bulge on the surface of your ovary, which then ruptures and, just like that, your mature egg is released.

Isn't your body wonderful?

Interesting Facts About Ovulation

- A human egg is the largest cell in the body, measuring in at 0.1mm (a sperm cell is the smallest).
- A female is born with all the eggs she'll ever produce. At birth, her ovaries contain approximately one million immature eggs, and by adolescence only 300,000–400,000 remain. During her reproductive years only around 400 will mature and be released, one and occasionally two at a time, at

ovulation. However, recent research has led to the discovery of ovarian stem cells, from which some IVF experts hope they might eventually be able to grow mature eggs.

- Ovulation largely happens in the morning in spring and in the evening during autumn and winter (50 per cent of women ovulate between midnight and 11am in the spring, and 90 per cent of women ovulate between 4pm and 7pm in the colder months).
- Younger women tend to ovulate from alternating ovaries, whereas women over the age of 30 are more likely to ovulate from the same ovary.
- Once an egg is released, it is only viable for 12–24 hours, but on occasion you can release two eggs within that time frame.
- A fallopian tube can pick up the egg released from the ovary on the opposite side of the body, so if you've been told that you have a blocked fallopian tube, or if you've lost a tube following an ectopic pregnancy, let this give you hope. One study found that around one-third of spontaneously conceived pregnancies were as a result of the remaining fallopian tube picking up the egg from the ovary on the opposite side of the body. That means that even if your right ovary *and* your left fallopian tube don't function or have been removed, your left ovary can release an egg that can be picked up by your right fallopian tube. How friggin' amazing is that?!

Luteal Phase: Ovulation to Menstruation

After releasing the mature egg, the now-empty follicle collapses, develops its own blood supply and becomes a temporary gland called the corpus luteum. It's the corpus luteum that produces and secretes progesterone, the dominant hormone of your luteal phase. Progesterone is the pro-gestation hormone and therefore supports pregnancy if it was to occur, but it has many other health boosting benefits such as: reducing inflammation, calming the nervous system, soothing mood and improving sleep (this is why it may be easier for you to fall asleep and sleep more deeply in the week after ovulation, or why you find yourself needing naps), stimulating the building of bone tissue, and keeping oestrogen in check by either supporting it if there isn't enough or opposing it if there's too much (high levels of oestrogen are associated with an increase in breast and uterine cancer, as well as a whole slew of menstrual cycle symptoms, which you can read about in Section Three).

Side note: if you're taking hormonal birth control with 'progesterone' in it, you won't receive the health benefits I've just mentioned. This is because you're taking birth control which includes progestin not progesterone, and they are different molecules. You only produce progesterone if you ovulate, which of course you won't do if you're on the pill.

My nickname for progesterone is The Great Sedater: it slows you down, making you more cautious and want to stay in and rest. It's essentially keeping you safe in case you're preggers. It not only slows you down, but you may find that it slows your digestion down too, causing constipation. Progesterone does this so that your gut has more time to extract and absorb nutrients from the food you eat in case you need to support a developing embryo. You'll also find that your appetite ramps up during your luteal phase because your body is gearing itself up to grow and house a baby. Go with it; if you don't eat frequently enough then unstable blood sugars will have you feeling hangry as hell. Just try to avoid reaching for comfort foods that are loaded with carbs and sugar, and instead reach for protein and complex carbs such as wholegrains and vegetables.

After ovulation, your cervical fluid dries up and thickens up overnight, becoming pasty and crumbly, perhaps with a slight yellow tinge to it. You'll really notice this because of how it looks and feels in your underwear; put simply, it goes crusty. Your cervix also lowers, closes and gets firmer. These changes are a sure sign that your oestrogen levels have dropped. If you experience a second bout of wet and egg white cervical fluid in your luteal phase, this isn't a fertile time, it's because your progesterone level may have dipped as oestrogen levels increased again (though not to the level they do prior to ovulation), and this relative ratio of high oestrogen to progesterone causes wetter quality cervical fluid.

Due to the warming effect of progesterone on the body, this sudden production of progesterone can be detected as a rise in your basal body temperature. If you've conceived, progesterone will continue to be produced, and 18 consecutive high temperatures should have you suspecting pregnancy.

As your uterus prepares for possible implantation – where a fertilised egg burrows itself in the lining of your womb – the cells in your endometrium swell with secretions and become so plumped up with fluid that they appear as one smooth surface and make your endometrium thicken to 18mm (if you recall it was a mere 4mm at the start of the cycle, so that's a heck of a lot of building that's gone on in there).

If implantation doesn't happen, your corpus luteum begins to disintegrate and by about day 26 of a 28-day cycle, its secretory function comes to an end and your endometrium begins to break down, initiating menstruation and the return to the follicular phase.

A Note About Ovulation Predictor Kits

I can't tell you how many times fertility clients have told me that they rely on OPKs to know when they're ovulating and therefore when to time sex or use donor sperm to conceive. And every time I hear it I take a deep breath and say, 'OK, I think I have a really easy way for you to up your odds of conceiving'. Folks, if you're waiting for a smiley face to appear on the window of your (costly) OPK, then you're likely to be missing out on a significant chunk of your fertile window. In the presence of egg-white quality cervical fluid, sperm can live for up to five days, so why not have his swimmers lurking inside you (they really do lurk). OPKs *do not* detect ovulation. They can pick up on the surge in luteinising hormone (LH) that occurs 12–36 hours before ovulation, and indeed, triggers it. But if you don't test frequently enough, you can miss the surge. You're really better off monitoring your cervical fluid, which by the way won't cost you a penny after you've bought a thermometer. After ovulation, your basal body temperature (BBT) rises by approximately 0.2°C thanks to progesterone, making BBT charting a highly effective way of determining if and when ovulation has occurred. Although this is a retrospective method, it provides a way of getting to know your cycle, which can then be used to predict your fertile phase in future cycles. Some people also experience a preovulatory dip in temperature known as a thermal nadir, which can be a clue that ovulation is about to happen.

SECTION TWO

THE CYCLE STRATEGY

Now that you know the inner workings of your body and your menstrual cycle, we're going to get into how the ebb and flow of your hormones influence your daily life, and how you can use them to improve your career, relationships, and health. Your energy, mood, appetite, sleep, sexual desire, creativity, productivity, ability to focus, interest in socialising, and need for movement and rest are all hugely affected by where you're at in your cycle. Life gets much easier when you get the gist of what typically goes on in each phase because you can understand what's going on internally and go easy on yourself.

In the following chapters you'll find that I've split the menstrual cycle up into four distinct phases, each corresponding to the four seasons of the year:

- The time of menstruation is your Winter.
- Your pre-ovulation phase is your Spring.
- The time around ovulation is your Summer.
- Your premenstruum (the week or so before your period starts) is your Autumn.

Each season of the cycle has its own set of superpowers and dangers, and as well as getting to know these, you'll become familiar with the scientific background to why we evolve so much through each cycle. From there you'll be able to look at your calendar and make adjustments to your work and social life to suit where you're at in your cycle, *to a degree*. There will be stuff that you can't change – perhaps a lot of it – but being in tune with your inner

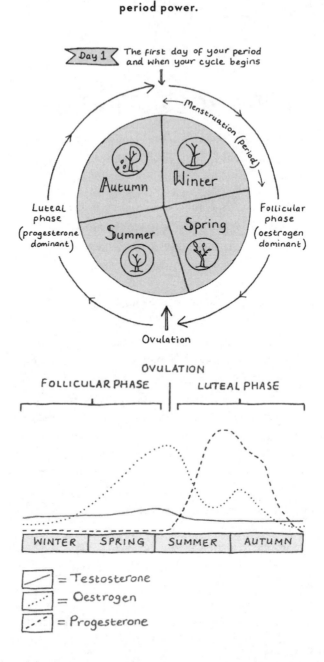

seasons will enable you to respect where you are in your cycle so that when it comes to the aspects that you can't move around or skip entirely, you can at least be aware of what's going on and take care of your needs so that there's less anguish and catastrophes. It's a bit like when it's cold, wet, and windy outside and you've got somewhere to get to. There will be times when you don't want to go outside and when you'll be able to change your plans, but there'll be plenty of times when you just have to dress appropriately, take an umbrella and get on with it, and that's exactly what The Cycle Strategy is.

Although there are typical powers and pitfalls associated with each season, this is about *your* experience of *your* cycle, which is why I'm starting off with stressing the importance of tracking your cycle from the get-go, as in *today*. What I describe in this section is brought about from my training and my clinical experience of working with menstruators for the past decade, but it's only a 346-page book, and it does not include every attitude and experience out there, so what you read in the coming chapters may well chime in with your personal experience of your cycle, or it may not, and that's okay. As with everything, it's your experience that counts, so think of The Cycle Strategy as a template to get you started; a flexible framework for you to play around with while you get to know the ins and outs of your cycle and collect your own data.

The Cycle Strategy isn't about having a perfect 'textbook' cycle. If your cycle is short or long, irregular or absent entirely, then this is still for you, in fact it's even more relevant for you. I can't tell you how many clients I've worked with who've found that once they start tracking their cycle conscientiously, it regulates to a set number of days. If you're someone who isn't menstruating – perhaps you're waiting for your period to return after coming off hormonal birth control or having a baby, or you're post-menopausal or a woman without a womb – then there's still a way for you to track and to bring the rhythm of the four seasons into your life. I've dedicated Chapter 7 to these specific times in life as well as the teen and perimenopausal years (the period of time before your periods stop when you experience symptoms such as hot flushes – see page 201), and how your experience of your cycle might vary if you're trans or non-binary.

The beauty of The Cycle Strategy is that you get to decide when each season ends and begins, and what your personal powers and pitfalls are in each phase (your experience of them and attitude towards them may also change throughout your lifetime). Once you've been charting for a few months, you'll be able to identify where your seasons lie. If your cycle is quite short you might find yourself with a season or two that's particularly short, and if it's long then you could be hanging out in your Spring for a while, wondering when the hell you'll transition into Summer and finally ovulate. If you have a hard time premenstrually then your Autumn might start immediately after ovulation and be long AF.

Ultimately I want you to value the data that you collect, to appreciate and respect what you discover, to recognise your own needs and to care for them. You know your body and your mind better than anyone else and tracking your symptoms and experience of your cycle will put you in the driver's seat of your health and life.

This is about your cycle. Your body. Your life. Most of us have been taught that our hormones and reproductive systems will hold us back in life somehow, but I'm calling bullshit on that because it's our cycles that will get us where we want to be in life – we've got them so let's use 'em!

I am eternally grateful to the co-founders of Red School, Alexandra Pope and Sjanie Hugo Wurlitzer, for teaching me about the seasons of

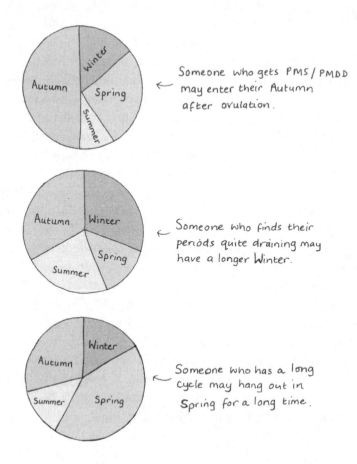

Someone who gets PMS / PMDD may enter their Autumn after ovulation.

Someone who finds their periods quite draining may have a longer Winter.

Someone who has a long cycle may hang out in Spring for a long time.

the menstrual cycle, which they have kindly allowed me to include in this section in addition to some of the qualities that, through their work, they have associated with each season. I highly recommend their book *Wild Power* and the trainings that they offer through Red School (*see* Resources).

Why Track?

Tracking and being aware of your menstrual cycle is the greatest act of self-care you can give yourself, and unlike joining a gym, starting a diet, or quitting coffee, it requires very little effort. When it comes to making healthy changes, cycle awareness has got to be the easiest habit to start, maintain, and implement. And it'll give you massive rewards very quickly. If you've got one minute to spare a day (it can even be whilst you brush your teeth or stick the kettle on), then this is a practice that you can do because it involves the simple act of noticing how you feel and writing it down.

Our menstruating years are when we are figuring out who we are, working through our vulnerabilities, developing our strengths, and coming to feel more at home in ourselves. You are in a continuous loop of being worked by your menstrual cycle, and each one that you move through gives you a chance to grow a little, or a lot, and outgrow the shell of the previous cycle somehow. You'll feel yourself growing outwards in the world, but also down into yourself more – gaining confidence about your right to be here on the planet as your true magnificent self. It isn't always pleasant, in fact it can feel hugely frustrating at times. But it can also be deliciously sweet and friggin' awesome to get to know yourself in this way.

Condensed into each and every menstrual cycle, is our experience from menarche (your first period) to menopause, so each cycle helps to prepare and refine you for menopause. It's the inner work that comes with cycle tracking that's vital if we want to make the psychological transition of menopause with ease, because landing in perimenopause and still not knowing what the hell is going on with your body makes for a rocky time.

Cycle awareness helps you to feel and respond to your changing mood and energy, which creates an inner stability and flexibility that allows you to be kind towards yourself. It gives you a way to create a menstrual map of your month and a way to plan your diary. It gives you instruction on how to care for yourself and capitalise on each phase of your cycle.

As you chart your own feelings and experiences you'll start to recognise your own strengths and struggles, adjusting The Cycle Strategy to suit your own patterns. With time you'll find that there are moments in your cycle where you're even able to predict your mood and energy down to the day. You'll get to know when you'll want to socialise and be out there in the world, you'll know when you need some time alone, and that predictability is good for relationships because it gives those close to you a blueprint for your unique rhythm. When you want to be on the couch with a takeaway and a box set on day 26, and your partner has booked a table at a nice restaurant, but you have no idea what to wear beyond sweatpants because you're bloated as fuck and not feeling all that fantastic about yourself, that's likely to lead to tension. If, however, they are clued up on your menstrual map (in whatever way you want to share it), they'll know that what you really want is a green chicken curry on the sofa and very little conversation, but some snuggling would feel good (as long as you don't have to listen to them eating).

Cycle tracking improves body literacy – your ability to read your body – which has tremendous knock-on effects in terms of self-esteem and mental health, so much so that I'm convinced that cycle awareness is the greatest untapped resource for improving the mental health of menstruating people. It allows you to recognise whether you feel depressed or anxious at certain points in your cycle, or most of the time, and if you do feel that way most of the time, whether your premenstruum intensifies these feelings – a phenomenon called premenstrual magnification. But although the cycle can exacerbate mental health issues, it can also provide moments of relief, and tracking your cycle will allow you to make the most of them.

Working with your cycle is a continual process of separating the wheat from the chaff, of saying, 'That doesn't feel good, neither does that, but this, this feels good, *I want more of this!*' It is a mindfulness practice which keeps you grounded in yourself. And acquiring the habit of checking in with yourself means you're better able to assess your own needs and desires and flex your muscles when it comes to boundaries and self-love. The cycle acts as a container; it's a way to know where you are and who you are, with everything you need to grow and evolve into whomever you damn well please. It grows you and it grows with you, and it allows you to come to rest more and more in yourself.

By the end of this section you'll know that variations in appetite, energy, mood, sexual desire, and sleep, as well as your need for company and time alone, are all 100 per cent normal, and they're usually pretty predictable too. You'll also know that your menstrual cycle does not need to be medicalised and treated, unless of course *you* feel that it needs to be. Tracking your cycle will help you to realise when your symptoms hit you and identify any possible triggers, and it will give you data that you can share with healthcare professionals so that you can advocate for yourself and so that they can treat you appropriately.

Always remember that you are the expert in you.

How to Track

Cycle tracking can take as little as fifteen seconds, or at times you might go deep and scrawl your feelings and experiences for half an hour or more. The aim with all of this is to do what works for you. Here are some ideas to get you started:

One word to rule them all

If you're dubious about all of this, unsure about how to go about it, or wondering how the hell you'll be able to fit tracking into your already-crowded life, this is the method for you.

Every day, just write down one word that encompasses how you feel. That's it. Yeah, it's really effing simple, but it's often the simplest and quickest methods that are easy for us to get on board with and commit to, and that's what we want here; a daily habit, so one word a day is great, truly it is, because it'll be enough for you to start to spot patterns, though I suspect that your curiosity will be piqued – why wouldn't it, you are fascinating – and you'll start writing more.

Even if you use another method for most of the time, there are likely to be days where you feel so amazing that you forget to track (confession – I've been there), so if you find that that's your tendency, go with one word a day in those feel good phases.

You can use the at a glance cycle dial on page 313, keep a note on your phone, or if you're into spreadsheets (apparently some people are) then you can easily create one that will give you a neat way of comparing things month by month. Actually, one word a day on a spreadsheet is a bloody great idea.

Use an app

Phone apps such as Clue, Kindara and Natural Cycles have many benefits and come in handy – they're very user friendly and the alerts help if you're prone to forgetting where you are in your cycle. But they do simplify and generalise experiences and it can be hard to make comparisons month by month. I want you to go deeper but it isn't a case of either/or, and you don't need to delete your menstrual cycle app. In fact, charting your cycle sits nicely alongside them. Do your research though, as some apps sell the data they collect to pharmaceutical companies, which is why I often recommend using Clue because they don't sell data, instead they work with research institutes at Oxford, Columbia, and Stanford universities. I'm also a fan of Clue's non-gendered interface.

Old fashioned pen and paper

This is my favourite method because you can write as little or as much as you like, colour code days (more on this in a moment), and if you're already into using a bullet journal (a system for using a notebook to plan, organise and track different aspects of life) then you can use it to rate some of the things you want to keep track of, such as energy, appetite and sexual desire on your daily pages, or have a chart in the same way you'd have a habit tracker and either use ticks or rate each item out of ten when they apply. When you keep track like this, I recommend including space for your non-ratable musings because there are bound to be some.

Because the menstrual dial is an easy way of looking at the whole of your cycle at once (see an example of a completed dial on page 313), you can glue or tape copies of the dial into your notebook or get creative and draw your own. A blank dial is available to download for free from my website (*see* Resources).

What to Track

Keeping track of how you feel physically and emotionally is a really straightforward way of treating yourself better, because it gives you a way to spot patterns and to identify what you need in order to feel nourished and resilient. This daily practice will make you stronger, and I don't mean improving things so that your mood and energy never dips, because newsflash, you are human. Sure, strength is about your physical capabilities, but there's also strength in being vulnerable, in softening and easing up on yourself, in recognising and respecting where you're at, and working with what you've got.

You can keep track of the physical side of things by noting the following:

- Energy level
- Trouble sleeping
- Libido
- Appetite
- Cravings
- Digestive upsets
- Bloating
- Breast tenderness
- Headaches
- Backache or other body pain
- Menstrual cycle pain
- Basal body temperature
- Cervical fluid
- Cervical position

You also need to note how you're feeling emotionally. The ability to recognise the emotions that we feel varies from person to person. It took me a long time and a whole heap of therapy to be able to name what was going on inside me, so in case you struggle to do so too, or need help on some days of your cycle, here's a quick list for you to refer to:

- At peace
- Scattered
- Hyper
- Grounded
- Restless
- Anxious
- Depressed
- Resilient

- Frustrated
- Confused
- Angry
- Resentful
- Jealous
- Excited
- Joyful
- Doubtful
- Strong
- Weak
- Capable
- Sad
- Happy
- Empty
- Full (can feel good or too much)
- Nourished
- Worried
- Content

You can also identify your needs for:

- Food
- Hydration
- Sleep
- Company and conversation
- Space and quiet
- Activity
- Intimacy and sex – with yourself or another
- Arts and culture
- A dishwasher
- Time to do what's important to you
- A hot bath
- Help

For the days when you want to explore your mood and experiences more deeply, here are some questions to reflect on. Depending on where you are in your cycle and your life some questions will feel more relevant than others. It's okay to answer one question or all of them:

- Is this a phase of your cycle where you feel at home, or at sea?
- What feels easy for you today? What feels hard?
- What needs do you have, emotionally, physically, spiritually, and practically? How can you tend to them in this cycle and in future cycles?
- What parts of your personality are in play during this phase of your cycle? How are they helping or hindering you?
- What, or who, are you drawn to or repelled by? How does that feel?
- How do you feel about your relationship with yourself in this phase, how are you talking to yourself?
- How do you feel about your relationship with others in this phase, how are you talking to others?
- Are you being kind to yourself, and if not, why not?
- How do the people around you react to you when you're in this phase, and how do their reactions feel to you?
- What challenges are you facing, how can you support yourself and how can you ask for support?
- What is your deepest desire today, how does that relate to where you are in your cycle and your life right now?
- What is your deepest fear today, how does that relate to where you are in your cycle and your life right now?
- If there was one thing you could somehow improve today, what would it be?
- What can you be proud of yourself for today?
- What are you grateful for today?
- Where do you get stuck or come undone?
- What are your natural talents in each phase, and how can you elevate them or make them seen/heard by others?
- What support can you give yourself or ask of others in each phase?

Putting it all Together

It's up to you how involved you get with tracking, but quite clearly you could end up with a lot of information, so let's take a look at what you can do with all of it.

At the end of each cycle, take some time to recap your experience of charting and of what you've tracked. What intention or plan did you set for this cycle and did it happen? What enabled that or got in the way? What insights have you gained and how can you practically apply them to future cycles? How can you love yourself more?

If you're using the menstrual dial or a diary then you can assess where each season began and ended by colour coding each day. By doing this you'll see within a few cycles how predictable your cycle is, and then you can colour code in advance so that when your best mate suggests a big night out, you'll know what dates to suggest. Hopefully the dates you give them will suit their cycle too!

To be forewarned is forearmed, so if you realise that there are days which are consistently tricky for you, write warnings about them in your calendar. I'm a fan of sticking 'slow down' as an all-day event on days 1, 2, 6, and 20, days when I can feel slightly depleted, and 'be alone' on days 21 and 24 when I really crave solitude and silence. That way, whatever I have to schedule for those days is done in mindfulness of how I'm likely to feel, and I'll try to move them to other days if possible.

Cycle tracking helps you to plan when to work hard, when to rest, when to hit the gym, when to be social, and when to take some time for yourself. Most of us are unable to live a life that's 100 per cent in tune with our cycle, so it's about bringing in awareness to those times where life doesn't sync up with the phase that we're in. When you have a full on day at work right in your premenstruum, make sure you get decent shut-eye the night before and don't skip meals, that way you can make the most out of your powers without being thrown off by exhaustion and low blood sugar.

Transition Days

If you notice that you're getting in the swing of a season but then have a day that's a bit off, it could be that you're transitioning from one season to the next. Transition days are days where it's common to feel a blip or a wobble, a slight falter which might manifest as feeling tired and emotional, or as intense as a rug being pulled from underneath your feet. They can be days where you feel too much, or not much, because sometimes they result in a sense of emptiness or numbness.

They come about because of resistance to leave a season that you feel at home in or that you haven't quite managed to express the powers of as you would have liked to. There may be anxiety about entering the upcoming season that could be about being seen, or your feelings around fertility – either because you want to conceive or really don't want to – and sadness if you want a relationship but aren't in one so there's an element of the missed connection. You might feel joy at leaving a season that you struggle in, but in rushing out of it without awareness, find yourself unravelling at the seams.

Your feelings about each season can change throughout your lifetime. For years I was an ovulation queen and couldn't imagine ever favouring another phase in my cycle, but once my cycle returned after becoming a mother, I began to shy away from the sunny side of the cycle as I experienced a detachment with my sexuality. With that, a distinct wobble on day 6 emerged, and with some exploration, I realised that it was my resistance to being seen and being visible as a sexual being, and of wanting to retreat and reclaim some time for myself, which made entering the phases which are typically about being out there and connecting hard to head in to. Then there's the matter of writing this book in five menstrual cycles – the intense pressure of needing to be highly productive in my Spring and Summer really affected my previous desire to be in them.

In a 28-day cycle these transition days are likely to be around days 6, 12, 20, and 28, but remember this is about your cycle and you may well notice the timing of them is different for you. They can also vary month by month and come earlier or later depending on your health and what's going on in your life. Get to know when these days happen in your cycle and if they disrupt your flow, plan around them; do you need to include a calming and grounding walk through a park on your way to work? How about making sure you've got a nourishing meal for your lunch? Do you just need to lie down for half an hour when you get in the door?

Without cycle awareness, transitioning seasons can hit you hard. They're unexpected and can leave you feeling as if the ground is going from beneath you, spelling catastrophe for your mental health, relationships and work life. And some people will find that they struggle throughout Spring and Autumn because they are transitional seasons, whereas Winter and Summer act as the poles of the cycle because they contain the two main events; ovulation and menstruation. A client of mine called Catarina experiences this with her cycle, 'I feel much more settled and calm in Winter and Summer, and also more grounded and connected to myself.'

With cycle awareness you know to expect these transitional days and seasons, and can soften the blow by landing on a mattress – which may be in a very literal sense in that lying down and doing nothing might make you feel a million times better – or it might be simply talking to yourself with kindness because you have an awareness of what's going on, stepping back from the daily responsibilities that you're able to, or bringing in other strategies to manage menstrual cycle issues. The key is to just get charting so that you know when to expect your period and how to care for yourself when you do.

Cycle tracking brings you into a more intimate relationship with yourself. It gives you the confidence to say 'yes' and to fully embrace your natural talents and opportunities, to develop healthy boundaries and confidence in all aspects of your life, to recognise your own needs and desires, and to cultivate self-respect and self-worth. It's the shit, so let's get into it.

Chapter 3

There will be blood (Winter)

Every mile is two in Winter
– George Herbert

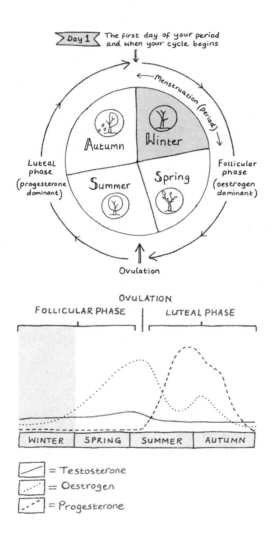

Here we are, at the start of your Winter. As one cycle is ending and another starting, it is both the moment of death and also of rebirth; which does it feel most like to you?

How do you respond to the knowledge that your period is starting? Do you feel the relief of not being pregnant, or of the build-up of PMT finally abating? Do you feel full of panic and dread because you suffer from menstrual pain, flooding, or other unpleasant symptoms? Does its arrival bring disappointment and a further dismantling of hope if you long for pregnancy, even in the absence of actively trying? Is it something you actively look forward to, an annoying inconvenience, or does your period simply pass by without much mention?

Whether you're greatly affected by your periods, or they don't trouble you at all, they do quite literally, rule our lives. They are one of the oldest systems of measurement and evidence of our internal tides, but they tend to get a bad rap and many of us would rather not have them at all. Periods are seen as a messy intrusion and an embarrassment; an inconvenience that can interrupt work and play. Periods are the only source of blood not caused by trauma but for the most part they are hidden, managed and minimised, which is ironic, given that they are a sign of a healthy functioning reproductive system and that menstrual blood is a rich source of stem cells – a type of cell that can develop into any other cell in the body and is therefore highly valued by the medical community.

The way you feel about your period is influenced by a whole host of factors; your past experiences of menstruation, the cultural and religious contexts in which you were raised, your experience of your first period (an event referred to as menarche), your family's attitude towards menstruation and the patterns passed down to you through generations, other people's reactions to your period (both currently and in the past), your current desires to avoid or achieve pregnancy, and the feelings you have about your body, gender, sexuality, health, and where you are in your life.

Why is it that when blood that comes out of a vagina is caused by a man 'taking' someone's virginity, the blood is celebrated – sometimes shown off – and he is admired and slapped on the back, but when it's a monthly natural biological process, it's repulsive and must be kept hidden?

Entering your Winter

The days around the start of your period are when your hormones collapse to their lowest levels. You may feel this hormonal drop off acutely and experience a state of collapse on some level as your period begins. Overwhelming fatigue, emotional vulnerability, teariness, anxiety and an unsettled spirit can all show up now, but it's often the case that you don't realise that's what's going on until you start bleeding, at which point it suddenly all makes sense.

You might find that you get a heads up that your period is about to start, either because the symptoms that you have a hard time with begin, or because you feel a slight separation between you and the rest of the world as the process of starting to bleed pulls you into yourself and you enter a void time. When you feel yourself pulling away from the world, that's your cue to do what you have to do in order to have a good experience of your Winter, whether that means stocking up on period supplies, or carving out some time for yourself. After tracking her cycle for a few months, my client Catarina spotted a theme around her Winter and is learning to work with how she feels:

> 'My Winter always starts in the evening or during the night. As I start to bleed I feel huge relief. Tension transforms and dissipates. I want to be alone and find questions annoying, specifically if they will involve a deeper conversation. I can't listen to music and have an aversion to physical contact (including breastfeeding). My partner likes to be physically affectionate but is learning to show his love in other ways such as bringing me a hot drink or allowing me some space.'

Here's how you'll know when you're arriving in your Winter:

- As oestrogen and progesterone decline, your BBT drops a day or so before your period starts, or once you start bleeding.
- It feels as if the bubble of premenstrual pressure has finally popped, and with it goes your bloating, breast tenderness and emotional tension.
- The safety valve in the cycle is released, your ego experiences a collapse and you're able to let go (tissues and teary film at the ready).
- The onset of your period brings emotional upheaval with it. It's not just a physically cleansing process – it can be an emotional clear out too.

- You develop a physical awareness that you're about to bleed or have already started.
- Menstrual pain. Joy of joys.
- You feel yourself drifting and disconnecting from the world around you as your energy becomes its most inward, making it hard to concentrate on the outer world.
- Instead, a deep inward focus is possible (and may be the only option if you're doubled over in pain).
- You enter a fog or dream-like state, perhaps an altered state of consciousness, where you feel a bit out of it.
- You might feel a sense of bliss as your body releases the natural pain-relieving hormones oxytocin and endorphins.
- Your boundaries dissolve, leaving you feeling more permeable and vulnerable to the world. This isn't the time to be doing a big food shop or have your in-laws visit.
- You might feel aroused as blood flow is directed to your womb and genitals.

If you have a hard time premenstrually, and particularly if you have an extreme form of PMS called premenstrual dysphoric disorder (PMDD), then the appearance of your period can bring instantaneous relief because it means that you're back in the half of the cycle where you feel like yourself again. Whereas if you have fertility or period problems and your period is unwelcome and unwanted, then this can make for a messy time, either in the form of actual leakage or emotional turmoil and physical pain that's best described as torture.

But even in the depths of misery, your period acts as an anchor. On a basic level it informs you that you're not pregnant, but it also gives you a chance to stop, take stock, assess, and let go. It's your monthly moment to check in with yourself, to assess the health of your cycle and your period, to read through your previous cycle of tracking and note how long the cycle that's just ended was, as well as what symptoms you experienced and when they occurred, and where you had peaks and troughs in energy, mood and sexual desire.

As you gather data from each cycle, you can compare them to previous cycles and begin to spot commonalities and patterns. For a lot of people with periods, this can be surprisingly specific. My client Gemma had been struggling with anxiety and depression and she'd been to see her GP who had prescribed her an antidepressant, but she was unsure whether she wanted to take it, so she'd held off on filling it out. She'd also attended one of my workshops and as she began to track her cycle, she was shocked to realise that she didn't feel this way all of the time – only on days 19–22, and then again just before her period started. Because Gemma was also prone to spotting a light amount of blood for a few days before her period started, I wondered if her progesterone was low and asked her to track her BBT as well as having a blood test so that we could look at everything together. She came back the following month and we could see that her BBT dipped noticeably at the same time as her mood dropped. The results of her blood test confirmed that although she was ovulating and producing progesterone, she wasn't producing enough to support the second half of her cycle. This was important because it was the calming quality of progesterone that she was missing out on that was probably leaving her feeling anxious, especially considering that she wanted to start trying to conceive. After discussing all the options available to her, Gemma decided to see a private doctor who was licensed to prescribe bioidentical hormones – hormones which are chemically identical to ones produced in the body – and she started taking bioidentical progesterone as well as using acupuncture and dietary changes to support ovulation and her luteal phase. In the next couple of cycles she noticed a massive difference to how she felt and her BBT temperatures became stable throughout her luteal phase. Her doctor suggested that she keep taking progesterone whilst trying to conceive and throughout her first trimester, and Gemma went on to have a healthy pregnancy. So for Gemma, it was very much a case of needing hormonal support, not antidepressants, and it was cycle tracking that allowed us to establish that.

Winter is the time to focus on your needs and to consider what's necessary for your upcoming cycle and for what you want more of in your life. In the same way Monday morning is when you think about the week ahead and make decisions about how you'll spend your time, who you need to speak to, and what needs your time and energy, your Winter is the season of your cycle where you can get clear about what you want in your life and what you need to work on in order to get there.

During your period, take some time out to ask yourself the following questions, both in relation to your cycle and your life:

- What am I battling with?
- What am I ready to let go of?

- What needs my attention?
- What do I want more of?
- Where can I bring energy and focus into my life?

These simple questions will help you to assess where you're at and what you want to change. I recommend answering them quickly and impulsively in order to get honest and perhaps surprising answers, and then consider what you want to work with for this cycle. Do you have a specific intention or goal for this cycle? Be truthful with yourself, write it down, and trust that the universe has got your back.

Winter's Superpowers

Set boundaries

Stake a claim in the ground for yourself and your needs – whatever they may be. If you feel permeable and vulnerable during your period then ask yourself what you can do to safeguard yourself while you're bleeding, and if there are things you need to say no to. Do you need time on your own or do you want closeness and intimacy? Are you able to ask someone to do the nursery run for you, can you eat dinner out after you finish work and get a quieter train home? If you don't feel you have any needs, that's awesome because it frees you up to think about what you want – what desires are burning inside you and how can you nurture them now and give them strength. My wise and wonderful menstrual mentor, Alexandra Pope, explains that menstruation is when the outer lights of the world turn down and our inner lights go up, and for our inner lights to be their most bright, they require darkness. It's this understanding that can help to inform the decisions about what you use your energy on in your Winter.

Nourish

Once you've cleared the decks, you'll be left with some space which you can either fill with a nourishing activity or leave as empty space. By nourishing activity, I mean doing something that is solely for you. You might do it on your own or share with other people, that's your choice, but the guiding principle is that it is something restorative, pleasurable and about you. Leaving space can be challenging and uncomfortable; it's all too easy to fill it with a 'quick' scroll through Instagram rather than sit with yourself in silence and see what's there, but give it a go. What's inside of you might be messy, but it's beautiful too.

Rest

Most menstruators that I've worked with find that the beginning of a period is the natural point in the cycle to rest in some way, and although this brings up the 'Am I a shitty feminist to suggest that we take some time off?' question in me, I do feel that some form of rest here, if you need or want to take it, can be hugely beneficial. Not only is resting in your Winter considerate of the process of menstruation (which does after all require some effort on the part of your body), but it allows your energy to build for the more outward and productive seasons of Spring and Summer.

Release

You can let go of more than blood during your Winter. It's the prime time to release pent up feelings, as well as people, situations, and beliefs about yourself that aren't serving you. Consider how you can clear out the old to make way for the new and shine the spotlight on what's important to you. Try freewriting, a technique where you write continuously for a set period of time without pausing to pay attention to spelling, grammar, or topic, and if you run out of things to say, you just write 'I don't know what to write' repeatedly until something else comes up. It's a great way of using ten minutes to dump all that accumulated mental chatter and give yourself some head space.

Receive

When you make space and are present during your Winter, you'll find yourself gifted with insights and creative solutions to problems you've been stewing on for a week or a decade. Learn to trust your instincts and the messages that come to you whilst you're bleeding. You've probably had revelations during this time before, but perhaps haven't tied them to the process of menstruation.

Winter's Dangers

Carrying on without awareness

If your period is light, short, or uneventful then you could find it hard to stay present in your Winter, in which case set things up so that you're reminded to move with awareness and remember to slow down, even if it's only by 5 per cent. Similarly, although painkillers thankfully numb pain, they can work so well that they also numb the process and you might miss out on the wisdom of your Winter. Bingeing on reruns of *Friends* is one way of resting and can be helpful because laughter gets feel-good hormone oxytocin going, but distractions can also prevent you from accessing a deeper part of yourself, so experiment with omitting them and seeing what happens. Could solitude and quiet for half an hour be that bad?

Ignoring the call to retreat
When you get the cue to take a step back from the world, get what you can in order so that you're able to follow this instruction, even if you have to step back into the real world pretty soon after. If all you can manage is twenty minutes, then really give in to that twenty minutes and then put your game face back on. Although there are times in life when pushing on is necessary and can't be avoided, recognise that that's what you're doing and make small adjustments to compensate. Not enough rest in your Winter can leave you feeling depleted in your Spring and Summer, and you'll miss out on the power of the most productive phases.

Guilt
Oh, how easy it is to feel riddled with guilt for easing up or taking time off, but take a look around. Has the world fallen apart because you removed yourself from it for an hour or a day? Do you not feel restored and more able to function in a fuller capacity because of it? Would you lambast a friend for doing the same? I thought not, so ease up on your self-inflicted guilt.

Rushing out
If you're sensitive to oestrogen slowly increasing while you're still in your Winter and probably bleeding, it's easy to feel a surge and go with it but try to hold back a bit and keep some energy for yourself, or you may well find yourself tired AF as you transition into Spring. After the depths and darkness of Winter, Spring can feel like a blessed relief, and it's all too easy to charge out of the starting gates and get back in the swing of things, but instead of burning off the energy that's only just getting going, experiment with letting it accumulate.

Menstrual Retreat vs. Menstrual Exclusion

Historically, menstruating women have been blamed for just about every misfortune going, from causing rivers and wells to run dry, to killing plants and flowers, preventing dough from rising, spoiling meat, curdling milk and mayonnaise, and making pickles rot. Some cultures and religions consider periods to be unclean and place prohibitions on menstruators whilst they are bleeding, to the point of being banished from their home. But there are also communities where menstrual blood is a sign of power, and menstruation gives girls and women access to the spiritual realm. For example, rather than be isolated, the women of the Kalasha people of North-West Pakistan gather in a large sacred building where they menstruate, give birth, and enjoy their time together.

In some religions – such as Orthodox Judaism, Islam, and Rastafarianism – sexual contact between a man and a woman is not permitted while she is menstruating, and some instruct that the couple sleep in separate beds. There are cultures which require the woman to seclude herself in a menstrual hut lest she contaminate the food and water around her. In the Hindu societies of Rajasthan, Bangladesh, Nepal and Bali, women aren't allowed to cook or come into contact with food and must refrain from visiting religious sites, which is also a feature of Islamic culture and the Shinto religion of Japan.

In some parts of Nepal menstruating women are seen as impure and are forbidden from touching other people, cattle and crops. Women are often secluded from their communities, and if they are allowed to remain in their own home then they are not permitted to enter the kitchen or worship room. In some rural areas of the country a tradition called *chaupadi* is still practised despite being outlawed in 2004, in which women are banished and forced to live in tiny sheds when they are bleeding, and poor hygiene and freezing temperatures have resulted in death.

At best, a menstrual retreat can provide respite from chores and responsibilities and create time to share in female company, but at worst they are detrimental towards physical and mental health and can risk death. Let's be clear in distinguishing that removing oneself from daily responsibilities to enjoy female company is inherently different from enforced segregation and neglect that is violent and oppressive and based on the belief that women are impure and dangerous.

Make Rest Radical

We live in a world where rest is rarely respected, and we're surrounded by ever-increasing pressure to do more and more. When we exist in a culture where growth at all costs is what's valued, rest becomes radical and your Winter is the perfect time to embrace it, if you feel called to.

Take your cue from nature; nothing blooms all year long so why would we bloom continuously? Winter is the natural time to hibernate, to rest and recharge, and to plan for the coming year, or in this case, menstrual cycle. It's when farmers take time off before the busy planting season of Spring begins and focus on important tasks such as fixing equipment and planning and preparing for the coming year. Similarly, your Winter is the time to rest and plan, to tend to important basics and to sack off whatever you can get away with (which is probably more than you think you can).

When animals hibernate in Winter, it allows for the conservation of nutrients that are essential for the rapid growth during Spring, and we aren't dissimilar to our furry friends; if you allow yourself adequate rest here, then you'll be firing on all cylinders in your Spring and Summer. That doesn't mean that you have to lie perfectly still in bed for three days, unless of course that's what you need or want to do, in which case, totally honour that. And if you can't because of adulting, then give yourself whatever you can, even if it's half an hour – you'll be amazed at what thirty minutes of purposeful rest will do for you.

Another way of bringing in some rest is to take time off from exercising. This is a great time to have rest days (even Olympic athletes have rest days), or to change the type of exercise you do to something gentler; walking instead of running, restorative or Yin yoga instead of a strong and fast-paced vinyasa class, a short and light cardio workout instead of high intensity interval training. Winter is where your energy draws inward and that can make physical activity feel like hard work, so don't squander the energy that you do have, focus it on whatever you deem as important.

Historically, rest was seen as something that the upper classes needed and that the working class needed to be steered away from, in order to prevent laziness and alcoholism, and the idea of taking time off now still smacks of privilege. As an able-bodied white woman with an education and a pretty stable life, I am certainly privileged, and yet there are times when I can find it hard to get the time out I feel I need when I'm bleeding. This means that for anyone less privileged than I am, the responsibilities of life will certainly create a barrier when it comes to taking time for yourself, especially if the demand placed upon you to earn an income and care for others is a heavy one. This may be the only time in the whole of your cycle where you feel that you can legitimately take some time for yourself, because, as another client Sandra has come to realise, being on your period may be the only permitted reason for you to slow down in life: 'I feel tired and want to hibernate, but I'm also at peace. I like my Winter because I feel like I don't have to force anything and that it's the only time in my cycle when I can allow myself to say "no".'

If you want to find ways to rest, consider:

- Retreating from social media. It sounds simple but I reckon it's the hardest kind of retreat.
- Hit the sofa with that book you've been desperate to read.
- Listen to a ten minute guided visualisation or meditation (there are lots of free ones online).
- Work from home so that you can at least stay in your pyjamas and slippers and strap a hot water bottle to your belly.
- Get an agreement in place with another parent where you can dump your kids with them for a bit and return the favour when they're on their period.
- Swan off to a spa for the day or recreate your own at home.
- Take your lunchbreak outside.
- Lie down and listen to a song or piece of music that moves you.
- Watch the grass or leaves move in the wind, or a candle's flame dance.
- Go to a restorative or Yin yoga class.
- Have a podcast or audio book downloaded so that you can disappear on your commute home from work.
- Chuck two decent handfuls of Epsom salts in a hot bath, light some candles and enjoy some peace and quiet.
- Go camping, even if it's in your own living room or garden.

Bleeding Liabilities

When men were sent to the front line during the world wars, women were needed in the workforce and we kept the ship sailing, quite literally. Research from this time concentrated on women's ability to perform tasks during menstruation, such as flying a plane (this particular study concluded that women were perfectly safe pilots *if* they had a 'healthy' cycle, as if they thought that bleeding might turn us into kamikaze pilots). But by the 1940s research shifted focus towards the possibility that certain types of work were associated with menstrual dysfunction, not because of occupational hazards and detrimental working conditions, oh no, being the fragile creatures that we are, this was about our inherent weakness and inability to cope with the working environment. Interesting timing. The men who made it home wanted their jobs back.

Periods have long been used to keep us out of positions of power, and that tactic is still in play today. In 2009, right-wing radio host G. Gordon Liddy expressed his concern about President Obama's nominee for Supreme Court Justice, Judge Sonia Sotomayor, 'Let's hope the key conferences aren't when she's menstruating or something, or just before she's going to menstruate. That would really be bad. Lord knows what we would get then', and when Donald Trump wanted to attack Fox News host Megyn Kelly for putting him under pressure during a Republican debate, he told CNN, 'There was blood coming out of her eyes, blood coming out of her wherever.' Classy, real classy.

We are not liabilities when we're working and bleeding, we regularly rise to the occasion and above it, we are not limited by our bodies – unless of course pain and/or heavy blood loss restricts you physically. Plenty of you will feel fine when you have your period and have no need to ease up on your workload, but for those of you that do, play to your strengths; if you know you can have a productive morning of work, do the important stuff then, and then switch to maintenance mode of replying to emails and tying bits and bobs up. Or do things the other way around if you're someone who gets hit with cramps and heavier blood loss in the mornings.

Contrary to menstruation being a physiological process that holds us back, I think we have a lot to gain from our bodies during this time. You can experience a coming home into yourself during your Winter, perhaps getting a sense of an inner direction or calling, or feeling the frustration of wanting to do something in the world but not necessarily knowing what that is. Allow your inner thoughts and emotions to rise to the surface. This is a time when everything is closer and accessible. Listening and being receptive are yin qualities that are associated with this deeply restorative phase – your period pulls you inward and provides a way to access a deeper part of yourself, and resting allows you to receive the wisdom that comes with your Winter. It gives you a chance to check in with yourself and assess where you are in life and if life is matching up to your dreams, and it's when solutions can come to you, but you need the space and stillness to hear them. During your Winter you have a deep and direct line to yourself, which is why some tribes such as the Yurok Indians treat the time of menstruation with great respect by upholding their tradition of women not working while they're bleeding. Instead, what they often refer to as their moon time is spent in meditation so that they can use this permeable state to be in contact with the spiritual realm.

While the vast majority of us aren't able to walk away from our responsibilities when we're bleeding, I do feel that there is power in doing so to whatever extent feels good to you *and* that you can get away with – but I've encountered a hell of a lot of resistance to this idea; it goes against the nature of being a feminist and it suggests that the only people who can indulge in this are the ones who are in total control of their schedules and who are financially independent. But when clients finally manage to carve out some time for themselves – and for some of them this has required more practical preparation than I had imagined – great things have taken place. I know, I know, I hear you when you say that you can't, and I get it, time is precious and so is your work and protecting your income. Time off can feel impossible and is a luxury that many cannot afford. But can you find ten minutes to give yourself and start from there? Can you gift yourself thirty minutes of quiet time, to turn away from the world and tune into yourself to see what happens, without scrolling on your phone?

Life is busy and whilst there are some responsibilities that you can't abandon, some projects can sit on the sidelines when you're bleeding. That doesn't mean that they aren't being worked on, often there's powerful work going on even in a dormant state, and ideas that were jostling, are able to settle and find their place. Have you ever battled your way through an afternoon meeting, struggled to come up with a solution to the mother of all problems, only for a cracking idea to absentmindedly come to you while in the shower the following morning? That's the essence of what can happen in your Winter. Stepping away creates space that is incredibly valuable when you're menstruating because it's a time when you can receive insights, perspectives and solutions – the answers to everything that you've been struggling with – but you won't be able to hear them if you don't make space for them.

Some work can absolutely not be left, and this can be a time in your menstrual cycle when you're able to do really awesome work, particularly if you're someone who feels tuned into what they're doing in the world, so do what you can to protect this time and prioritise the work which is most pressing and/or valuable to you. That means addressing all the bits and pieces that don't fall into either of those categories and putting them to one side for now. And if you've been struggling with a piece of work, this is the time to step away from it, either by sending it out into the world and letting go (along with any need to hold onto it in a continual quest for perfection), or by leaving it be for a day or a few if you're not feeling it. Rest assured that from day 3 onwards, as your hormones start to climb again, you'll feel increasingly energised and motivated.

Menstruation is a time when your intuition is high, so if you find yourself unsure about your path in life or what education/training to undertake, or if you're considering a career change, this is the time when suggestions will drift in and you might receive clues about your calling in life. Though it needn't be large scale, a calling is about your big work in the world and how you'll use your unique perspective and talents to address a particular problem. Pay attention to what you're drawn to during your period; make notes and just sit with them for a little while. You don't have to uproot overnight (unless of course you want to), but you can let ideas about your callings in life sit on the edge of your periphery. Being called to do something can feel inspiring and exciting, but also terrifying and overwhelming. Start with simply being aware and sitting with things for a bit. Your cycle will act as a fertiliser and each time you head into your Spring and Summer your hormones will help you to develop the roots and shoots that will bring your ideas into reality. And because callings don't go away, they just become painful on a spiritual level if they're not acted on – typically in your Autumn – it will get to the point where you have to take action. Learn to trust the instincts you have when you're bleeding – they hold a power that the world needs.

The Politics of Period Leave

Some companies and countries have menstrual leave policies, where menstruators can take paid time off work without it affecting the time they can take off for sick days or holidays. As someone who used to have extreme period pain that was debilitating and made walking pretty hard, let alone working, I think this is flipping fantastic because there are plenty of us who have a bloody hard time when we're bleeding, and it is high time that the workplace took this into consideration. Not to mention the fact that women do the bulk of unpaid work in society, so given that we are likely to be doing several days' extra work a month when compared to men, I think it's reasonable to have a day or two off when we're bleeding.

Yet there's also part of me that shrinks away from the idea of it; we've spent so long dismantling the incorrect idea that we are the weaker sex, incapable of controlling our hormones but somehow able to destroy crops and pollute water, that menstrual leave feels like a massive step backwards. Like after all the protests, we're finally admitting and accepting that we aren't as able as the penis owners and, as Emily Martin, vice president for workplace justice at the National Women's Law Center in America told the *New York Times*, 'It suggests women are uniquely handicapped in the workplace by the fact that they have periods ... and that every person who menstruates is ill.' In fact, plenty of menstruators have no issues with their periods and a lot of those who do, continue to excel in their work when they're bleeding. But what about those who do struggle? After all, an online survey conducted by YouGov found that 30 per cent of women have taken time off work because of menstrual cramps (although the same study showed that 68 per cent of those that had did not share the reason for this with their employers).

Surely the simple answer is to have an all-inclusive policy for ill health, which includes period problems, pregnancy loss, issues related to perimenopause and menopause (when your periods stop), as well as long-term health issues and mental health conditions in all humans, not just people with periods. That way the very real potential for discrimination – for lower salaries, less opportunities and generally using our bodies against us, *again* – would be removed. But how about we get down to the root of the issue, and while we're at it improve menstrual cycle education, the diagnosis and treatment of menstrual disorders, and the availability and accessibility of health and wellness models. Not much to do then.

Period Poverty

Menstrual supplies are an absolute must for anyone who has a period, but bleeding is a billion-dollar business and as prices go up, the number of menstrual products per packet goes down, making them increasingly inaccessible to those who can't afford them.

While this undoubtedly affects those living in the developing world, it is very much an issue in the developed world too. The charity Plan UK reports that one in 10 girls aged 14 to 21 in the UK have been unable to afford menstrual products, one in seven have struggled to afford them, and 40 per cent have had to improvise and use other methods to catch their menstrual flow. Taping tissues or whole rolls of toilet paper to underwear is the most common replacement, followed by socks, clothing rags, newspaper, and doubling up on underwear in a desperate attempt to contain blood.

The same report states that 49 per cent of girls in the UK have missed an entire day of school because of their period, and a report by the charity WaterAid and UNICEF found that more than a third of girls in South Asia don't attend school when they have their period. This has devastating consequences, as Meghan Markle, Duchess of Sussex, pointed out in 'How Periods Affect Potential', her 2017 article for *Time* magazine: 'When a girl misses school because of her period, cumulatively that puts her behind her male classmates by 145 days. And that's the mitigated setback if she opts to stay in school, which most do not.'

This is not okay. With astonishing figures like this, it's clear that improving the availability of menstrual products by making them free, improving menstrual health education and the health of teens' periods, is a vital early intervention when it comes to addressing gender equality in education and the workplace. As Chella Quint, menstrual educator, comedian, author, and founder of the #periodpositive campaign states: 'Period poverty is not just financial poverty – sometimes it's poverty of knowledge, confidence, sustainability, or access and schools can address this right now.'

In the UK almost 70 per cent of girls aren't allowed to go to the toilet during school lesson times, which results in 16 per cent of them missing school because they're worried that they won't be allowed to use the toilet – and so begins our education in needing to obtain permission from those in authority to simply do what our bodies require of us, something I see play out in pregnancy and labour when women tend to talk about what they'll be 'allowed' to do. Of those that do attend their classes, almost two-thirds worry about leaking in class which is hardly conducive to learning. Now imagine coming on in the middle of an exam. Quint is currently leading a campaign in the UK to encourage schools to keep a supply of menstrual products in the toilets nearest the exam halls in order to alleviate this additional worry. Imagine the massive difference this basic provision would make to menstruating students.

One in three women worldwide don't have access to a safe place to go to the toilet, and of these an estimated 526 million have no choice than to go to the toilet out in the open and are therefore at an increased risk of disease, shame, harassment and attack. Periods aren't dirty, but when period products are unattainable the very normal act of bleeding that affects half of the population becomes a risk in terms of hygiene and personal safety. And I haven't even got into how being unable to care for oneself by simply having a period product and somewhere safe to use it impacts on someone's self worth.

There are some fantastic charities and organisations around the world working to improve education and access to menstrual supplies, including:

- Binti International work in the UK, the USA, India, and Africa to improve access to pads, as well as educating about menstruation in order to break the taboos and stigmas that surround periods.
- Bloody Good Period work to end period poverty on the ground by giving these products to those who can't afford them and providing long-term menstrual education to those less likely to access it. They rely on public donations of menstrual supplies which they redistribute to asylum seekers, refugees and those who can't afford them.
- Days for Girls supply reusable menstrual kits to women and girls in over 116 countries, as well as menstrual health education.
- Femme International distribute reusable menstrual products, and run an educational program in schools and community groups across Kenya and Tanzania.
- #HappyPeriod provide menstrual products to anyone with a period that is low-income, homeless, or living in poverty. They use public donations of products and money to do so and have several chapters across the USA.
- Huru International work across Africa to reduce the number of days that girls miss every month because they lack the resources and information they need to manage their periods, by supplying them with reusable pads and information.
- Irise International work in East Africa and focus on developing a replicable and sustainable solution to the challenges girls face in engaging in school during menstruation.

- I Support the Girls collect and redistribute donations of tampons and pads (as well as new and gently used bras) to women and girls who are in need in the USA and other countries.
- Plan International UK campaign for girls' rights around the world and have launched a menstrual manifesto to address period poverty.
- The Cup Effect is a charitable NGO and social enterprise that campaigns to raise awareness about menstrual cups and make them more widely available. Through projects with local partners in Kenya, Malawi and the UK they provide training sessions about cups and distribute them to people living on low incomes.
- The Cup Foundation empower underprivileged girls worldwide by providing them with sustainable menstrual cups and comprehensive education on sexuality and reproductive rights.
- The Red Box Project are a community-based initiative in the UK who place red boxes of period products in schools for those who may not be able to afford them.

First Blood

Experiences of menarche – your first period – are as varied as we are, but there are common themes that weave through our stories, of unease, curiosity, surprise, horror, shame, celebration, fear, disgust, pride, relief, loss, and joy. There's a lot bundled up in that first blot of blood.

Your first period may have been met with celebration; some of you will have revelled in the attention it brought and some of you will have squirmed and wanted to disappear from view. For others it will have been less significant, and that might have felt okay, or not. If the arrival of your period signalled a further financial burden for your family, it may not have been welcomed. The awareness that your body was now capable of reproducing might have led to you being viewed in terms of your body's now dangerous potential, something to fear and be wary of because it could now get you in trouble, and that could have provoked conversations and shifts in your family dynamic. It's commonplace for the start of your first period to signify that you have become a woman, but what if you weren't ready or had no interest in becoming a woman? What if you really wanted your period to start but you had to wait years for it to finally arrive; what did this mean for how you viewed yourself?

Research shows that when a girl's first period is acknowledged positively or celebrated as a rite of passage instead of being ignored or expressed as a negative, they are more likely to have a positive body image and to engage in healthy behaviours such as seeing a gynaecologist. Think back to your first period (if you can remember it); how did it feel and how did those around you react? Consider what was imprinted on you in this phase of your life, not only because it's astonishing how behavioural patterns are replicated in each generation so it's worth considering if there's a pattern that you want to break with your own children, but because your experience of menarche and that time in your life can also show up in your menstrual cycle month after month, making it worthy of investigation and thought. The emotions of people who have periods are frequently blamed on their cycle. Were your feelings as a teenager heard and validated or dismissed as being down to 'rag week' and PMS, and have you internalised these attitudes and learned to ignore what you feel?

You'll find a list of questions below to help you explore your memories of your first period. They've been adapted from Jane Bennett's *A Blessing Not a Curse*, which I highly recommend (*see* Resources), and I suggest setting aside some time where you won't be disturbed. Doing this exercise can bring up grief, rage, sadness, and of course love and joy, so give yourself privacy and space to get into this in whatever way you want to.

- How did you find out about periods? How did you react to this knowledge?
- How did you feel as you anticipated getting yours, was it something that you looked forward to?
- How old were you when you got your first period?
- Do you remember where you were?
- What happened?
- Were you excited, worried, proud, ashamed?
- How did you feel physically and emotionally?
- How did you feel about 'becoming a woman'?
- Whom did you tell? How did they respond?
- Who found out? How did they respond?
- Did you feel celebrated?
- Was it a rite of passage that was framed positively by your mother/sister/ father, or was the message that this would be a cyclical struggle for you, and a cross to bear as a woman?

- What spoken and unspoken messages did you receive about your developing body and about menstruation (from your family, peers, magazines)?
- In your adolescence/teen years, do you feel that your boundaries were respected, or were there transgressions?
- Can you see any pattern or relationship between your menstrual cycle as an adult woman, and your experiences as a newly menstruating adolescent?
- Is there any correlation between how others respond to you now and your menstrual history?
- What do you know about your sister/mother/aunt's experiences of menarche and their menstruating years?
- What messages about menstruation do you retain today?
- Are there things that you would have liked to have heard from your mother at this time, but didn't? What about your father?

If you have trouble connecting with this phase of your life or your memory is sketchy, dig out some photos and see if you can get a sense of who you were then, and of what was going on. I also recommend talking to your family members about their experiences of their first period, and about their memory of you around the time that you got yours. You may well be surprised at what they share.

Bad Blood

You probably already know if your period is a time when you feel like connecting with others or if you prefer some time alone. If you feel worn out from caring for loved ones, parents, kids, friends and even colleagues, then embrace this as your time, to care for yourself and be cared for – if there are people around to help and if you're able to let them. Retreating not only gives loved ones an opportunity to develop and grow without your help but it can also create a better balance of household chores and encourage independence in your offspring (and possibly your partner too). If you're used to being needed by all and sundry, you'll probably relish this freedom, but if there's a part of you that no longer knows who you are when you're not in relation to someone else, or that needs to be needed, then this empty space could feel way too empty, but sit with it and get into it.

There will be blood (Winter)

Contemplate what you would do if you didn't have to think about others, care for them, or worry about what they might think of you. What would you do with all this mental space and freedom? Your response will suggest what you could do as a nourishing activity in your Winter and believe me when I say that if your answer is 'doing nothing', that is a perfect activity.

As you head towards your period, and during it, increased blood flow can make your genitals tingle in the same way they can around ovulation, and although some people like intimacy with another during their period, I commonly find that it's a time when clients prefer to masturbate and to keep pleasure and orgasms for themselves.

Orgasms are one of my top professional recommendations that I give clients for relieving menstrual cramps, and they're a personal favourite too. They relieve tension of all kinds, aid sleep, and boost feel-good brain chemicals such as serotonin, dopamine, and endorphins, all of which help to improve mood and decrease pain. When I've mentioned this on social media it's created some very interesting responses from people of all genders, so let me address the points that come up:

'The last thing I want is a dick inside me when I've got my period.'
My response: Fair enough, but sex doesn't have to involve a penis or penetration.

'I don't want to put my dick inside her when she's bleeding.'
My response: Great news, you don't have to! There's this wonderful anatomical feature called the clitoris, you might have heard of it?

'I don't have a partner' or *'I don't want to have to be intimate with my partner when I'm on.'*
My response: There's this incredible thing you can try out called masturbation, I really recommend it. #girlswanktoo

'What about the mess?'
My response: If the idea of seeing blood or staining your bed linen concerns you, you can put a towel underneath your pelvis, or try Soft Cups®, a menstrual cup that sits beneath your cervix and moulds to your shape, and which can be worn during sex.

Self-care Essentials

The more self-care you can bring in now, the more you'll get out of your Winter, and to quote Alexandra Pope, 'how you care for yourself here sets the tone for the rest of your cycle'.

If you struggle with pain or just want to feel good when you're in your Winter, listening to or making music, having a massage, being outdoors, laughing, and exercising (particularly with someone else) can all boost your happy hormones – dopamine, oxytocin and serotonin – but it's not the ideal time to start a new exercise plan. Your body may not be that co-operative and feel heavy and uncoordinated, leaving you feeling down about your fantastic efforts. But hold that thought because exercise is a great thought to have, it is after all well known for being the magic bullet that improves mental and physical wellbeing, just save starting it for your Spring, particularly if you're prone to feeling depleted during your period.

For those of you who get hit with migraines, keep track of when you get them because there's a strong correlation between the occurrence of them and the start of a period; up to 70 per cent of menstruators who get migraines notice an association between the two, and there are two theories on why they occur:

- The hormonal withdrawal in the days before your period can trigger headaches and migraines, which may be exacerbated if you have an imbalance between your levels of oestrogen and progesterone at this time.
- The release of prostaglandins as your period starts triggers inflammation and pain (you can read more about this process in the section on period pain on page 277).

Forty-five per cent of menstruators who get debilitating migraines have been found to have a deficiency in magnesium, so it's worth considering supplementation along with eating a magnesium-rich diet in order to reduce the frequency and severity of them. Foods which are high in magnesium include spinach, chard, avocado, almonds, cashews, black beans, pumpkin seeds, sesame seeds, sunflower seeds, bananas, and dark chocolate.

Unlike migraines that strike around the start of a period which are related to oestrogen withdrawal, end menstrual migraines (EMM) that come towards the end of your period are thought to be related to blood loss and low levels of iron.

If you're keen to start tracking your basal body temperature, now is the perfect time to do it as you'll get a full cycle of data.

Stamp out Cramps

Cramps can be debilitating enough to interfere with your personal and professional life and require painkillers, yet many people, including some doctors, don't take them seriously enough. Severe menstrual pain should *always* be investigated, not only is suffering unnecessary because it can often be resolved fairly easily, but it can be a sign of reproductive disorders such as endometriosis, adenomyosis, and fibroids. You'll find 20 of my favourite suggestions for dealing with cramps on page 279, and one of my favourite methods is to use abdominal castor oil packs throughout the menstrual cycle.

Castor oil packs

Castor oil is extracted from the seeds of the castor plant which, when taken orally, is known for its ability to get bowels moving due to its laxative effect (it's this motion that can irritate the uterus and stimulate contractions to induce labour). But there's a much gentler way of using it, and that's by using a castor oil pack on your lower abdomen. Although there isn't much research out there on castor oil, it's a traditional remedy that's been in use for over a century and it remains an affordable and effective way of treating reproductive complaints.

I recommend them for menstrual cycle problems such as period pain, ovarian cysts, fibroids, endometriosis, and adenomyosis, as well as when healing from an unsuccessful round of IVF, miscarriage, or a termination. Castor oil packs provide a gentle way of improving blood flow to the organs in your pelvis and can be used to soften well-healed scar tissue after a caesarean birth or laparoscopy. Two and a half decades after I had an appendectomy, they really thinned and softened the chunky scar I was left with. They're incredibly relaxing and a great excuse to get horizontal but should not be used after ovulation if you are trying to conceive, during pregnancy, or in the immediate postpartum when you're still bleeding. Some people like to use them when they have their period, and others prefer not to, but I recommend using them with caution during your period if you're prone to heavy flow or flooding, and as with all oils, you should apply a small amount to your skin and wait 24 hours to see if you have a negative reaction to it before going the whole hog. To make your own DIY castor oil pack, you will need:

- A 250ml bottle of high-quality cold-pressed castor oil (preferably organic).
- A piece of cotton or wool flannel that's large enough to cover your lower abdomen when folded in half (muslin baby squares work well).
- A hot water bottle or heating pad.
- Another muslin square, small old towel, or cling film to cover the pack with while you're using it.
- Old clothes to wear and an old towel to place underneath you as castor oil does stain.
- A glass container with a lid to soak the flannel in the castor oil, and to store it between uses (glass Tupperware® or a jar are perfect).

Your first castor oil pack could be a slightly messy affair, so don't do it on your favourite sheets. Once you get the knack, it gets easier and there won't be any mess. Here's what you do:

- Fold your piece of cotton or wool cloth so that it is a size that will cover your lower abdomen.
- Place the folded fabric into your glass container (you can fold it up further so that it fits in there), then saturate the cloth with your castor oil. It doesn't need to be dripping wet, castor oil is very thick so once you use it the increase in temperature from your body heat and the heating pad will make it runnier.
- Stick some relaxing music on or enjoy some silence.
- Lie down somewhere comfortable, with an old towel underneath you, and your hot water bottle/heating pad and your glass container with castor oil-soaked cloth in it all next to you.
- Turn your phone off.

- Carefully remove the cloth, unfold it, and place it across your lower abdomen.
- Then, cover the saturated cloth with another folded muslin or an old towel. You can use cling film (saranwrap) but this isn't ideal because it's plastic.
- Place the heating pad or hot water bottle on top of the cloth.
- Take some deep breaths, meditate, read a book, watch *Queer Eye*, or if you're anything like me, fall asleep.
- Keep the pack on for 30–60 minutes.
- When you're done, store the saturated cloth in the glass container. It can be reused around 30 times, though you may need to top it up with extra oil occasionally.
- Wipe off any excess oil, and if you prefer to wash your skin afterwards, a diluted solution of baking soda and water will remove it easily (1 tsp to a pint of water).

My recommendation is to do the pack for three consecutive days a week (it's lovely to do before bedtime), for 1–3 months and assess if you feel they're helping you. One word of warning: oil gets hot easily and can burn you, so don't use a just-boiled hot water bottle.

It's Trippy, Trippy, Trippy

When people used to tell me that they got really high on their period, I assumed it was because they were self-medicating with cannabis to manage their cramps, so it came as a shock when they explained that they hadn't used any drugs to reach this state – it was simply how they experienced their period. To be honest I was incredulous that someone else could have such a joyful experience of bleeding when my uterus felt like it was waging war with itself, and yet, a couple of years down the line, I found myself having the same experience.

To begin with, I started noticing that I would feel slightly out of it an hour or two before my period started which in those days was very helpful because it meant I had some warning to chuck some painkillers down my throat and dash home. Then, I realised that if I was able to seclude myself and rest, the gentle high would progress into a dream-like state where I would experience visions. I was still in horrendous pain, but I'd manage to hold off on taking pain meds for an hour so that I could get the most out of it, then relent and take painkillers which sadly prevented me from continuing with this interesting experience.

Then, as my period pain subsided over the course of a year, it became harder for me to experience this natural high. The pain had helped me to access this liminal state, and without it I had to work harder at getting there and doing less was the key to this. Eating food would bring me out of my head and into my body, so I stuck to water and herbal teas in the morning and did what I could to be alone, because feeling or hearing someone around me would pull me back into the world in the same way that hearing someone snoring prevents you from drifting off to sleep, or at least this was how it was with my experience of menstrual tripping.

WTF is all this about?

When you start to bleed this can trigger a release of endorphins – the body's natural painkillers. There are two points in the cycle where endorphins are highest; at ovulation, and at onset of menstruation, and specifically the first day. Period pain can stimulate endorphin secretion, but research has found that endorphins are produced even in the absence of severe pain.

Menstruation can bring with it a pleasant high that the practicalities of daily life can prevent you from attaining, but because it's a state of consciousness that requires you to stay present with it for it to happen, you need to move slowly and with awareness. It can be hard to access when riddled with pain, although the enforced rest can help to get you there.

When I suggested this to my client Sara, not using painkillers and cracking on with life the next time she came on, she was initially mortified at the idea because she'd relied on them to make it through her period for years. But because I'd been treating her for a few weeks and her next period was due to start on a weekend, she decided to give it a go. Sara's period was still painful, but not like it used to be, and as she laid in bed with a hot water bottle over her womb she kept waiting for the point to arrive where she'd have to take the painkillers already laid out on her bedside table. But that point didn't come. Instead she found herself feeling deeply connected to the process of bleeding and discovered that it allowed her to let go of the emotional build up that had accumulated over the previous weeks. The following period was even better and came with the physical awareness of bleeding, but without her usual pain, so that Sara was able to do what she described as bed-based yoga and truly experience the physicality of her menstruating body in all her glory.

You have my wombfelt sympathies if your period is a hardcore ordeal, and if you're in that camp, as I once was, it's hard to believe that bleeding could ever feel reasonable, let alone pleasurable, but it can. Just know that it's possible and park the idea that it might be one day for you somewhere in your head.

Wings and Things

The average tampon contains several types of chemicals and given that tampon-users put approximately 10–12,000 tampons inside their vaginas during the menstruating years, it's worth picking which product you use wisely. The average tampon contains:

- Rayon, a highly absorbent synthetic material.
- Chlorine, used to bleach tampons and disruptive to your vaginal microbiome.
- Dioxin, an endocrine disruptor that the Environmental Protection Agency have determined that there is no safe level of exposure to. It's produced as a result of chlorine processing used to bleach tampons, and some research has found a link between dioxin and endometriosis in non-human primates.
- BPA is another endocrine disruptor and it's commonly found in tampon applicators.
- Fragrance. Would you spray perfume inside yourself? No, so stick to fragrance-free tampons.
- Non-organic cotton. Cotton is one of the most genetically modified crops on the planet, and pesticides and herbicides are often sprayed on cotton, which increases the risk of them ending up in your tampons, so buy organic tampons if you're able to.

In the UK and Europe, manufacturers aren't legally required to disclose their ingredients, and Leah Remfry-Peploe, one of the co-founders of Ohne, a 100 per cent organic tampon subscription service, makes the point that there are stricter regulations for the labelling of hamster food than there are for tampons and pads. How is this even possible?

If there's one thing that the ridiculous blue liquid tampon adverts have taught us, it's that tampons are highly absorbent, which is great when you're bleeding heavily, but if you're prone to vaginal dryness or a lack of cervical fluid, is it wise to put something highly absorbent inside your vagina? I recommend that you don't, and instead opt for another method.

Pads, in some form, are as old as time. Modern versions are varied in size and absorbency and can be single-use or reusable. Single-use pads are more absorbent because of the high-tech ingredients used in them. Unfortunately, these modern ingredients are likely to carry a long-term environmental impact as it's hard/impossible for them to break down once they end up in landfill, and some people find that they react to the chemicals and plastics in them, including fragrance. There are other disposable pads on the market that use organic cotton from companies who are more transparent about the ingredients that they use, such as Freda, Dame, Sustain, and Natracare who manufacture organic tampons and/or natural pads.

Companies like Lunapads and GladRags manufacture cloth pads that are washable and reusable. They have no fragrance or weird additives in them, and they're breathable too, which means that if you're prone to eczema or skin reactions, you could find that you get on better with cotton reusables. They are more economical in the long-run than disposable pads, and also save millions of tampons and pads from ending up in landfill sites. Cloth pads come in an extensive range of shapes, sizes, colours, and prints, and there are pads designed specifically for heavy flow too. After use they can just be chucked in the washing machine with your regular coloured laundry, though in the same way using fabric softeners on towels can reduce their ability to absorb moisture, so can using them with cloth pads.

Menstrual cups are a great option for a lot of people. Worn inside the vagina, they collect menstrual flow but don't absorb vaginal moisture, which is particularly relevant if you're prone to vaginal dryness. They can be worn for up to 12 hours at a time because they hold significantly more blood than a tampon and there is no established link between cups and increased risk of toxic shock syndrome. They only need to be lightly washed with soap and water before reinserting them (buying two can make using public bathrooms easier), and they can be reused for 10 years, saving you a small fortune as well as reducing the environmental impact of menstrual products – each cup replaces approximately 2000 disposable menstrual products. They're usually made from soft medical-grade silicone and are free of the problematic chemicals found in tampons, but it's worth thinking about what soap you use to wash your cup because it's those chemicals that could end up inside you.

Mandu Reid from The Cup Effect tells me that, 'Despite the immense individual and environmental benefits of menstrual cups, they have remained largely unsung since the 1930s when they were first invented. The main reason for this is commercial, they are a terrible business idea! The big companies do not manufacture or market cups because if they were more popular and more widely available, profit margins would take a huge hit. Most people can use a menstrual cup – with the exception of those who prefer not to or are not able to insert things into their vagina such as those with vaginismus or uterine prolapse. When used correctly, cups are more reliable and discrete than pads or tampons – if your cup does leak it's usually because it has not opened properly or is positioned wrongly – simply remove it and try again, all it takes is a bit of practice!'

In recent years a new menstrual product has finally entered the market; period-wear. Companies like Lunapads, FLUX, WUKA, Sustain, Modibodi, Pyramid Seven, and Thinx all make underwear that absorbs menstrual flow. They're designed to be used on their own and are capable of absorbing 2–4 tampons' worth of blood, but some people prefer to use them as back up if they're prone to flooding. I bought one pair and fell for them hook, line and sinker. Using them can be nerve-wracking at first, but once you're able to trust them and if you find they work well for you, it's worth investing in a few pairs as they can take a while to dry. They can be worn for up to 8 hours which means they're also a great overnight option, and they're also suitable for use after giving birth or if you're prone to bladder leaks. Styles vary across brands and some seams are smoother than others so if a VPL bothers you, you might want to opt for a skimpier style or one that has a smooth seam. There are numerous boxer-style options, which means they're a great option for trans-men and non-binary folk or if you're someone like me who just finds boxers incredibly comfy, and, like other reusables, they're more environmentally friendly than single-use products.

Switching the type of product that you use can help to relieve menstrual pain. If you have vulvodynia – a chronic pain syndrome which affects the vulva, see page 127 – then period-wear may be the least aggravating for you. Period-wear can work brilliantly as a primary way of catching your flow, and also as a back-up if your flow is heavy and you find that you need to use tampons as well.

Reusable menstrual products such as cups, cloth pads, sponges, and period-wear all reduce the environmental impact of menstruation, and if you prefer to use tampons with applicators, check out D, the world's first reusable tampon applicator. Manufactured by DAME, it's designed to be washed between uses and reduces environmental waste and pollution. Over half of tampon-users in Britain flush their tampons and applicators down the toilet, which is why nine applicators are found per kilometre of beach along the UK's coastline.

Top Tips to Get the Most out of your Winter

- Assess what per cent your internal battery is at and let that dictate what you're able to do and not do in this phase.
- Take time out to do something that nourishes you.
- Ask what, or who, do you have to say goodbye to in order to retreat in this phase.
- Do what you have to do but see what you can get away with not doing. We put ourselves under tremendous pressure most of the time, far more than other people would expect of us. Do less for an afternoon or a few days, you'll be able to pick up the pace soon enough.
- Ease up on responsibilities where you're able to and ask for help if you need it.
- Don't rush, strip your days back so that you have time to get from one place to another.
- Prioritise self-care, even if all you can manage is ten minutes.

- As you come out of Winter you may experience a quiet knowing, an inner focus and resolve, making it a great time to get clear about what you want to bring attention and energy to in this cycle – an intention. Write it down somewhere visible and keep coming back to it to stay on track.
- Connect to the 800 million menstruators who are bleeding with you at the same time, many of whom don't have access to menstrual products or education, so if you're in a position where you're able to donate money or menstrual products, give to organisations such as Bloody Good Period, the Beauty Banks, and Red Box Project.

Chapter 4

Let's get this party started (Spring)

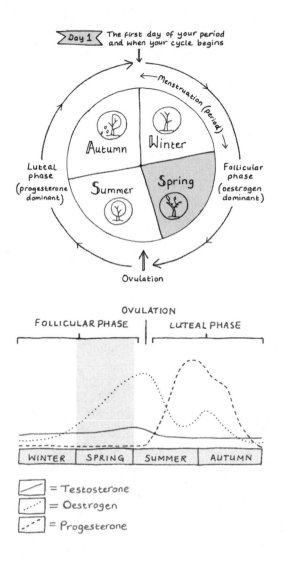

And breathe, your Spring is here. It's time to shake off the slump of hibernation and step into the sunny side of your cycle. As you emerge from your cocoon, can you feel life getting lighter and brighter again?

This is the season for new beginnings and for starting over, of possibilities and potential. The lead ovarian follicle for this cycle is developing and growing, and as it heads towards ovulation it pumps out increasing amounts of oestrogen – your Beyoncé hormone – leaving you feeling energised, motivated, and interested in the outer world again. You'll feel an enthusiasm for life and its possibilities (unless your period has left you feeling wiped out that is) and find yourself increasingly in your groove.

Transitioning from Winter to Spring

You might find yourself racing out of Winter, delighted to leave the cyclical darkness behind and any suffering you experienced along with it. But if you're at home in your Winter and get a lot out of being there, then you might find it hard to leave this powerful time and cross over into your Spring. Perhaps you feel some trepidation around the superpowers associated with being in the sunny side of your cycle? This is, after all, where you step back into the light, and with that comes visibility. Do you welcome it, or shy away from it?

If you realise that you're sensitive to the gentle upswing of oestrogen from day 3 (the third day of your period), pay particular attention to the days that follow as it may be that you either have a fairly short Winter season that you come out of around day 3 or 4, or, if you go on to feel depleted and emotional a few days later, you probably need to appreciate that you're still in your Winter and need to ease up a bit while you're technically still there rather than jumping back in. I know that when you're feeling good that it can be irresistible to get back in the swing of things but try to keep something in the tank. When my client Azizah is in her Winter she feels exhausted, but in her Spring she says, 'I begin to feel like I can do anything and begin to take things on. It's probably when I'm at my most vulnerable and I'm likely to take too much on.'

This is the season where oestrogen really gets going, bringing positivity and energy along with it, but as your energy begins to move upwards and outwards, you might feel like you've got a jetpack on your back. And although it's mighty tempting to let go of all control and see where this propulsion takes you, try to keep control and hold back by 20 per cent. This can be tricky if you're bursting at the seams and ready to get yourself out there, but if you can rein yourself in and contain some of that energy, it will ground and propel you through the rest of your cycle. One way to do this is to maintain a connection to the anchor of your period. This can be as straightforward as recalling the intention you set at the beginning of this cycle. Your Spring is going to give it a whole lot of impetus, so you'd be wise to keep it present in your mind. Write it on a sticky note and stick it on your mirror so that you see it alongside your beautiful self every day.

It's common for those that struggle with their period to rush out of the gates, put the depths of their Winter behind them and get lost in the hedonistic high of their Spring and Summer, but holding on to your experience of Winter will motivate you to keep up with the self-care practices that will improve your period and overall health in future cycles.

You'll know you're in your Spring because you'll feel:

- An inner spark
- The glimmer of possibility
- Lighthearted and playful
- Increasingly resilient
- Enthusiastic
- Social
- Curious
- Creative
- Experimental
- Energetic
- Motivated
- Increasing self-esteem and a stronger sense of self
- An inner surety of yourself and your place in the world
- An increase in cervical fluid and vaginal lubrication, possibly sexual desire too
- Happier with your reflection – your skin clears up and your features take on a more symmetrical appearance

Spring is nature's birthing season, so take some time to reflect on what is emerging in you. What are you creating and bringing into the world, and what do you need in order for what you're doing to grow?

Your renewed interest in the world could leave you feeling like a kid in a candy store; drawn to every pretty thing and playfully skipping from one thing to the next. This is the time to enjoy the possibilities that are available to you without getting serious about them, or where none exist, to create them because you could find yourself buzzing with ideas. As oestrogen increases, your memory and mental agility will improve and once testosterone gets in on the act you'll want to take on challenges. You're capable of doing more now that your hormones are getting going, but see if you can hold the tension until you're well and truly in your Spring, it'll be worth it.

Spring's Superpowers

Potential
Your Spring is where you'll get a sense of the spaces where you can grow – in your body and mind, but also in the world. Can you feel the potential within you, in the spaces between your joints, the space between thoughts, the space between where you end, and others begin? It's these spaces that contain possibilities. Spring is when shoots pop out from the ground overnight, and your transformation in your Spring can feel this sudden, because all the while you were resting in your Winter, your energy and potential was gathering deep inside, building tension in order to be ready for this burst of life.

Build and expand
Your energy, stamina and self-esteem are all on the up. From potential comes expansion. Once your level of oestrogen gets going, it acts as fertiliser on the shoots that have poked their way through the ground, giving you the energy and momentum that you need to build and expand. This might mean building muscle, self-esteem, or a new habit. Or expanding your work and social networks now that you're interested in the world again. Take up space and be more visible.

Be curious and explore
Spring is when lots of pathways emerge, and different opportunities present themselves to you. You've got options here and nothing is set in stone so allow yourself to be curious and explore them. What and who interests you?

What would you do if you could get away with it? Now is the time to try something different and experiment with a new approach, style of clothing, or form of exercise. Take a chance and risk something, I dare you.

Play

Embrace the child-like quality of this season and play! Physically you could find yourself craving more movement, and when it comes to mental activity, know that you don't have to move from an idea to a fixed solution. Sit with it, let it grow and play around with other options. My other half always knows when I've entered my Spring because I joke around, take the piss, and generally wind him up – markedly different from how I am in my Winter when I crave quiet solitude.

Spring's Dangers

Exposing yourself

You're buzzing with ideas and your self-confidence is soaring. Naturally, it's tempting to reveal yourself to the world when you're feeling this good, but you'd be wise to keep your cards close to your chest for a few more days. Like new shoots in the Spring, you're vulnerable to sudden frost even if you're feeling strong and capable, and exposing yourself too soon can be detrimental to your projects and self-esteem. Keep your ideas in a greenhouse and let them proliferate alongside the lining of your womb.

Succumbing to pressure

If you've successfully managed to move slower or have a period of rest in your Winter (high five to you), then you could be feeling the pressure to be serious and crack on again, but there's tremendous value in the playful nature of your Spring, so try to leave a bit of a buffer zone between you and the world.

Tiredness

If you're tired in your Spring, then something has gone seriously awry because this is the time when your energy should be picking up quite rapidly. Fatigue here suggests that you're doing way too much throughout the whole of your cycle, and that you need to prioritise strengthening yourself by eating well and resting well.

Distraction

As you move towards the end of your Spring and oestrogen is close to peaking, you could be left feeling distracted because in this phase oestrogen is keen to get you on the move so that you seek out a potential mate. You might have had lots of wonderful ideas come to you, but if you don't focus on something now, you'll miss out on the productivity of your Summer.

When Spring is Where you Struggle

If you feel drained and tired during or immediately after your period, consider if you could have iron deficiency anaemia, and don't underestimate the effects on how you feel both physically *and* emotionally. Being deficient means that you might miss out on the powers of your Spring, because your body is busy trying to recoup energy, not expend it.

Ask yourself: how are you over-extending yourself, what's weighing you down, and how can you receive more nourishment in your diet and relationships? Are you respecting your need for rest in your Winter, do you keep going or charge out of the gate too soon? When my client Sandra began tracking her cycle, she found that rather than feel energised and playful in her Spring, she was feeling stressed; 'I feel the pressure to be a social butterfly after taking some time for myself in Winter, and I put too much in my schedule which leaves me feeling chaotic and clumsy.' I suggested that she create buffers of time in the first few days of her Spring so that she wouldn't overload herself, and encouraged her to find some softness in this phase so that she could hold off on getting serious so soon in her cycle and enjoy the playful aspect that's possible here instead.

When you're utterly exhausted and thoroughly deficient, it's easy to look at those around you and wonder why you're struggling so much, and start making unhealthy comparisons about how useless you are. Take it easy over there and give yourself a break. Look at your health in the context of how challenging and demanding life is for you and begin to appreciate that even the smallest of tasks can be overwhelming when you're feeling weak. There is a strength in you, I know there is, and if you give yourself a few months of living in tune with your cycle and prioritising self-care that nourishes you, you'll be able to tackle the tasks that daunt you now with ease.

When you're learning to care for yourself, particularly during and after your period, it can be helpful to treat yourself as a child and prioritise your basic needs. Children do not respond well to having to wait to drink/eat/wee/poo/sleep, but somewhere in the growing up process we don't just learn how to control our orifices, we override and ignore them to our detriment. Go back to basics and listen to what your body needs.

Are you able to live with a little childlike naivety in your Spring, or do you come down hard on yourself and act as an overbearing parent might? When comparing the menstrual cycle to the life cycle, your Spring equates to your childhood and teen years and in the same way you can't rush a child, you can't rush in your Spring. Rushing in your Spring can take on the quality of growing up too soon, of getting serious too quickly and missing out on the explorative play where it's okay to mess things up and get it wrong. Imagine the potential you could find in yourself if another part of yourself wasn't watching over your shoulder and judging every move to the point that you felt you couldn't try things out? This is exactly the kind of behaviour that you don't want lurking around in your Spring.

I'm Coming Out

The sense of possibility in your Spring makes this a great time to explore different avenues available to you, both in terms of the day to day (a project you're weighing up, a task you're getting started with), and the bigger picture (further education, a new job or career path). This is the phase of your cycle where you'll feel that the world really is your oyster, making it the perfect time to explore different ideas, perspectives and ways of working.

During this time of expansion, you'll be gifted with a helicopter vision that allows you to see all the possibilities that are available to you. Experiment with them. You don't need to fully commit to anything just yet, and you might not have the focus required of you to do so due to the playful nature of Spring, so embrace where you are and mess around with ideas. Take a few steps along each path and see where you get. This is when you're most open to new ways of thinking and working; try reading articles and books by people you admire and use them to inspire a different approach.

As your creativity bubbles away, you might come up with a big idea or ten, but it wouldn't be wise to start shouting about it just yet. Keep your cards close to your chest for a while, protect those new shoots of yours and let them harden before you share them with the world. Exposing them now could be detrimental to both your big idea and your sense of self. Towards the end of your Spring, when you've sat with your seedlings for a few days and they're sufficiently developed and strong enough to be released into the world, think carefully about whom you'll share them with. Will your friend truly get what you're trying to do, or will they frown in confusion as you try to explain, leaving you disenchanted and doubtful? Is your slightly clueless workmate best placed to offer an opinion or would it be better to speak to someone influential whose opinion you respect? Speak with people from your target audience; who will buy your product or read your book, which colleagues or investors do you need to sell your idea to and get on board?

It's not just the outer world that can kill your creative genius, your internal quest for perfection can continually fuck things up too. It's pretty much guaranteed that as soon as you raise your head above the parapet by doing something bigger, bolder or riskier, you become a target for your inner critic. And if you're not careful it will devour you, and your incredible life-changing, profit-making big idea will be killed off before it's even got legs. Get ready for it and tell it to F off. Tell that critic of yours that you know it's trying to do you a favour and protect you in what's probably a very misguided and outdated way, but you're having fun in the playground of potential for now, so you'll see it in your Autumn where it belongs. Autumn is the home of your inner critic, and if the thought of this scares the crap out of you, fear not, I've got tools for you to handle them when you get there.

Spring is not the time for perfection, in fact, sod perfection and aim for incompetence. Be liberated by your naivety, feel the freedom of having options and risk something. Just start something, anything.

It can be hard to concentrate once the come out and play vibe hits, so keep in mind that you can work with your daily cycle too – when are you most productive, when can you ease off so that you can play? Or can you create a day where you're working and being social? Maybe that's the day you meet with people you want to do business with, so that you can present yourself and your work in a strong light.

Relationships

Annnnnd you're back in the room. Hello, hi, how you doin'? Yep, that spark and interest in other people is here too which means Spring is when your relationships truly flourish. So, make space for play and for cheeky flirtation, pencil in dates, and generally be out in the world trying All The Fun Things with All The Fun People.

When you're hanging with friends, opt for socialising away from your home; go for a hike or to the beach, try a dance class together and that new restaurant you've been talking about trying for weeks. Or, if your best mate is in their Autumn, do them a solid and offer to cook dinner at their place (on the condition that they'll return the favour when you're in yours of course).

If you've been desperate for time away from your partner and kids for the last week or so, perhaps preferring your own company or that of your friends, then the start of your Spring can see you returning to the summery phases of your cycle where you actively seek out connection with your other half and your children. This is when to book in fun activities with your kids that you can't be arsed doing at other times. Your energy in this phase is child-like, matching perfectly to the energy of your offspring, and your natural curiosity and patience in your Spring makes spending time with your kids feel easy and enjoyable, which makes a change if you've spent the last two weeks trying to hide in the bathroom. Your Spring is when you can find yourself being the kind of parent you wish you could be all the time and can be a valuable time for bonding activities – enjoy it.

Self-care Essentials

Spring is your chance to start afresh, to commit to a new plan for self-care or recommit to one that you previously abandoned. Between your period and ovulation there's a perfect window of opportunity for you to switch things up and form a new habit. After ovulation healthy habits are harder to maintain, so do the groundwork here when change is easier, and you'll be more likely to keep it up.

If you've been tracking your cycle diligently and managed to move with awareness during your Autumn and Winter, then you're probably gaining an understanding of what you need to do in order to improve your health, support your hormones, and feel better about your life. Now is when you want to put those nuggets of wisdom into action and implement changes. As you accumulate data on the nuances of your particular cycle, you'll become increasingly attuned to what you need to have a happy and healthy cycle.

Want to bring in some self-care but not sure where to start? You'll find my list of suggestions in Section Three of this book. Remember that it's always easiest to start with adding things in before moving onto cutting the bad stuff out, and a simple place to start is staying hydrated, eating healthy food regularly, moving more than you do, and respecting when you need to switch off and rest. And cycle tracking, don't forget cycle tracking!

If you find yourself prone to feeling distracted and scattered as you move towards ovulation, play around with using techniques and movement that ground your energy – such as breathing techniques, yoga and tai chi – and movement that's intensive and burns off excess energy. See what works best for you. If you've been left feeling depleted from your period, then prioritise resting and eating nourishing food, and speak to your GP as they can help you to figure out why you're feeling so wiped out.

When it comes to digestion, as oestrogen rises it increases the contraction of the smooth muscle in your intestines, creating the wave-like movement known as peristalsis that keeps things moving along. It also increases the diversity of your microbiome – the ecosystem of microorganisms housed inside you – which is great news for your immune health as a strong immunity starts with a healthy gut that's full of fantastic gut bacteria. If you are prone to irritable bowel syndrome (IBS) then oestrogen can cause increased hypersensitivity to pain and spasm.

Seed Cycling

If your hormones and menstrual cycle are out of whack, then seed cycling is for you. Consuming different seeds during each half of your cycle helps to boost oestrogen levels in the first half, and progesterone in the second. If you have absent or irregular cycles, light/heavy flow, a short luteal phase, PMS, perimenopausal symptoms, or if you're post-menopausal, then seed cycling is a great option for you.

Seed hulls contain lignans which bind up excess hormones, and seed oils contain essential fatty acids which are the building blocks for making hormones.

Here's how you do it:

- In the follicular phase of your cycle (days 1–14 of a 28-day cycle), or from new moon to full moon if you're not currently menstruating, eat 2–4 tbsps of both ground flax seeds and pumpkin seeds per day to gently and naturally increase oestrogen levels. Pumpkin seeds are high in zinc which supports progesterone production and release in the second phase of your cycle.
- In the luteal phase of your cycle (days 15–28), or from full moon to dark moon, eat 2–4 tbsps of both sesame seeds and sunflower seeds per day. The zinc in sesame seeds and the vitamin E in sunflower seeds both help stimulate the production of progesterone. The lignans in sesame seeds help to block excess oestrogen, and sunflower seeds provide selenium which assists the liver in its detoxification role and improve overall hormonal health.

Buy whole organic seeds and use a coffee or spice grinder to get a powder which you can add to porridge, soups, salads and smoothies. Or just eat them whole if you prefer. You can grind enough for the week ahead and store them in the freezer. Stay clear of pre-ground seeds as they oxidise rapidly and go rancid.

You might experience a change in your cycle within the first month of seed cycling, but it usually takes 3–4 cycles to see a noticeable difference because that's how long it takes for a follicle to mature and be released at ovulation.

Push it Real Good

When it comes to exercise, this is the time to really push yourself by doing anaerobic exercise – anything that makes your heart thump in your chest and sweat pour off your face. Anaerobic exercise is classified as being high intensity or carried out at your maximum level of exertion, making high-intensity interval training (HIIT) perfect, especially if you're a busy bee as HIIT workouts are usually capped at 25 minutes. Weightlifting, kickboxing, spinning, running, swimming, dancing and even walking are other examples that can get your blood pumping, and because rising oestrogen can turn you into a social butterfly, Spring is the perfect season for doing exercise that's social and that involves other people. Want to try CrossFit or yoga? Get yourself along to a class in your Spring. The playful nature of this season, and the willingness to take risks that's common here, makes it the perfect time to try a new form of exercise so that you can gain some momentum to keep it up during the rest of your cycle.

Your Spring is when you have a higher tolerance for endurance and pain, your uptake of oxygen is increased, and you can also recover better, so it's when you can make a lot of training progress. But towards the end of Spring and as you get closer to ovulation, high levels of oestrogen can make you more prone to injury so be sure to focus on your form.

Go hard or go home: A word of warning
A go hard or go home approach might get you the physical gain that you want, but reproductively it can turn you into a graveyard. It's common for some top-level athletes to stop getting their periods, but I'm seeing an increasing number of clients who are exercise enthusiasts who have stopped getting theirs too. This is not okay! Your period is a sign of health and that you are ovulating. Ovulating is a good idea because when you ovulate you produce progesterone, the hormone that keeps oestrogen in check and helps to prevent breast cancer and endometrial cancer. Progesterone is anti-inflammatory, it regulates your immune response, supports the health of your heart, breasts and bones, and soothes your nervous system by reducing anxiety and aiding sleep. In other words, it's a rather fantastic hormone. But if you don't ovulate, you don't produce it and you don't get all those wonderful benefits. The International Olympic Committee (IOC) have highlighted a condition called Relative Energy Deficiency in Sport (RED-S) which is caused by insufficient energy intake and/or excessive energy expenditure. It was previously known as the Female Athlete Triad and one of its features is menstrual dysfunction, along with low bone mineral density.

If your period is very light or has disappeared altogether, then it's time to get real about what you're eating and how much you're exercising. Chronic energy deficiency, which arises from inadequate calorific intake in relation to energy expenditure can cause a condition called hypothalamic amenorrhoea (HA), where your periods stop coming because the hypothalamus gland up in your brain stops sending out a signal to your ovaries to ovulate. Overexercising, sudden weight loss, not eating enough healthy fats and/or carbs, and disordered eating can all make your brain decide to shut down ovulation. Why does it do this? Well, it's a really smart way of preserving energy; when your body recognises that your energy input is low in relation to your energy output, it decides that it's a lean time, one where it wouldn't be wise to conceive and undergo the high-energy requirement of pregnancy, and instead it slams on the reproductive brakes. In these circumstances an 'eat more, exercise less' approach is what's needed, as well as addressing any underlying stress that can contribute to this absence of periods. This can result in weight gain, which for some people is a good thing because it's associated with the return of menstruation (#strongnotskinny).

Many of the clients that I see with HA use exercise as a way to support their mental health, and the idea of greatly reducing, and usually stopping exercising altogether for a period of time, can come as a shock. It's important in situations like this to bring in other mood boosters and soothers to compensate while you adjust to dropping your exercise routine.

My client Laura came to see me after going through a round of IVF which had been abandoned because the clinic had told her that she hadn't produced enough eggs in response to the drugs. They were about to head straight into another round and she was hoping that I could help her to produce more eggs. I took one look at her lab tests and immediately wondered what her menstrual cycle was like because her hormone levels suggested that she had hypothalamic amenorrhoea (HA). Laura told me that she had always had a regular 28-day cycle with no menstrual issues of any kind, but that over the past year her cycle had lengthened to being three months long, and that this change happened shortly after she got into CrossFit, which she did up to four times a week in addition to yoga and Pilates. Knowing that fans of CrossFit often change their diet, I asked her if she'd made any dietary changes, and she said that she'd also gone low-carb. I explained that I thought she had HA and that the amount of exercise and her diet had caused it. Astonishingly, her IVF clinic had not mentioned any of this to her and wanted her to go straight into another round in which they'd use more drugs. I explained that I'd prefer them to wait so that we would have time to get her cycle back and that doing so would likely result in a more favourable response to the IVF drugs. Thankfully, although their IVF clinic were a bit bemused, Laura and her partner both saw the sense in this and agreed to hold off.

We started with two acupuncture treatments a week to help her recover from the IVF, and to regulate her cycle by stimulating her ovaries, which we then reduced to weekly sessions in subsequent cycles. I also gave Laura the following recommendations:

- Eat more carbs, and to include protein, healthy fats, and complex carbs in every meal (she was already eating plenty of vegetables).
- Avoid intense forms of exercise, including CrossFit and more strenuous forms of yoga, until her cycle became more regular, at which point we could discuss gradually reintroducing them, though not to the same frequency. I told her that she could continue with Pilates and working on her pull ups but suggested that she try forms of exercise which built her energy up instead of depleting it, such as restorative yoga, tai chi and chi gong.
- Start supplementing with a pregnancy multivitamin, Omega-3 Fatty Acids, and vitamin D. We discussed other supplements but felt they could be brought in at a later stage if we felt that they were needed.
- Track her basal body temperature and cervical fluid so that we could assess when she ovulated.

Laura found reducing the amount she exercised hard, and although the acupuncture helped her to feel good, we had to find other supportive measures, such as going for a walk in the morning, and using yoga nidra – a relaxation technique that involves listening to a meditation which guides you into a not-quite-asleep state and leaves you feeling thoroughly rested. I also gave her a moxibustion kit to use at home; moxibustion is a gentle form of heat therapy which involves burning the dried leaves of a herb called mugwort on or above acupuncture points in order to stimulate them and is a great way of boosting energy and thereby supporting ovulation.

In her first cycle of us working together, Laura ovulated on day 23 and her cycle was 35 days long instead of 90 days – a massive improvement and a real testament to her willingness to commit to improving her menstrual cycle and supporting her fertility. Her next cycle was 31 days, and the one after was 30. At this point they decided to contact their clinic to plan their second round of IVF and they're currently waiting to start their cycle. Needless to say, they are really pleased that they decided to wait and feeling really prepared for this round.

Is Spring your Dry Season?

Spring is when cervical fluid begins to increase and helps to keep your vagina lubricated, but if you're prone to vaginal dryness, then your level of oestrogen could be low. Low oestrogen is common postnatally and during perimenopause, but I see more and more of it in young clients who don't have children, so what gives? Low oestrogen can be caused by:

- Getting older
- Peri-menopause and menopause
- A full hysterectomy
- Premature ovarian failure
- Having a baby
- Breastfeeding
- Reduced blood flow to the ovaries
- High stress levels
- Disordered eating/lack of nutrients/low cholesterol
- Being underweight
- Over-exercising
- Some medications, including hormonal birth control
- Polycystic ovarian syndrome (PCOS)
- Gluten intolerance
- Thyroid problems

Signs and symptoms of low oestrogen include:

- Absent or irregular periods
- Lethargy

- Depression
- Low sexual desire
- Vaginal dryness or loss of feeling
- Painful sex
- Wrinkles
- Night sweats or hot flushes
- Disturbed sleep, waking in the middle of the night
- A leaky or over-active bladder
- Bladder infections
- Joint pain
- Dry skin and eyes
- Depression, perhaps with lethargy or anxiety
- Melasma (sun damage)
- Poor memory
- Feeling fragile emotionally compared to how you used to feel (hi mums with babies)

Ways to improve oestrogen production:

- Bring some routine into your day by eating regularly and getting to bed at a decent time.
- Include lots of healthy fats in your diet – wild salmon, olive oil, grass fed butter, coconut milk, nuts, seeds, avocado, olives etc.
- Lay off strenuous forms of exercise.
- Use acupuncture and abdominal massage to improve blood flow to your ovaries.
- Avoid coffee and stimulants.
- Cut out gluten.
- Avoid alcohol or limit it to a couple of glasses of wine per week.
- Try seed-cycling.
- Supplements to consider: Vitamin E, Pomegranate, Maca, Black Cohosh, Dong quai, Shatavari, Red clover, Collagen.

The Perfect Time to CoppaFeel!

Breast cancer is the most commonly diagnosed cancer in women under the age of 40 in the UK. One in 8 women will receive a breast cancer diagnosis in their lifetime, and around 400 men are diagnosed every year, so checking your boobs every month is an important healthcare habit. While getting to know what your boobs are like all cycle long and what's normal for you is always a fabulous idea, checking them in your Spring (post-period and pre-ovulation) can be a good time to assess them for any changes as pre-menstrually and during menstruation, hormones can cause swelling and tenderness.

Charity CoppaFeel! recommend being aware of:

- Changes in skin texture such as puckering or dimpling that can resemble orange peel.
- A lump or area that feels thicker compared to the rest.
- A sudden, unusual change in size or shape.
- Nipple discharge (fluid that comes from the nipple without squeezing it).
- A change in nipple shape or the direction that it points in, or if it's become inverted.
- A rash or crusting of the nipple or surrounding area.
- Pain that's constant/unusual for you.

Breast tissue can be found all the way up to your collarbone and around in your armpits, so it's vital that you assess all of your chest and not just your boobs. Although some breast changes are normal and a result of hormonal fluctuations in your menstrual cycle and the ageing process, all of the above are signs and symptoms of breast cancer, which is why it's important that you get to know your boobs throughout your menstrual cycle, and if you notice an abnormality, don't hold off on speaking to your GP.

Half of invasive breast cancer cases in the UK are diagnosed after symptoms have been self-detected and reported, and regularly checking your breasts means you get to know what's normal for you and seek out help if you notice any changes. CoppaFeel! make it easy for you by sending you a free reminder by text every month. Sign up at www.coppafeel.org/remind-me.

It's never too late to start checking!

Top Tips to Get the Most out of your Spring

- Keep track of your ideas and plans.
- Dream big and feel your potential.
- Plan social occasions for your Spring and Summer.
- Pick something towards the end of your Spring to focus on during your productive Summer.
- Nurture yourself.
- Let your ideas grow before you expose them.
- Try something new or recommit to a previously abandoned plan. Go on, you can do it!

Chapter 5

Don't stop me now (Summer)

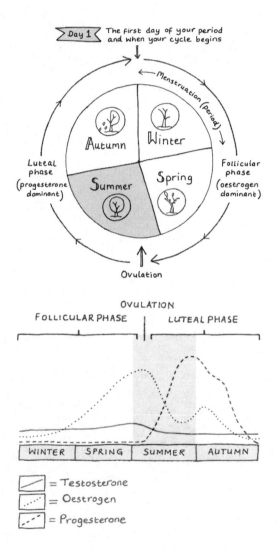

The arrival of your Summer heralds the final hormonal push towards ovulation. Oestrogen reaches its peak, triggering LH and testosterone to arrive on the scene and boy, don't you know it; the cumulative effect of all three hormones can be intense in an oh-so-awesome way.

You're in a state of flow, and with that comes an inner strength and flexibility that enables you to adjust and move with what life chucks at you, all with a dazzling smile on your face. You're oozing capability and confidence, not to mention some serious sex appeal, and because you'll feel both productive and playful, this the ideal time to stretch yourself and make the most out of your professional and personal life. And why not? You're feeling good and looking good, so werk it.

In the run up to ovulation, your hormones are trying to get you laid and knocked up. They make us look good and feel good (so that you'll wear *that* dress), interested in exploring the world (so that we seek out a mate from a different neighbourhood and different gene pool), talkative and confident so that we put ourselves out there (hi, fancy going for a drink sometime?), and horny (wanna come home with me?), because whether we want kids or not, it's undeniable that the biological purpose of ovulation is about procreation and populating the Earth. We've really excelled at that, but even among those of you who do want kids, I don't think there are many people who would want ovulation to be about conceiving on a monthly basis. Great news folks! You are more than a reproductive vessel and can use the ovulatory spike of hormones for a whole host of other exciting possibilities; pleasure, both in and out of the bedroom; improving your athletic abilities; and nailing it in your professional life. However you choose to use it, your Summer is all about raising your game and enjoying life.

Transitioning from Spring to Summer

As your hormones climb rapidly towards their summit, life suddenly feels easier and more enjoyable, and you'll find yourself taking more on. My client Azizah really enjoys her Summer: 'My whole being is at peace and I wonder why I thought anything was difficult. Everything seems to come together and I am my best self.'

This is the season to jump in with both feet (or ovaries) and say a big fat yes to what comes your way, and you'll no doubt have plenty of choices of things to say yes to, because this is the season where you're likely to be inundated with opportunities. It's as if the universe is on your side and everything and everyone you need to take life to the next stage is drawn to you. This is why getting clear on what you want for each upcoming menstrual month during your period is key, because what lands on your lap around ovulation is likely to be linked to your intention for the month.

In the same way appetite and need for sleep are often reduced in the summertime, and we're somehow able to do more, on less, so it is during your Summer. Similarly, just as before electricity we worked longer hours in the summer to take advantage of the increase in daylight hours, this is your time to really capitalise on feeling productive, as Kate does. 'Summer is my season! My mood is really positive and I feel like I can do anything I want to, and I can get so much more done in my Summer than in other phases. It's when I try to work on important projects because when I leave them till my Autumn they don't seem to have the same level of impact. I prefer to use my Autumn to tweak and amend things.'

You'll know you're in your Summer because:

- You're firing on all cylinders and feel unstoppable.
- You feel level headed and able to articulate your thoughts and feelings clearly and confidently.
- You've got some serious sass going on, and when it comes to flirting you're on fire.
- You're in the mood for pleasure and feel turned on by life.
- You find yourself getting tingly and wet at the thought of you know who.
- As oestrogen reaches its maximum, your cervical fluid increases in volume, fluidity and slipperiness before drying and thickening up after ovulation.
- Your capacity for giving and receiving love increases, and so does your desire to seek out union and joy.
- If you were to feel your cervix, you'd discover that it's soft, high, open and wet (though it will return to being low, firm and closed once you're in your luteal phase).

Summer's Superpowers

Invincibility

In your Summer you are the queen of your domain (or king if that suits your gender identity better) and you feel like you can do it all: run the show at work, impress the hell out of your clients, and fly through your to-do list. Well guess what, sweet cheeks, you can. Your communication and parenting skills are on point, you can take on the most ardent of opposition and even handle your passive-aggressive colleague and your patronising father-in-law with grace. Wanna use this phase to challenge patriarchy? Be my guest.

Productivity
This is the time to do work which is challenging and audacious. Your hormones can help you to break new ground without breaking a sweat, so decide what you want to do and get to it.

Expansion
Can you feel yourself expanding? Maybe you're walking tall instead of slouching or looking up at the skyline that surrounds you and making eye contact more than you do at other times. Perhaps your self-esteem is soaring and you're able to take ownership of your work in a way that exceeds expectations. Expansion is happening somehow; your Summer is the time where your energy moves upwards and outwards as oestrogen seeks to expand our world in little and large ways. Remember, oestrogen is your Beyoncé hormone and the run up to ovulation is when she goes on her sell-out world tour and slays, so there's every chance that this is the season where you'll perfect your bootylicious moves.

Connection and communication
Oestrogen wants you out there chatting potential mates up, making your Summer an ideal time for first dates and rekindling long-term relationships. You can use your natural ability to communicate with others in this phase to enjoy your friendships, and to take the lead in your classroom or workplace and really make an impression. Summer is the phase to put yourself out there, share yourself and your ideas, and connect with the people who can help you achieve what you want.

Pleasure
Life can feel so damn good in Summer. The hormonal high of ovulation courses through your body like a gloriously long orgasm. For me ovulation feels like amazing sex in the middle of the afternoon on a warm Summer's

day followed by a delicious nap as the sun streams through the window; there's something active about it (sex, orgasm), but also passive and receptive (lying down, feeling open to connection, orgasm), and that encapsulates the duality of the energy of Summer – we are active agents making great strides in our lives, but also experience things coming our way without much effort. Pleasure isn't just about physical intimacy, it can be about enjoying a meal or reading a really great book, looking at an incredible piece of artwork, or listening to music that gives you goosebumps.

Summer's Dangers

Feeling too visible
If you feel more at home in the shady half of your cycle, the bright light and visibility of Summer can feel intense and make you want to hide away from the world. And although it can be where you feel the most positive about your body and your work, that doesn't always mean that you want to share them with the world. It's also a sexually-charged moment of the cycle, and if you feel uneasy about inhabiting your sexual power or have experienced trauma, then it may be hard for you to embrace all of what the season has to offer, particularly when it can sometimes seem like every man on the street is able to pick up on your pheromones – chemicals which we excrete that play a role in attraction, particularly round ovulation – perhaps making you subject to unwanted attention.

Saying 'yes' to everything
I know, I know. I told you this is the season to say yes, and it is, but the almighty caveat is to consider where in your cycle you'll be when you have to fulfil what you commit to now. Are you loading your diary up smack bang in the middle of your Autumn? Because that's unlikely to work out well, so say yes, but be judicious with your timing.

Getting giddy
Okay, I love oestrogen, I truly do, but she can make even the most focused of us a bit scatty. If you find yourself motivated and ready to knuckle down to do some work that isn't physical in nature, i.e. it's desk-based, but once you sit down you find yourself unable to concentrate and get the job done,

you can blame oestrogen. That minx just wants you out strutting your stuff to attract a mate, in fact she wants you to walk further than you usually do in order to find someone genetically dissimilar to you (research shows that we do walk more around ovulation), so it's thanks to oestrogen peaking that you feel restless and unable to concentrate as you approach ovulation.

Wasting opportunities
You get that this is the season to stretch yourself and be productive. You also know that this is the season where you could conceive. But what if you've got no idea what you're meant to be doing with your life, or aren't conceiving and you want to? Then there's a very real possibility that sadness, anxiety, frustration and depression can all decimate the natural positivity and productivity of your Summer.

Summer is Where you Struggle

For some menstruators (usually those who are sensitive to the effects of oestrogen), Summer can be a bit of a wild ride. As oestrogen hits its apex, you can feel too high to concentrate on anything, and some people will experience a bit of a collapse at ovulation or immediately afterwards – in the middle of Summer – because the energy required to ovulate has left them feeling a bit depleted, and also because there's a short period immediately after ovulation where hormone levels are low; oestrogen, LH and testosterone all bottom out, and progesterone is only starting to rise. If you're sensitive to this rapid decline post-ovulation then you might feel similar to how you feel later on in your cycle, just before your period starts. Once progesterone and oestrogen begin to climb, this cloud should lift, and you'll begin to feel the serene quality of progesterone towards the end of your Summer.

If you suffer from PMDD then your Summer is likely to be all too brief, perhaps ending soon after ovulation, and the time that you are there will be bittersweet, because while you love who you are and how you feel in the first half of your cycle, the awareness that in the coming days you'll land in the second half fills you with dread and anxiety.

My client Ericka had been battling with PMS for years, and because the extreme feelings she experienced after ovulation were normal for her, she thought that's what everyone felt when they were PMSing. It wasn't until she came to one of my workshops, and over the course of the day everyone shared their menstrual stories, including their experiences of PMS, that she realised that things were more intense for her than they were for others. Ericka started tracking her cycle meticulously, and she quickly realised that her Summer was short-lived, lasting from day 11 to 14, at which point her mood would plummet and she'd feel quite low, then around day 18 to 23 she would feel anxious and irritable and experience intrusive thoughts that really disturbed her, and which usually coincided with an argument with her flatmate. Then, from day 24 to 26 she'd feel teary and sad, but once her period started she would be crying with relief because she felt like herself again. Ericka got in touch with me to share what she'd collected and told me that she was wondering if she had PMDD, that she wanted help but didn't know what she should do. Because she lived far away, we had our sessions together online, and I recommended that she keep tracking her cycle so that we'd have more to work with and explore, as well as booking an appointment with her GP which she should take her cycle tracking notes to and discuss the possibility of her having PMDD. I also referred her to a nutritionist who was local to her.

By this point Ericka was in her Spring and starting to get nervous about what would happen in her Autumn. Her GP was impressed with her cycle notes and agreed that she met the diagnostic criteria for PMDD (which you can find on page 275), and she gave Ericka a prescription for an antidepressant called citalopram which she could take throughout her luteal phase. But Ericka was unsure about taking it and wanted to know what I thought. I told her that there are times when medication is appropriate, and that while she was working on other treatment strategies, she might find it useful to have it as an option to use on her hardest days. Ericka's nutritionist recommended that she start taking magnesium and B-vitamin complex, and we both felt that the combination of exercise and keeping her blood sugar level balanced would improve her symptoms.

That first cycle, Ericka found that not skipping meals and eating more protein made a difference to how she felt after she ovulated, but when her anxiety hit on day 19 she decided to give the citalopram a go and it helped immensely, which meant that she had the headspace to arrange to go to a yoga class with a friend. She felt such an improvement that she decided to keep going to yoga with her friend and instructed her friend to hold her accountable to this commitment. Because the weather was warm, she also started walking home twice a week while she listened to an audio book. The next cycle followed a similar pattern, and in the one after I floated the idea of using less citalopram, but Ericka, who was now enjoying feeling much more like herself for the first time in years, quite understandably wasn't ready for this, so we agreed that we'd give it two more months before discussing it again. In that time, Erika realised that underlying the arguments that she was prone to having with her flatmate in the middle of her Autumn, was that she really wasn't happy with her living situation and she decided to move in with a close friend instead. Before I could ask Ericka if she was up for going without citalopram for a cycle, she told me that now that she had better support around her, she was ready.

Without the citalopram, she still experienced some mood swings and anxiety, but it was significantly less than it had been, and Ericka decided that she wanted to try cognitive behavioural therapy – a talking therapy which focuses on how your thoughts, beliefs and attitudes affect your feelings and behaviour, and helps to develop alternative ways of thinking and behaving – which, along with cycle tracking and the other supportive methods Ericka had employed, helped her to continue to manage her PMDD.

Who Runs The World?

Summer is all about raising your game, taking risks, and pushing yourself. This is the ideal time to dedicate long hours to a project and crack on with things that you might put off during the rest of the month when your energy shifts.

In the beginning of your Summer, specifically the days leading up to ovulation, your oral ability is at its greatest, making this the ideal time to say your piece in a meeting, be interviewed, carry out public speaking engagements, and ask for a promotion or raise (given the despicable gender pay gap and low numbers of women in upper management and CEO positions, I highly recommend that you do this). I'm convinced that every single one of you reading this has an opinion or idea that at least one other person in the world needs to hear, but if you're sat there thinking to yourself that this isn't you and that you have nothing of value to say, consider where you are in your cycle. If you're not currently in your Summer, come back and read it when you are.

If you still don't feel that you have anything to say (and even if you do), you could use this time to look at whose voice isn't being heard in the world and use your voice to amplify theirs. This might be your colleague who has an incredible mind but is so introverted that nobody pays attention to what she's trying to say, or a community that's subject to oppression and violence. Let's face it, our society is set up so that it's the opinions and work of rich white men that are seen and heard – hardly representative of our diversity is it? This is the season to challenge yourself and to challenge authority; shake the apple tree and see what gives.

If you're in an educational or work setting that's traditionally been the preserve of men, where women are ignored and talked over, use the 'amplification' strategy that female White House staffers used during President Obama's time in office: when a woman makes a key point, another woman repeats her point and gives her credit for it. This ensures that points made by women are heard, and that ideas aren't stolen by the men in the organisation. We have plenty of ideas, skills and talents, we're also good at being polite and dedicated A grade students, but for our voices to be heard we need to be noticed, and that means we have to be visible. So, how comfortable are you with visibility? Is it something that makes you squirm or are you happy being in the limelight? Or, could it be that you're comfortable being seen at a particular time in your cycle? Your Summer is the time to be seen and to be your own cheerleader, a skill which I'm currently learning from my two-year-old son who exclaims loudly and proudly, 'I did it!' when he conquers a task … and goes on to show his new talent for peeling an orange to everyone in the room. This is exactly what we need to be doing for ourselves, drawing attention to how fabulous we are and praising other women publicly and specifically, so that we draw attention to one another and lift each other up.

In *The Cancer Journals*, Audre Lorde shares the words she spoke at a talk she gave in 1977, capturing the essence of what holds so many of us back from speaking up, as well as how vital and necessary it is that we do:

'I began to ask each time: "What's the worst that could happen to me if I tell this truth?" Unlike women in other countries, our breaking silence is unlikely to have us jailed, "disappeared" or run off the road at night. Our speaking out

will irritate some people, get us called bitchy or hypersensitive and disrupt some dinner parties. And then our speaking out will permit other women to speak, until laws are changed and lives are saved and the world is altered forever. Next time, ask: What's the worst that will happen? Then push yourself a little further than you dare. Once you start to speak, people will yell at you. They will interrupt you, put you down and suggest it's personal. And the world won't end.'

When it comes to planning our progress in a linear fashion, we're highly skilled, too skilled in fact. How often do you tell yourself that in order to start doing X, you need to do Y and take a course in Z, then you might be ready to finally move up in your organisation or career by, oh a whole 1 per cent? But your Summer is when you can make great leaps. Despite your detailed and neverending plans, progress does not have to be incremental and dependent on you becoming ridiculously qualified. Instead, you can skip ahead and get further quicker. Go on, I dare you.

If you're prone to imposter syndrome – the belief that you're inadequate, incompetent and a fraud – and find that it keeps you small because you're continually telling yourself, 'Shit, shit, shit, shit, someone's going to realise that I have no idea what I'm doing or talking about, so I can't possibly step up to the plate', then how about adopting an attitude of, 'Ah fuck it, I'm just gonna see what I can get away with'? I'm here to tell you that this is the way forward. It's how I got the book deal that led to what you're holding in your hands.

Ovulation is an ideal time to receive constructive feedback so if you have regular meetings with your boss, mentor or teacher, this is a great time to schedule them for. You'll be more inclined to listen and take their thoughts on board without attaching emotions to them or getting defensive and be able to calmly and confidently defend your position if necessary. This is when you can master the art of defending without being defensive.

When you're soaring in your Summer it can be bloody annoying to be held back by other people and the practicalities of daily life. When you've got an inner drive to get shit done, it can be utterly frustrating to be held back by colleagues who haven't pulled their weight or having to take time off work because your kid is ill. You want to unleash all that determination and energy that's rising up in you – this is your time to shine godamnit!

Similarly, if you haven't landed on your path in life yet then this can make for an unsettling time, because while you feel the surge of hormones, and an urge to do something with them, you don't necessarily have a sense of what to actually do. If this is sounding familiar then remember that this is the time in your cycle when you're likely to be at your most adventurous and social, making it the ideal time to start a blog, go on a weekend-long course, and attend a mentoring or networking event. My suggestion is to do something which brings you pleasure and gets your juices going.

Inherent in risk-taking is a chance of things failing, but if they don't work out, have you really failed? Nope, nope, no, not at all. I won't have you berating yourself because you've taken a chance. Celebrate your courage, tenacity, and abilities and keep track of what's worked well, especially if a plan hasn't panned out as you wanted it to. Write that shit down so you don't get chewed up in a week's time when your critic comes out to play. I guarantee it's more painful to have nothing to show because you were intimidated and fearful, than to have something to show which didn't work but can be adjusted, developed, and learnt from.

If, at the beginning of your Summer, the 'hey good looking, why are you working when there's a world out there waiting for you to explore it' vibe of oestrogen messes with your ability to work, and you can't sit at your desk for a minute longer, try working in short fastpaced bursts, take breaks to walk around your office or go outside when you're on a break, speak to colleagues about projects, and have lunches with clients to fulfil your need to move and socialise, that way you can satisfy your oestrogenic urge to explore the world, and then get back to it. Try not to beat yourself up if you don't finish things up, this isn't the time for details, it's for brave broad strokes that can be finessed in a few days if you're afforded the luxury of time, because once progesterone begins its ascent, it'll bring with it the calm focus to attend to the nitty gritty details that would quite frankly bore you to tears right now.

Welcome to the Pleasure Zone

The combination of oestrogen and testosterone as you head towards ovulation can be a game changer when it comes to sexual desire. Oestrogen increases blood flow to your genitals, making you feel all tingly (skinny jeans and a bike ride, anyone?) and causing your cervical fluid to become profuse, slippery, and stretchy. Though if you're low on oestrogen then your vagina might feel less Niagara Falls and more Mojave Desert, in which case lube is your best friend whilst you work on increasing your oestrogen.

Sex in the run up to ovulation can often be the most enjoyable in your cycle because you're more likely to feel horny and lubricated, your cervix has moved upwards making penetrative sex more comfortable, and orgasms can come easier and quicker. But rather than being the sex-crazed ovulators that we're often portrayed as, who will jump on anyone hot that's in front of us, the hormones of ovulation can make us want to masturbate more, because although there's research showing an increase in sexual desire around ovulation, it also shows that it doesn't always translate into sex with someone else, and whether you're in a relationship or not, you may prefer masturbation to having sex with another.

Plenty of people find that our sexual desire 'only' appears at certain times of the month, usually when oestrogen is high in relation to other sex hormones – in the lead up to ovulation and perhaps in the days before menstruation too, and when testosterone is on the scene. This is entirely common and normal, but there are plenty of people in this category who feel that there must be something wrong with them, that they're defective somehow – you're not.

Humans are described as being *concealed ovulators* – we don't exhibit clear signs of ovulation to everybody else by running around in heat displaying massively swollen red genitals to all and sundry – and because of that there's a sense that we might be up for it at any given moment, when in actuality your libido can be as flat as a pancake for some of the menstrual cycle when oestrogen and testosterone aren't around. When I speak to clients about this I often wonder if it would be easier for us to accept the prevalence of desire appearing around ovulation if we were like the female guinea pig, who only permits penetration when she's in heat (aka ovulating), the rest of the time a membrane seals off the opening to the vagina. What if women were like this? Perhaps it would solve the issue for those of us who are disinterested in sex during sections of the menstrual cycle, because it would not only be acceptable but expected.

If you find the lead up to ovulation is the only time when you feel a blip of interest in being intimate, then for heaven's sake make sure to keep some space in your diary to have some fun with your partner or just fly solo. And if you're someone whose sexual desire is present all cycle long, then more power to you.

When it comes to ovulation we do exhibit some subtle cues though; our features become softer and more symmetrical, skin often clears up, and our body odour is even perceived as being more pleasant around ovulation. The pheromones we emit in the ovulatory phase of the cycle may send out a signal that males pick up on to subliminally identify when we're fertile, thus explaining the reason scientists found that female strippers earn the most tips when they're ovulating (and those on the pill earned the least).

Your Spring and Summer are when you might really feel and be able to embrace your sexual power, though if you feel an unease around yours then it might feel uncomfortable, and if you're anxious about conceiving, either because you want to or really don't want to, then Summer can present a challenge because in the moment of connection, an uneasy tension also exists, preventing you from fully embracing intimacy and your other half.

Lost Desire

It's common to feel a dip or disappearance of libido in Summer after ovulation as oestrogen and testosterone decline. Interest in physical intimacy can be fleeting after ovulation, so if the urge is there, get to it before you miss the moment. Post-ovulation your cervical fluid loses its slippery quality so it's normal to feel quite dry in the second half of your cycle, though if there are days where it's wetter in quality, it usually indicates that your oestrogen is higher in relation to progesterone, either because you have excess oestrogen or not enough progesterone. Your cervix will be lower in the second half so if you have penetrative sex it may be uncomfortable in certain positions or in all of them, so you may prefer to skip penetration. Masturbation, non-penetrative sex, and lube are all good ideas to help sex to be more enjoyable post-ovulation and at all other times too.

Is it rare for you to want sex and initiate it, but if your other half gets their timing right, you can get in the mood and wonder why you didn't feel like this before they got you going? Guess what, this is also normal! Renowned sex educator Dr. Emily Nagoski estimates that around 85 per cent of women don't experience spontaneous desire as their dominant style when it comes to desire (spontaneous desire being when out of the blue you think to yourself, 'I feel like having sex'), and 30 per cent of us rarely or never experience spontaneous desire for sex. Yup, you read that right and no, it doesn't make you dysfunctional, although the pharmaceutical giants would love for you to believe that you are. Instead, women are more likely to experience responsive desire, in which interest in sex develops once we are in a scenario where we begin to feel aroused, such as kissing (and you've managed to stop thinking about work stress, the pile of dishes, and the state of your bank account). And a reminder that the vast majority of us require clitoral stimulation to feel turned on and have an orgasm, that's just how our anatomy works. Do educate your lover if they're not clued up, especially if you're someone who experiences responsive desire. #moreorgasmsplease

I'm purposely avoiding using the phrase 'sex drive' to describe your interest in sex because I'm in agreement with Nagoski, who states that thinking of sex as a drive isn't accurate or helpful. In her book *Come As You Are*, she explains that biological drives are about survival (i.e. our need to eat, drink and sleep), but sex is not a drive because you cannot die from the lack or absence of it. Instead, Nagoski describes it is an incentive motivation system that makes us seek out sex and enables us to thrive. If you're someone who doesn't experience spontaneous desire, and you view the lack of that *type* of desire as a low sex drive, then it's easy to conclude that you're broken and abnormal. Whereas if you view your sexual desire with the lens of understanding that almost a third of us don't experience spontaneous desire regularly and most of us have responsive desire, you are in fact perfectly normal. That feels much better, right?

Now that we've established that it really is very normal for, a) your sexual desire to be spontaneous and/or responsive, and b) that your sexual desire can fluctuate throughout your menstrual cycle, let's look at specific issues that can interfere with a healthy sex life.

If your libido is MIA after coming off the birth control pill, then I am not surprised. Consider that the pill works by putting hormones in your body in order to suppress ovarian function which screws with sexual desire. When ovarian function is suppressed it reduces the testosterone output of your ovaries, and testosterone is a major player when it comes to desire. The introduction of synthetic hormones also means that your body has to compensate somehow to prevent your body from being harmed by excessively high levels of hormones. It does this by increasing your production of a protein that's produced in your liver called sex hormone binding globulin (SHBG). SHBG's job is to mop up excess hormones in your blood by binding to them so that they can be excreted before they cause problems, and pill users have four times the amount of SHBG that non-pill users do in order to achieve this. Sounds good so far, right? I mean, your body is just keeping you safe.

The trouble is that all that extra SHBG is binding up your already diminished level of testosterone that you have circulating in your blood, rendering it useless, so it's no wonder that some pill users report a loss of libido. It's nice to think that when you come off the pill, your SHBG level simply returns to normal, but this is where it gets depressing. While SHBG levels *do* decline, research which assessed levels of SHBG for 4 months after participants stopped taking the pill found that at the end of the study they still hadn't returned to the baseline level of someone who had never taken the pill, which some experts believe has the potential to affect your libido and sexual health for life. I bet your doctor never told you that when they wrote out your prescription.

Sexual desire can also do a runner when you're in a depleted and/or stressed state. Let's say you have a one-year-old who doesn't sleep through the night, which is perfectly common and developmentally normal for a child of that age, but not for you. Maybe your diet is a bit disordered because you're so busy doing All The Things so that you either forget to eat or just eat whatever is easy and quick (usually crappy carbs), or you're trying to lose weight and are restricting your intake of calories and fat. And let's not forget that you're surviving on caffeine and sugar, plus dealing with whatever relationship, work, health, family, and financial stresses that you've got going on. Okay, are you with me? You're sleep deprived, your hormones are struggling because your diet and healthy fat intake is inadequate to support hormone production (because you need fats to make hormones), your sexual desire has been shunted down the priority list because your body is so busy trying to regulate your blood sugar level and your stress hormones that the idea of procreation (the whole point of desire according to your body) is quite frankly preposterous. In addition to this you've probably spent so much time in physical contact with your child, caring for them, providing affection, and being used as a human climbing frame, that you're feeling thoroughly touched out so the idea of any more physical contact is enough to push you over the edge. And let's not forget that if you're breastfeeding then the hormones used to make milk will be suppressing the hormones involved in sexual desire. Plus whatever relationship and life factors you have in the mix. *Can you see why you have no interest in sex?*

If you're not a mum, my bet is that for you a lot of the above still applies. Is your sleep shit, are you doing way too much and producing high amounts of cortisol, are you so busy running around or trying to lose weight that you're neglecting your need for food, do you survive on caffeine and sugar to make it through your working day, and need booze to wind down at night? *Can you see why you have no interest in sex?*

When you're repeatedly tired/stressed/hungry/undernourished, your body dials down desire because in this depleted and stressed state, sex and procreation is not a priority, survival is. Think of desire as the star on top of the Christmas tree (or angel, maybe you're an angel person); it's only ceremoniously placed on top of the tree once the lights, baubles and tinsel are in place, i.e. you're taking good care of your basic needs for healthy food and drink, are getting enough sleep and have a handle on stress, and if you're in a relationship, that you're happy in it.

If you've experienced a decrease in sexual desire, also consider if any medication you're taking could be to blame. Medications that treat depression, anxiety, mood disorders, blood pressure, epilepsy and multiple sclerosis (MS) can all impact on desire and ability to have an orgasm, as can alcohol, lack of good-quality sleep, hypothyroidism, and just about everything else in your life, both in and out of your relationship.

It may be the case that singletons experience a heightening of desire at ovulation more than people in long-term relationships because your hormones are driving you to seek out connection with another, whereas when couples transition from the lust phase of a relationship to attachment in long-term relationships, there can be an overall lessening of desire that involves non-hormonal factors.

Think about who you're getting jiggy with around ovulation. Once you start kissing and hugging, you produce oxytocin which promotes bonding and suddenly the person you just fancied getting it on with but wouldn't want to meet your parents, becomes the one you want to stay for breakfast, and while there's nothing wrong with that, bear in mind that your hormones can lead you to form a deeper connection than you had planned. Some research has found that women who are attracted to men are more likely to be attracted to a 'cad' – a man who is charismatic and physically attractive, but not necessarily reliable – at ovulation, rather than a 'dad' – a man who is nice and reliable and more likely to be a committed partner and father to a child – who you're more likely to shack up with in the latter half of your cycle when progesterone makes you want safety.

When it Hurts so Bad

Pain during sex can really get in the way of having a good time and can impact on your relationships and how you feel about yourself too. Painful sex is not acceptable because it robs you of a vital part of you that deserves to be expressed and experienced. If you experience any of the following, which according to the American College of Obstetrics and Gynecology, 75 per cent of us will experience at some point in our lifetime, then please, please, please speak to a healthcare professional about what's going on. If they dismiss you, don't accept it – your sexuality is deserving of healthcare.

Dyspareunia

Aka pain during sex. Unfortunately, too many sufferers are told that it's all in their head and that they just need to relax and have a glass of wine – an appalling suggestion given that what they really need is to be taken seriously, assessed, and offered appropriate treatment. Pain during sex can be caused by a number of things – for instance endometriosis, a hormonal imbalance, pelvic floor dysfunction, prolapse, adhesions and scarring from surgery, infection, as well as a history of episiotomy, cancer treatment, or pelvic trauma. All can be helped by appropriate treatment, such as seeing a women's health physiotherapist. If you find sex painful, as well as getting to the bottom of why you do, I recommend checking out Ohnut, an intimate wearable that resembles a stack of squishy stretchy donuts, which is designed to be worn around the shaft of the penis and allows users to customise the depth of penetration. Pelvic floor exercises (aka kegels) involve clenching and releasing the layer of muscles that support the pelvic organs and spans the bottom of the pelvis, but when these muscles are too tight (hypertonic) they can aggravate pain during sex, as well as urinary issues such as incontinence.

A women's health physiotherapist can assess your pelvic floor and provide treatment and advice.

Vaginismus
This is where the pelvic floor muscles that surround the vagina, bladder, and uterus involuntarily spasm and tighten, making penetrative sex, vaginal examinations, and the use of tampons painful or impossible. Anything that triggers the body into anticipating pain can initiate vaginismus, such as anxiety, stress, birth or sexual trauma, back/hip injuries, and menopause. After experiencing a negative painful experience where the pelvic floor muscles shorten and tighten, the fear of recurrence then causes the pelvic muscles to brace as they try to protect further pain, thus perpetuating and confounding the pain–spasm cycle. Treatment should include seeing a highly-specialised women's health physiotherapist and might include the use of vaginal dilators, sex therapy, relaxation techniques, and injections of Botox to the pelvic floor.

Vulvodynia
This describes pain in the vulva which can occur when it is provoked (during sex, use of tampons, wiping after going to the toilet, having a vaginal exam), and also when not provoked (pain from any form of touch, clothing, or even simply sitting down). Pain can be generalised and affect the entire vulva, or be specific to one area, such as the clitoris or the entrance to the vagina. When symptoms are limited to the entrance to the vagina, it's known as vestibulodynia. Treatment options include: working with a highly skilled pelvic floor physical therapist; addressing any underlying hormonal imbalances that reduce lubrication; calming the nervous system by improving sleep, and reducing infections, emotional stress, and intake of inflammatory foods; following an elimination diet to identify any dietary triggers; improving gut function and nutritional deficiencies, and getting support for issues such as exhaustion, abuse and birth/sexual trauma.

Interstitial cystitis
Also known as painful bladder syndrome, interstitial cystitis (IC) can result in symptoms which are similar to a urinary tract infection called cystitis, but the latter is caused by an infection, and IC is not. Frustratingly, the

actual cause of it remains unclear. IC features symptoms such as; abdominal or pelvic pain; persistent, unpleasant sensations in the bladder; discomfort with bladder filling and partial relief upon emptying; bladder pressure; urinary frequency and urgency and frequent urination at night. Seventy-five per cent of people with IC experience pain with intercourse and 90 per cent of women with it report low sexual desire, difficulty with arousal, bladder pain during sex, and an urge to urinate during sex. In one study 87 per cent of participants with IC experienced pain associated with pelvic floor dysfunction – the inability to use the muscles of the pelvic floor to control bladder and bowel movements. There's also a strong correlation between IC and a digestive disorder called small intestinal bacterial overgrowth (SIBO) in that the majority of patients with IC who also had gut issues tested positive for it, and treatment of SIBO resulted in a 47 per cent improvement in IC symptoms.

The Big O

Ovulation of course. Do you know when it's happening? If you pay attention to your cervical fluid, you'll notice that your peak flow occurs in the couple of days before ovulation as oestrogen hits its high note. If you're charting your BBT it may dip around this time before jumping up after ovulation, and if you're using urine strips to detect the LH surge and help determine when you're about to ovulate you'll hopefully get a positive result. You might get a sense that it's happening purely because you feel so darn good.

Some people experience sensations such as a pop, twinge or twang in the lower abdomen as ovulation takes place, and in some ovulators this escalates to pain which can either be felt as a dull throbbing ache, or sudden, severe and stabbing. Pain at ovulation, known medically as *mittelschmerz* is often dismissed, but it's a medical red flag and should be investigated by a doctor to find out what's causing it as it can suggest the presence of ovarian cysts, endometriosis, or a sexually transmitted infection called chlamydia. Pain at ovulation can be improved and relieved with pelvic massage, acupuncture, and exercise.

Chlamydia

Chlamydia is a bacterial infection which causes inflammation and scarring to the fallopian tubes which can narrow them and cause pain as the egg released at ovulation tries to journey down a fallopian tube. Other symptoms include pain when weeing, an unusual vaginal or anal discharge, abdominal pain, and bleeding after sex, although most people who contract chlamydia won't experience any symptoms of it which is why it's been dubbed 'The Silent Disease'. It's treated easily with antibiotics but left untreated it can cause pelvic inflammatory disease (PID) the complications of which include scarring to the inside and outside of the fallopian tubes which can block them and therefore cause infertility and ectopic pregnancy, and long-term pelvic pain. You can be tested for it at a sexual health clinic or at your GP surgery, or you can buy your own test kit to do at home which you then send to a laboratory for testing.

Spotting a light amount of blood at ovulation happens to around 4.8 per cent of menstruators and is likely caused by the sharp fall in hormones after ovulation before progesterone climbs to an adequate level. Spotting can be a normal event with nothing sinister behind it, but it's worth knowing what's normal for you and speaking to your doctor if you regularly bleed between periods or after sex, or experience irregular bleeding or spotting.

While research suggests that anovulation – the lack of ovulation – occurs in around a third of all clinically normal menstrual cycles and is more common during teens and peri-menopausal years, not ovulating regularly is an indicator of a hormonal imbalance such as hypothalamic amenorrhoea, polycystic ovarian syndrome (PCOS), and excess production of prolactin – a hormone which suppresses ovulation. If you have irregular or long cycles, or your period has gone AWOL then ask your doctor to test your hormones. You can find suggestions of what to have tested in Section Three.

Not eating enough calories and carbs, drinking caffeinated soft drinks, and taking prescribed or recreational drugs can all mess with your ability to ovulate. Drugs which interfere with ovulation include:

- Non-steroidal anti-inflammatory drugs (NSAIDs) such as ibuprofen, naproxen and mefenamic acid can prevent the follicle rupturing so that no egg is released.
- Anti-depressants classified as selective serotonin uptake inhibitors (SSRIs) such as citalopram and fluoxetine.
- Steroids such as those used to treat allergies and asthma.
- Medications used to treat high blood pressure and ulcers.
- Recreational drugs such as cannabis and cocaine.

Self-care Essentials

Your Spring and Summer are your most social seasons, and in contrast to socialising in your Autumn and Winter, which might go against your natural inclination and leave you feeling depleted, socialising in your Spring and Summer can feel essential and rejuvenating. The first part of your Summer is the time to load your diary up with all the fun things. If there's something or someone that you like to avoid, then this can be the ideal time to fulfil your obligation, as what usually ruffles your feathers is more likely to be water off a duck's back. But make it a lunch rather than an overnight visit – you don't want to lose out on your fun time.

As oestrogen peaks in the lead up to ovulation it can suppress your appetite for food but at the same time it stimulates your sexual appetite; in fact, decreased appetite before ovulation often coincides with a peak in sexual desire because oestrogen wants you horny and searching for a mate, not wandering the supermarket aisles and hiding away in your kitchen.

However, once you ovulate you'll probably notice an increase in appetite as progesterone (the nesting hormone) begins to rise. You're more prone to blood sugar instability in the second half of your cycle, and with that comes mood swings and that delightful state of feeling hangry, so now is the time to ramp up your intake of protein and fat to help stabilise your blood sugar and mood.

If, in the middle of your Summer, you find yourself prone to a post-ovulation collapse in energy and mood, take some time to evaluate how well you're caring for yourself around this time. In my practice I find that there's a direct correlation between an insufficient foundation of self-care, largely around not eating regularly or well enough, and struggling in the few days after ovulation. The cumulative effect of oestrogen suppressing appetite and it working with testosterone to make you get more done, means that you can do more on less, but the downside of this is that you can get swept away by feeling on top of things and neglect to take care of your most basic needs, and if you're prone to feeling deficient, this can set you up for a problematic second half of your cycle, leaving you tired and down in the dumps.

Alcohol intake around ovulation, particularly binge drinking is known to increase oestrogen levels (and sometimes testosterone and LH too), perhaps making you more prone to the hormonal drop off post-ovulation. And let's not forget that alcohol is a depressant too.

You have less need for sleep at the beginning of your Summer before you ovulate, so this is the time when you can probably get away with a few late nights, but once progesterone begins to rise post-ovulation, falling asleep and staying asleep will get easier, so be good to yourself and use this stage of your cycle to catch up on restorative sleep, particularly if you're prone to insomnia premenstrually.

When oestrogen suddenly drops off after ovulation and then again just before your period starts, it can cause spasm and fast motility in your digestive tract, which can result in diarrhoea. Once progesterone begins to rise, it slows down the wave-like movement called peristalsis in your gut by relaxing the smooth muscle that lines it, resulting in a slower transit time and mild constipation as progesterone peaks in the middle of your luteal phase (this is why constipation is so common in the first trimester of pregnancy, when rapidly increasing progesterone – the pregnancy hormone – slows everything down). In the upper part of your gut, progesterone causes the sphincter at the top of the stomach to relax, which can cause reflux and heartburn.

A Tribe Called Sweat

Thanks to the sharp rise in testosterone pre-ovulation, when it comes to exercise the start of your Summer is when you're likely to hit your PBs. This is the time to raise your game and go for it. It doesn't matter if that means walking an extra length of your local park or smashing your 10k time, carrying your shopping home or powerlifting an additional 10kgs. Pay attention to your form though as one study found that the anterior cruciate ligament of the knee (ACL) is 4–8 times more likely to be injured now than at any other point in the cycle.

Midway through your Summer, after you ovulate, make the switch to low impact cardio and conditioning forms of exercise to focus on stretching and fat-burning. Aerobic exercise is perfect if you're prone to oestrogen excess as sweating is one way of excreting excess oestrogen, but keep it at a pace where you can hold a conversation – remember that the second half of your cycle isn't the time to push yourself to your limit, it's about maintaining what you've built in the first half.

If there's tension in your relationship or there's an absence of desire, try working out together. Not only does exercise cause a state of physical arousal that mimics those created in the thrill of having the hots for someone – sweaty hands, a racing pulse, and shortness of breath – but research shows that couples who do physical activities together report feeling more satisfied in their relationships, and the non-verbal matching of each other's physical behaviour, such as throwing and catching a ball or keeping the same pace whilst jogging, helps couples to feel emotionally attuned and bonded to each other.

Top Tips to Get the Most out of your Summer

- Leave space in your diary for having fun.
- It's the perfect time for a first date or to reconnect with your partner of 14 years.
- Lean in and do the work that'll get you further. Your hormones are behind you.
- Embrace the 'ah, fuck it, why not?' nature of rising testosterone at the start of Summer. Take a chance and have a go at something.
- Try to do any public speaking in the few days leading up to ovulation.
- Get some batch cooking done once oestrogen and testosterone have simmered down after ovulation and stash them in the freezer for your Autumn and Winter.

- The beginning of Summer could be when you feel most confident and happy with how you look. Try a new outfit or style, and get your photograph taken.
- Perfect time for a holiday.
- This is the time when you'll be able to tolerate your in-laws (or your own family) visiting.
- Say yes.
- Keep track of your successes; you might be feeling so awesome that you don't bother tracking but write that shit down – you're gonna need an account of what you've got up to this month in your Autumn when the time rolls around to deal with your inner critic, and I don't want you hiding your head in the sand, you're too gorgeous for that.

Most (but not all) of the menstruators I work with prefer the sunny half of their cycle to the shady side, but you can't hang out here forever; it's time to get ready for your Autumn.

Chapter 6

Highway to hell (Autumn)

*What may look like on the surface to be uncontrolled anger, destruction
and rage may actually be truth, justice and love.*
– Layla Saad

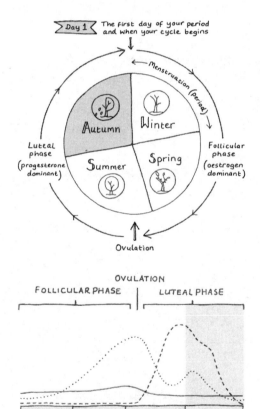

Welcome to the less glamorous half of your menstrual cycle!

At some point after ovulation, you'll notice a subtle or dramatic shift in how you feel and behave. The high of your Summer might extend beyond ovulation for several days, perhaps even a week (lucky you), though you might notice a subtle shift and feel a bit quieter and more introspective. Or, if you're sensitive to oestrogen taking her first nosedive (you can look forward to a second one just before your period starts) then you might find yourself unceremoniously dumped in Autumn the day after ovulation and feel cranky/agitated/sad/tired/all of the above. It's not all doom and gloom though, because if you find your energy collapsing after ovulation, you may well experience an Indian Summer before you land in your Autumn proper – a bit of a fifth season – as your levels of oestrogen climb again, along with progesterone, the dominant hormone of the second half of your cycle.

Transitioning from Summer to Autumn

The transition from Summer can be problematic for a lot of people, so identifying the day that you move into Autumn can be one of the most important aspects of charting your cycle. For some people it can fluctuate in each cycle by a few days, and is often a consequence of increased stress and/ or decreased self-care. Pinpointing your transition day(s) is essential because this alone has the potential to revolutionise how you feel about yourself in your premenstruum. They're often the days where you feel like crap and give yourself a hard time, but don't realise what's going on until your period arrives, at which point you look back and go, 'oh that's why!' By charting your cycle you'll be able to predict when you'll feel the wobbles and make plans to handle them. I can't emphasise enough how doing this one thing will mean that you'll move from meltdowns and misery to compassion and dignity. By using cycle awareness you'll cultivate an inner kindness towards yourself, which is sorely needed in your premenstruum.

> 'I began charting my cycle on a daily basis and a pattern began to emerge of days 20–23, the start of my Autumn, being very problematic. I experienced low mood, strong emotions and extreme feelings of not being good enough. I always knew that I suffered with symptoms of PMS, but I had no idea that the days were so specific and predictable. Using The Cycle Strategy has been

a huge game-changer: I've realised that I'm not a highly depressive crazy woman, and I finally have a reason as to why I feel so low at this time in my cycle and can now plan my life accordingly for those tricky days and stop giving myself such a hard time.'

Just like my client Natalie above, you'll be able to recognise the day, or days, that you make the switch within a few months of charting your cycle. What crops up in your Autumn is incredibly important and being diligent with charting your experiences and feelings here can really serve you. In fact, when it comes to charting your cycle, you might find that this is one of the seasons where you get the most data.

You'll arrive in your Autumn at some point after ovulation, often around day 20 or 21 in a 28-day cycle. Here's how you'll know when you're there:

- The flow and productive energy you experienced in your Spring and Summer is interrupted.
- You feel yourself detaching and withdrawing.
- Your energy slumps and turns inward.
- You're more sensitive to criticism, whether it's how you chat to yourself internally, or comes externally in the form of your boss, your partner, *your mother.* In your Summer everything was rosy, but now you view things with a critical eye. All you see are faults and what needs to change.
- As you track your cycle, you might find that nagging questions keep cropping up in your Autumn. This is a season where your gut feelings and intuition can really serve you by helping guide you towards choices which serve you rather than everyone else.
- The way you communicate shifts, and instead of responding, you react. If you're not sure when you're in your Autumn, you might want to ask your best mate or other half!
- You become more assertive and want to focus on what's important to you. Last week you were happy to visit your distant relatives, help your friend out, or cheer your kid on at their weekly swimming lesson, but now you feel the pressing need to do something for yourself, whether it's to rest, to enjoy a coffee and an opportunity to daydream, or see that film that nobody else is interested in.
- Your libido does a vanishing act and so does your natural lubrication.

Although some people will feel right at home once they land in their Autumn, this premenstrual phase of the cycle is typically where we fall apart a little or a lot – our energy and positivity disappear, our emotions spill out, our frustration leaves us feeling like tightly wound coils, and of course the physical side of things such as sore boobs/bloating/dodgy digestion/night sweats/headaches/backache can all make for a really fun time.

Coupled with this full-on assortment of symptoms, the start of Autumn marks your arrival in the hemisphere of the cycle that isn't validated. Society favours who we are in Spring and Summer; fertile young women who are nice and kind and polite, not to mention up for it. Autumn is where we grow up and get real, it's where you move into the mature half of your cycle. The rose-tinted glasses of Summer are replaced with X-ray specs, granting you the power to see through things with laser like clarity, which, in addition to a lowered tolerance for putting up with bullshit, can either feel altogether freeing or dangerous.

Try to maintain a curiosity about what appears for you here. When something comes up, ask yourself, what's really going on here, what's this about? It's likely that the angst, anger, exasperation, irritation, sadness and tears that you feel here are about what you experience *throughout the whole of your cycle*, but in the first half, oestrogen does a stellar job of glossing over the little, and sometimes very large, niggles. In the first half of our cycle, oestrogen is there to make us chatty and horny, with the aim of getting us to have sex and procreate. This outward energy makes us care about our loved ones' happiness, and commonly results in us going to great lengths to help them out, often to our own detriment. Fundamentally, oestrogen makes us oblige others. It's what Julie Holland, MD refers to as 'the veil of accommodation', a phrase that perfectly encapsulates the social coherence that oestrogen seeks to create.

Autumn is where you can take a step back and assess your responsibilities towards others. You begin to step down as your energy turns inward. Far from being awful, this is in fact wonderful, because you are in the half of your cycle where your hormones will help you to truly prioritise your own needs and desires. But if you don't manage to move with awareness, and you try to maintain the 'go get 'em tiger' feeling of Summer, then you're likely to burn out quickly, and instead of this being a gradual process, it'll be sudden and disastrous. After the productive nature of Summer, Autumn may not feel particularly purposeful or helpful, but it is – *if* you know how to work with it.

Autumn's Superpowers

Deep thought and focus

The day that you transition into Autumn is your cue to zero in on what your target for this phase is. It's when you shift from the outward expression of Spring and Summer and move into the inward focus of Autumn and Winter. Your energy levels will be declining, so it's crucial that you be purposeful with the energy that you do have. It's in your Autumn that you have an ability to go deep and concentrate, so don't squander your last chance to bring a project through to completion before this cycle ends.

Reviewing

You'll also find yourself equipped with helicopter vision, which means that in the same way you can spot every household chore that hasn't been completed by your housemate as soon as you walk in the door, you're able to consider the bigger picture with a project that you've been working on, or situation that's been on your mind. You have the ability to scrutinise and reconsider here, so take a step back and approach things with fresh eyes.

Deciding

This is a time of great insight and you have the clarity to make a decision about something you've been mulling over for a while. Autumn can be where you feel most in touch with your intuition and you'd do well to trust it. This might sound woo-woo to you, but it's backed up by scientific research which demonstrates that your first response – your gut instinct – is astonishingly accurate 90 per cent of the time. This is the phase to take advantage of your instinctive prowess, so learn to trust your instant response before you moderate it with critical thinking and reason, especially when it comes to saying no. Decide what's important and what's not; what's important enough to take with you into menstruation and your next cycle? Are you going to leave your job or relationship, or stay? If you're still not sure about something then I recommend sitting with it for a while, and consider it whilst you have your period, as that's often a time when answers can come to you.

Editing and organising

Just like pruning your garden in the Autumn creates vigour and more fruit in the following Spring and Summer, some clever pruning here will create more pleasure and balance in subsequent cycles. Autumn is the phase to examine, take stock, and get rid of what isn't working for you. That might apply to a work project, your relationships, or your clothes. Organise, tidy, and clean. This is the time to clean out your fridge and sort out your inbox. Rising progesterone can produce a nesting feeling similar to what pregnant people often feel towards the end of their pregnancy, and the premenstrual urge to finish things literally and metaphorically is nature's way of getting you ready to drop your responsibilities so that you can go to ground in some way when your period arrives.

Speaking candidly
The key to this phase is to trust your inner bitch and the messages she's whispering to you. When I say inner bitch, I mean your uncensored internal voice that gains momentum in your premenstruum. If you don't listen to what that wise bitch is saying, then she'll start screaming at you, and that's when things can get *very* stormy. So, before you lose it, and there can be power in losing it, but before you do, figure out what she's asking you to do. What does your inner bitch require of you? Does she want you to get better at saying no, to spend some time on your own, to stop letting others step all over you, to stop being so attached to your inbox when you're not meant to be working (and not getting paid to), to spend less time on social media and save your sleep and thyroid in the process (more on this in Section Three), or to do what brings you pleasure, to put your needs first? And if, for some reason – let's say you're sat next to your good-for-nothing, mouth-breathing colleague in a meeting, and they dare to suggest that you haven't pulled your weight – you go all Mother of Dragons, then it's worth remembering that from time to time, scorching the Earth is important because it clears the way for new growth and acts as a fertiliser.

Autumn's Dangers

Pain and catastrophe
If Autumn is where you struggle, and you don't pay attention to what's going on, then you're likely to find yourself in emotional and physical pain of some kind. Ideally your experience of your premenstruum is grounded by healthy

ego development in your Spring and Summer, but if you haven't managed to banish your critic to this phase of your cycle, then you may well enter your Autumn in an already vulnerable state.

Chucking out the baby with the bathwater

We can get really into the spirit of pruning and become a tad overzealous. There can be a tendency to undo all your good work, so find some softness and space before doing something radical. Hit pause. Take a walk around the block and come back to it with fresh eyes. Is this something, or someone, that you really want to get rid of?

Truth-talking

The raw honesty you find flying out of your mouth can become disrespectful and damaging. If you find yourself being brusque, then consider when it was that you last ate. Low blood-sugar levels have the potential to turn speaking matter-of-factly into fuck-you-very-much.

Overloading your schedule

If you've embraced feeling invincible in your Summer and said yes to every opportunity and request that's come your way but forgotten where those commitments will fall in your diary, then death by schedule is a real possibility.

Hating on yourself

Your inner critic will run riot if you allow it to, so if you haven't developed the beneficial skill of speaking to yourself with compassion, then this is your cue to start.

Working with your Inner Critic

'You're useless'
'You're pathetic'
'You're disgusting'
'What's wrong with you?'
'You're such a mess. Look at you!'
'Everyone else is so much better than you'
'Nobody wants you, I don't know why you bother'

Your inner critic is capable of put-downs that would rival Simon Cowell. They have a knack for showing up when you really don't want them to, are great at nitpicking, and they're capable of bringing you to a standstill in a heartbeat. This inner part of yourself can bring about intense feelings of shame and inadequacy, leaving a path of destruction in its wake.

Your inner critic remembers all your past hurts, all the times you were told off, ignored, rejected, laughed at, embarrassed, abandoned, and shamed, and it just wants to keep you safe by protecting you from further pain. It's worried you'll make a fool of yourself or be rejected, but it's using outdated software to do so.

Autumn is the natural home of your inner critic, so remember one of my top tips from Spring: if your critic shows up in any other phase, tell them to piss off and that you'll see them in your Autumn where they belong. During your premenstruum, research shows that you're more likely to interpret other people's expressions negatively, which gives your inner critic the fuel it needs to go on an all-out rampage. A slight frown or tilt of the head from your boss is all your critic needs to convince you that you're really crap at your job and that you won't get that promotion, when the reality is they were just wondering what to get for their lunch.

Feeling overwhelmed, anxious, depressed, and defensive are all tell-tale signs that your critic has shown up, and they're likely to appear any time that you move out of your comfort zone. This is something worth celebrating because their appearance means that you are doing something right, that you are moving into a place of great potential and growth, but you do need to find allies who will support you and help you to step into the light.

Your critic is highly observant and there to take care of you, so don't dismiss them. That being said, they have a tendency to play dirty, so here's how to work with your inner critic:

- Harness the energy of your Summer and do something, anything, that you can use to give your inner critic something to work with or stand up to; create something, cross off some tasks on your to do list, start a project or complete one.
- Your inner critic is more likely to show up when you're tired, hungry, or otherwise vulnerable. This is another reason why basic self-care in your Autumn is non-negotiable: Eat decent food, stay hydrated, sleep. Avoid hangovers.

- Slow down. When you're rushing around without awareness your critic is more likely to jump on board.
- Be aware that your critic is calling you to account in your premenstruum, by keeping a close tab on you they're keeping you focused on what's important to you and helping you to improve what you do.
- Figure out who your inner critic is. Close your eyes and consider all the hurtful words and phrases that fly around that beautiful brain of yours that hold you back. Got them? Okay. Now, what does the voice that you hear sound like? Do the words they use, or their tone of voice remind you of anyone? You might discover that your internal voice and phrases are connected to someone from your past – a parent, a teacher, a narcissistic ex – and in doing so, you can start to identify where these voices came from, allowing you to distance them from your more up-to-date version of yourself.
- Remove yourself from the vicious cycle of repetition. Jump off the hamster wheel and decide to have it out with your critic. Don't let communication with them be a one-way street where you sit there with your head in your hands, tears and snot streaming down your face, absorbing all their insults whilst they let rip. You're better than that.

Instead of collapsing at the mere sight of them, you have several options:

1) **Hunt them down.**

   As you go about your day, quietly observe your thoughts and reactions to situations. Be on the lookout for your inner critic and when you have them in your sights, let them know that you've spotted them and that you're wise to their every move: *'I see you critic and I know what you're up to, so whatever you're about to attempt, just know that I've got my eyes on you.'* In doing so, you'll start to separate their voice from your own and be able to change your internal dialogue.

2) **Stand up to them.**

   'Well, you know what, critic, I'm not taking that. I'm looking back over my diary and noticing all the wonderful things I've done. I know you think I'm lazy because I'm on the sofa in my joggers, but that rest is well deserved because in my Summer I totally smashed it, so now I'm prioritising rest. You do know that at the moment my dominant hormone

right now is progesterone, don't you?' (whilst giving your best don't-you-know-anything scathing look).

3) **Grill them.**

Your inner critic is great at making headlines; attention-grabbing generalisations that are easy to take on board as a statement of fact but dig into the details and a headline rarely stands up to scrutiny, and that's what you need to do with your critic. After each statement your inner critic makes, stop them before they can make another, and ask them a question that forces them to get specific; *'Hold on a second, critic, let me get this straight – you're saying that I'm useless, well okay, let's run with that for a moment, useless at what, specifically? 'Cause if you're gonna make statements like that, I need details.'* This provides you with an opportunity to put up a boundary and gives you a chance to scrutinise the answers from a place of confident composure.

4) **Challenge them.**

All your critic cares about is criticising, they'll continuously switch perspective in their attempt to keep you down, so call them out on their behaviour and get ahead of the game. *'Come on, what else have you got for me? I bet you're about to tell me that I do this, and that, and that too – you're so predictable, and quite frankly, boring. You say it all like it's a bad thing and we both know that that's not the case, and yeah, I know you're just trying to protect me, but how about you help me instead?'*

5) **Kill them with kindness.**

Try genuinely asking your critic for help, that is what they're trying to do after all, and if you speak from the heart they'll have nowhere to go. *'Ugh, I think you're onto something there, inner critic. I'm really struggling to get anything done, things just aren't flowing for me today and I'm feeling so frustrated and down about it. What's going on? Can you help me figure it out? Oh yeah, you're right, I did skip breakfast this morning … maybe I should make a note of how that's affected my mood today and put a warning in my diary for next month. And yeah, I agree, I'm tired and could have done with someone else cooking dinner, or just ordering takeaway. Thanks for having my back.'*

If you find yourself struggling with your inner critic, and even if you don't, then I really recommend watching social psychologist Amy Cuddy's TED talk 'Your Body Language May Shape Who You Are', and adopting the power pose she describes at every opportunity, but particularly before moments when you tend to collapse and feel down about yourself. Though you might want to find a place in private to assume the full position, or moderate it when you're amongst others. You don't want to do what the leaders of the Conservative party have done in recent years and take it to a bizarre extreme whereby your stance is so wide that you look like you're attempting the splits, or doing the Ministry of Funny Walks Monty Python sketch.

When Autumn is Where you Feel at Home

As with all the seasons, everyone has a place where they feel most at ease, and for some people, that's their Autumn. The calming nature of progesterone can be a soothing relief after the intensity of Summer, when, if you're sensitive to oestrogen peaking, you might be left feeling scatty and unable to exploit its productive nature.

Summer is the brightest season and it comes with a charge of sexual energy that others can pick up on whether you want them to or not. Summer's when you might find yourself receiving attention from strangers as you walk down the street, and this visibility can leave you feeling vulnerable – too seen. If that's true for you then you might welcome the shady side of your cycle, preferring the feeling of coming down and into yourself.

Slow and Low

Autumn can still be a productive time to get stuff done, but the tasks and your environment have to match this phase, and it's often the case that what's needed is time to focus and go slow, and a chance to fly under the radar so that you can work without being interrupted. Where possible, shift your diary around to suit where you're at. For example, you might struggle to come up with new ideas here but find yourself excelling at reviewing and making decisions about what's good and what needs to be reworked or chucked out. If you're unable to move things to a different day, then try to schedule them for the period of the day where you naturally peak in energy and concentration.

When I began writing this book, I made the classic mistake of trying to start a chapter at the start of my Autumn and found myself incapable of typing more than ten words without deleting them because I thought they were utter tripe. My inner critic was having a field day. *'Who are you to try and write a book? You've got nothing to say, you can't even finish one sentence.'* I was ready to give up, until I caught myself and realised it was day 18, which for me is classic floundering time, and therefore my energy was better suited to reviewing the first draft of another chapter. Until days 20 and 21 that is, when, as progesterone peaks, I find myself able to do work that requires a deep inner focus ... but *only* if I have the stillness and space to achieve it.

Reflect on what *you* need in order to work at your best. Look at your menstrual charts and see what's got in the way during previous months. Do you need to work with headphones on, so that you don't have to listen to your colleague jabber away whilst you try to focus? Can you find some stillness in your day so that you can do what's necessary and potter the rest of the time? Or does working with others help you to feel energised here?

Autumn is the perfect phase to push a project through to completion, something to take advantage of so that you give yourself a big pat on the back, tame your inner critic, and gain some well-deserved downtime whilst you bleed. You'll find yourself capable of deep thought and focus, and your ability to examine and make decisions lends itself to leadership roles – if you've built your confidence up enough during your Summer.

Editing is one of the superpowers of Autumn, but you need something to actually edit, and if you've struggled to create and produce something during your Summer, you could come unstuck here. For instance, high oestrogen in the run up to ovulation may have made you a bit scatterbrained, so although you were sharp and at your most articulate, you may have been too 'up' and jittery to knuckle down and get things done, and although, as oestrogen dips post-ovulation, you may experience a bit of a brain fog, as progesterone rises it can help you to focus because it slows your brain down, lessening the likelihood of distraction.

If you haven't landed on your path in life yet, then you could find yourself unravelling in the Autumn. It's hard to feel a gratifying sense of achievement if you're not really sure what you're doing, and your inner editor has nothing to edit. In fact, you're likely to give yourself a really hard time, so if this is you, I suggest working on something that interests you. It doesn't matter if it's something you think could lead to a new and fabulous career or not, this is about building up your self-esteem. If you're not working or are in a job that isn't for you then pay attention to what pops into your head during Winter as that's the time to recalibrate and connect with your place in the world, as well as Spring, when ideas that come to you are worth trying out and exploring.

Rolling in the Deep

Back in the heady days of Summer there was nothing wrong with your lover, but now they're rubbing you up, and not in a good way. Or you might still feel great about them – from a distance.

The two halves of your menstrual cycle might present you with the classic love them/loathe them dichotomy you're likely to have experienced in at least one relationship. In the same way your first trip to Ikea with your new partner can determine whether your relationship will continue or not, Autumn is the proving ground of your menstrual cycle.

When you're in your Spring and Summer your body wants you to see past your partner's faults and only see how great they are so that you'll have sex with them and conceive, but without the feel-good hormones of ovulation, you could find yourself wanting to stab your other half with a fork because they're talking with their mouth full of food. According to professor of psychology, Martie Haselton, PhD, repeatedly not conceiving also has an impact on relationships in the premenstruum – even when you're not trying to conceive and have no desire to have a baby, because your body doesn't get the message that you're avoiding pregnancy, it just reckons your other half isn't up to the task and writes them off as a dud. It then creates ways for you to recognise this so that you move on to the next stud, which is why Haselton states in her book, *Hormonal*, that this is a time when tension and conflict appears in – presumably heterosexual – relationships.

A lot of what we experience with our partners here is about us testing them. How present are they, will they be able to enter the depths of our Winter with us, are they up to it? Do they disappear, or do you feel you have been met, supported, and seen?

Perhaps not surprisingly, research investigating women in lesbian relationships found that although their experiences of premenstrual distress were similar to those reported by women in heterosexual relationships, rather than what researchers Jane Ussher and Janette Perz describe as, 'the lack of understanding or support, rejection, and pathologization commonly found in heterosexual women's accounts, lesbian interviewees reported awareness and recognition of premenstrual change, responsiveness to needs, open communication, and responsibility sharing' that had a significant positive effect on the experience of the premenstruum, and supported an open expression of needs, self-care, and prevented feelings of guilt and self-blame.

We could all do with working on being conscious of what is going on with ourselves and being willing and able to share our experiences with our loved ones, because when we don't understand or aren't able to name our experiences, we can become indignant. Charting your cycle is your best tool to self-awareness. It can wake you up to the reality that a relationship isn't good for you and that something needs to change.

Autumn can be a hard time to communicate; truths can either fly out of your mouth or, because your energy is turning increasingly inwards, you can end up conversing with yourself but not with your loved ones. We assume what we're thinking, and feeling is obvious and that they should know what it is that we want. Well guess what, they don't. More than likely though, they really want to know! The truth is that they'd love to have some insight into what's going on with you because they also experience the fluctuations of your cycle. Sharing your experience of how you move and evolve throughout your menstrual cycle is a great way to do this. Not convinced? I get it, but if you asked your partner the following, how do you think they'd respond?

- Would you like to know when I'm most likely to be up for going out and having fun?
- What about when I'm at my horniest?
- And when I'll be tired, a bit cranky, and would prefer to be left on my own?
- How about when I'd love to hang out on the sofa in silence, but you'll know it's not because you've done anything wrong, I'm in my own head and I don't really want to talk?

Do you seriously think that your loved one would say anything other than, 'Erm, of course I would!' to this? Can you see how getting to know your cycle has the potential to revolutionise your relationship?

Naturally, you're going to need to find a safe way to share, a way that feels good for both of you. You could sit down and have a chat, or go with a note on the fridge, a heads-up email at the start of the day, a midday text …

whatever works for you. Just get on with it because all of our relationships could do with this boost.

Now, this next bit is for those of you with partners who have no clue about what goes on for us throughout every menstrual month (by the way, that's not their fault, how can we expect them to get it when we're only just beginning to?).

Your other half's experience of your cycle may be that they feel you're an entirely different person at different times, and this feeling might even echo your own experience. You're not. In the same way someone's energy, mood, behaviour and skills change throughout the day, so do yours as you travel through your menstrual month. If your partner doesn't get how or why you change so much, here's how you can break it down to them.

> 'You know how you wake up in the morning and you're a bit fuzzy, and you're only capable of taking care of the basics like showering and making coffee, but then once you're on the move your thoughts start to come together and your energy picks up, and you feel really positive and productive. But then you hit a slump in the afternoon and might feel a bit flat/agitated if your day isn't going very well or if you haven't had time for lunch, so you're best left to get on with work on your own, and then later on you need to finish things up before the end of your day, so that you can relax and do something nice before you fall asleep? Well that's what it's like for me in every menstrual cycle.'

Explain that you *are* the same person, but there are different energies and tasks suited to each part of your cycle, just as there are during their day. When it comes to your relationships, remember:

- You're more sensitive to noise and smells in your premenstruum. This isn't a time to eat in silence, because your fork is likely to become a weapon.
- Communicate preemptively. Don't wait till you're in the thick of your Autumn, give them a heads up that you're heading there and explain what that means practically.
- Stay away from accusatory language: 'You do X, you're such a X', etc., and stick with, 'I feel X when X happens, so what I'd like is if X could happen instead'.
- Ask for help. Instead of glaring at them when they ask what's for dinner, send them a midday text saying, 'Day 21 alert! It would be incredibly

helpful if either you cook tonight, or we get take out and watch *Grey's Anatomy*, which by the way will not only provide you with a way to have a good cry, but you'll potentially be left alone if they don't want to watch it. Bonus.

- If you experience a rise in libido during your Autumn, get on it because sexual urges here don't tend to hang around. It's also the phase of your cycle when it can take you a while to climax because you've got less oestrogen and testosterone, so do what you can to relax and get in the mood before you get down to it.

Self-care Essentials

There's a striking parallel between some of the symptoms of PMS and low blood sugar: fatigue, irritability, headaches, anxiety, palpitations, dizziness, poor concentration, and feeling moody and/or tearful. Progesterone diminishes insulin sensitivity, so in the second half of your cycle you're more susceptible to blood sugar and insulin imbalances.

As oestrogen declines, so does serotonin, causing a dip in mood and an increase in appetite. To balance blood sugar be sure to eat regularly and eat well. Prioritise protein and healthy fats in order to keep cravings for caffeine, crappy carbs and sugar at bay. You'll also want to make sure you're eating enough fibre to keep your bowel movements regular. Constipation is traditionally defined as three or fewer bowel movements per week, but I prefer my clients to have at least one satisfying and complete poo a day. Pooing on the regular is essential when it comes to balancing your hormones because it's a key way of getting rid of oestrogen, and with oestrogen you really do want to use it and lose it. When it lingers in your body it can cause excess oestrogen and lead to heavy periods, breast tenderness, bloating, PMS, fibroids, headaches and migraines, insomnia, anxiety, as well as breast and uterine cancer. Another way to ensure your bowels keep moving is to up your intake of water. There's a Chinese saying about digestion that I love, which is, 'You need enough water to float the boat'!

When it comes to booze, a higher intake of alcohol is associated with an increase in oestrogen, which we've established is not a good thing (if you suspect you don't have enough oestrogen, this is not your cue to drink a bottle of prosecco). Alcohol intake is associated with an increase in premenstrual anxiety and mood changes, and smoking is associated with menstrual cramps and back pain. Plus, although alcohol may help you to fall asleep initially, a review of 27 studies concluded that it reduces REM sleep, which is the most restorative phase of sleep.

Although your energy is likely to be lower in your luteal phase, be wary of using caffeine to see you through the day. One small study suggested that caffeine elimination is slowed in the late luteal phase, and is therefore more likely to negatively impact on sleep if you're sensitive to caffeine.

The good news is that once progesterone and oestrogen start to rise after ovulation, falling asleep gets easier and quicker, taking you into sleep that is deep and restorative. This is the time to get to bed earlier and stock up on some z's, as the bad news is that when progesterone and oestrogen start to fall as you approach menstruation, sleep becomes lighter and you can find yourself in the #wideawakeclub because it gets harder to fall asleep and stay asleep. If you battle with insomnia, then check out the guide to successful slumber in Section Three.

Trouble falling and/or staying asleep increases your production of the stress hormone cortisol, and just one night of interrupted sleep can mess up your blood sugar level the following day, which means you'll be flagging and more likely to seek out caffeine and sugar to get you through the day, which then screws with your mood and sleep and before you know it you're in a vicious cycle. As if that wasn't enough, sleep deprivation in the second half of your cycle increases premenstrual mood disturbances. So, you have lots of reasons to prioritise eating and sleeping well post-ovulation, because if your self-care isn't up to scratch then your blood sugar, mood, and sleep will be all over the place.

A better way to improve both the quality of your sleep and give yourself an energy boost, is to get moving. It doesn't matter what you do to get some exercise but be aware that feeling sluggish in your Autumn may mean that you really struggle with that HIIT workout, so opt for some gentle yoga, swimming, a brisk walk outside, or dancing around your kitchen to Madonna. Whatever you can do, just do it. Movement gets your energy flowing, and a lot of the unpleasant side of your premenstruum, physically and emotionally, can be about your energy being stuck. Though if you tend to feel depleted post-workout, then it may be that resting and replenishing yourself is more important and any exercise you undertake should be moderate.

Exercise makes you feel good by releasing endorphins, the neuro-transmitters that cause euphoric highs associated with running, laughing, and orgasms. Studies have found that regular aerobic exercise greatly reduces the symptoms of PMS, and that low levels of physical activity correlate to the incidence of PMS. Exercise that makes you sweat is a great way of excreting oestrogen, so if you suspect you have excess oestrogen (see page 235 for a checklist of signs and symptoms) then sweating is going to be a helpful self-care strategy for you to bring in.

It's not just movement that's important, actual rest is too. If you can't rest – and although I know some of you think it's impossible, I'm here to tell you that it's not – just start with ten minutes or half an hour. If you don't think you can, then do activities which are about the self; a guiding principle here is to do what nourishes you. If you're a bit deficient, prone to exhaustion, feeling down, and possibly seeing unstable higher temperatures post-ovulation on your BBT chart, then resting and eating well is going to be really key. I think we all feel the stay at home on the sofa vibe of progesterone, so go with it on the days that you need to and don't give yourself a hard time about it. You might feel like you're doing nothing but you're actually doing a lot; you need time to stare into space, to drift, this emptiness is necessary for thoughts and energy to gather internally, and it's better to embrace this instead of staring at your screen, berating yourself for not achieving anything. Though it might not be measurable, rest is constructive and productive.

If there's adequate rest in your Autumn, then you'll be feeling energised in your subsequent Spring and Summer. But if you don't rest here then you'll be depleted in your sunny seasons, and that means low energy and low libido, effectively turning the whole of your cycle into a rather 'meh' state.

Avoid running yourself into the ground in your Autumn by:

- Taking care of the basics: eat well and regularly, stay hydrated, sleep, exercise if it feels good, rest when you need to.
- Avoid lunch meetings. Instead, go for lunch on your own with a book, people watch and daydream. Take a break from your day.
- Don't plan a big dinner out with friends when you've been slammed during the day. Hanging out with friends is a great way of raising the soothing nature of progesterone, but invite them over instead, and chuck them out at a reasonable time.
- Nap if you need to, or just get horizontal for twenty minutes.

The Power of 'No'

It's going to be hard for you to get any rest if you aren't able to say no, in fact you'll be overstretched and overwhelmed, and that ain't good for anybody.

In the past, our survival was dependent on getting along with each other, and the fear of saying no can be because we fear damaging our relationships and we want to avoid the social awkwardness of letting someone down. We want to please but saying yes can come with great sacrifice and end up causing more harm than good because we either let ourselves down or the other party down.

If you find saying no hard, then remember that the more things you say no to, the more you'll be able to say yes to what's important to you. Trust your instinct; what's your gut response when someone requests something of you? If it's not a resounding 'hell yes', then it's a no. Let it be that simple. Sure, there are some responsibilities that you can't get away from – important meetings, the school run – but that only jacks up the importance of saying no when you're able to. If we don't manage to do this then resentment builds and becomes corrosive.

Our inability to turn down offers and people is often based on what others will think of us and our fear of missing out. But saying no can be beautiful and earn us the respect and admiration of others; in fact, when I think about my own practice and all the occasions when I've told clients that I don't give treatments on such and such a day because my period is due – something that scared the shit out of me initially – they've always understood, and even been inspired to somehow incorporate this way of doing things into their own lives. In saying no, you are respecting your own boundaries and needs, and asking that others do the same. Do you want to get trodden on again and again, or do you want to raise the bar by saying no with grace and determination?

Get clear about what's important to you and use this list to determine what you agree and commit to. Know that when you say no you are creating more space for your yeses.

Anger is an Energy

When we feel frustrated, upset, angry, and filled with rage in the Autumn phase of the cycle, there's a tendency to believe that it's our hormones that are making us 'crazy'. You might let these feelings out, perhaps venting at the objects and people around you, but later on might feel the need to exonerate yourself by blaming it all on PMS. While your hormones, or in some cases the lack of them in this part of your cycle, can impact on your mood, they're simply shining a light on issues that are there all the time. If you blame how you feel on PMS then you're doing yourself a disservice. Why? Because those around you will take their lead from your cue and won't take what you're saying seriously. You'll miss an opportunity for your grievances to be heard and then bring about change.

We have come to dread the emotions of the premenstruum and most of my clients want me to take their anger away. Although I can help to calm the storm, I don't entirely want to. That's because anger is there to alert and instruct us. As women we are conditioned to bite our tongues, to hold it all in, but doing so causes psychological and physical harm. How many menstrual cycle issues are caused by swallowing our feelings and taking deep breaths instead of voicing them? The mental switch you need to make is to realise that your feelings here are very real and have nothing to do with your hormones, but your hormones are helping you to give voice to them, and it's on you to do something about them. Passive aggressive huffs and puffs won't get you anywhere, nor will subtleties. Be clear, be direct. Use your words. You have to tell your partner that you're done with being the one who does the bulk of the chores, you have to ask your parents to respect your space, you have to ask your boss why you didn't get promoted and be prepared to go to their boss to be evaluated, you have to tell your friend what you're unhappy and unsatisfied with.

There might be occasions where it's appropriate for you to apologise if you express your feelings in a malicious way – because self-care also means taking responsibility for your words and actions – but do not apologise for feeling angry, do not apologise for feeling upset, do not apologise for feeling, full stop. The sadness and rage you feel in your Autumn is important; it must be recognised, named, and expressed.

Anger is a reaction which psychologists refer to as a secondary emotion because it comes, usually quickly and unconsciously, after feeling a primary emotion such as fear or sadness. Anger is there to serve you, screaming at you to wise up to a personal or social injustice. It's there to instruct you, to stop you in your tracks and alert you. It's there to tell you that's it's not up to you to do the dishes night after night, that it's not okay for your parents to ignore the boundaries that you give them, that it's not okay that you're passed up for promotion when you are talented, experienced and more than qualified for it, that you don't have to make do in your relationship. We have a lot to be angry about; we're paid less than men, the #metoo movement has shown the appalling degree to which we experience sexual harassment and assault, a third of us have experienced violence at the hands of men, in some countries our reproductive right to access abortion is legally denied and therefore we're subject to legally enforced pregnancy and childbirth, there's a distinct lack of decent and affordable childcare options available to us, we do the bulk of unpaid work and emotional labour in society and living under patriarchy is fucking exhausting. And that's just if you're white, straight, cis-gendered (your gender identity matches the sex you were assigned at birth), and able-bodied.

The world doesn't want us to be angry, the world wants us to be nice and polite and always fucking smiling, and there's no group more affected by that restriction than Black, Indigenous and People of Colour (BIPOC) because of the entrenched racism and pervasiveness of tone policing in our society. As writer Layla Saad explains:

> 'Tone policing is a tactic used by those with privilege to silence those who don't by focusing on the 'tone' of what is being said, rather than the actual content. It is when white people ask BIPOC to say what we're saying in a "nicer" way. It's saying (or thinking) things like: I can't take in what you're telling me about racism because you sound "too angry". Or your tone is "too aggressive". Or the language you are using to talk about racism is making me feel "ashamed". Or the language you are using to talk about racism is "hateful" or "divisive". Or you should address white people in a more "civil" way if you want us to "join your cause". Or the way you are talking about this issue is not "productive". Or if you would just "calm down" then maybe I might want to listen to you. Or you're bringing too much "negativity" into this space and you should focus on the positive. There are so many direct and subtle ways that tone policing takes over. Essentially, it is a request that BIPOC share our experiences about racism without sharing any of our (real) emotions about it. It is also a demand that racism be presented to you in a form that is more palatable to you and doesn't make your White Fragility flare up.'

In a medical setting, tone policing is life-threatening because it's used to silence the symptoms and pain of women of colour, who are already subject to race-based discrimination and poor health outcomes that education and income do not offer protection from, such as:

- Black couples are twice as likely as white couples to be infertile, yet assisted reproduction is not promoted for black couples in advertising.
- Black women are more likely than white women to have unnecessary surgeries such as hysterectomies.
- Black mothers in the USA die of pregnancy or birth complications at 3–4 times the rate of white mothers. And if you think we're doing better than that in the UK, we're really not: black women are *five* times more likely to die in the childbirth year than white women, and Asian women are twice as likely to.
- In the UK, black women are twice as likely to have a stillbirth as white women.
- Pain is undertreated in black women.
- A 2012 review of endometriosis research found that only two articles were devoted to endometriosis in black women. They were published in 1975 and 1976 and found that black women with endometriosis tended to be incorrectly diagnosed with pelvic inflammatory disease – a disease caused by sexually transmitted infections.

Throughout history, women have been subject to mistreatment, harassment, and abuse, but none more so than women of colour. Feminist discourse is dominated by the voices and needs of white women, when the bodies that are suffering the most are the bodies of colour. We need to acknowledge that we have benefitted from the exploitation and torture of black, indigenous women of colour. These crimes were not committed with our hands, but they have been and still are aided by the silence of white women.

In the American South there is a history of medical students practising medically unnecessary hysterectomies on poor black women without their informed consent – so commonplace that they were nicknamed *Mississippi appendectomies* – because women who went into hospital with common ailments wound up having their wombs stolen from them. And it was the experimental reproductive surgeries performed on black enslaved women in the 1920s and 1930s that gave birth to modern American gynaecology.

These surgeries were performed without anaesthesia because black people were incorrectly believed to be 'stronger medical specimens' who didn't need it, a belief that is unbelievably still rampant today and results in the physical pain of black patients being overlooked and of black people receiving less pain relief than white people, including black children who are less likely to receive pain medication by emergency room doctors than white children. In the US, researchers analysed data from the medical records of over 900,000 children with acute appendicitis, a condition which medical professionals agree warrants the use of pain relief. They found that 56.8 per cent of children received pain medication of any kind in the ER, but that black children experiencing moderate pain were less likely than their white counterparts to receive pain relief, and when it came to those with severe pain, white children were given opioid pain medication 33.9 per cent of the time, but black children received them significantly less frequently at just 12.2 per cent.

It's often the bodies of women of colour that are exploited in the name of 'progress'. In the 1950s, Puerto Rican women were deceived and exploited into being the first human test subjects of the birth control pill, and a US state-backed sterilisation program there also resulted in over a third of Puerto Rican women being robbed of their reproductive rights.

The development and use of the Depo-Provera® contraceptive injection is also steeped in racism: Dorothy Roberts reports in her book *Killing the Black Body* that a '1978 FDA audit of a Depo-Provera trial at Emory University in Atlanta discovered the reckless disregard for the health of the 4,700 black subjects'. Roberts goes on to state that the South African government pushed Depo-Provera® on black women during apartheid as a method of population control by providing it for free at factories and other places of employment, and sometimes threatening women with the loss of their jobs if they did not consent to it. The injection continues to be pushed on black girls and women today. Eugenics programs were in place long before the Nazis came to power, and 32 states used federal funding to control what they declared 'undesirable' populations, including people of colour. In 1974, Judge Gerhard Gesell found that an estimated 100,000 to 150,000 federal-funded sterilisations were performed on poor women annually, most of whom were black.

It's vital that contemporary feminists be mindful of how they exclude the needs of black women from their political agendas, especially when white women often get upset at being left out of the spaces created solely for black women. Instead of respecting these boundaries, those of us with white privilege so often exert it and insist that we join in. Pamela Merritt, co-founder of reproductive justice action group Reproaction points out that, 'Black women have always been at the forefront of the fight for reproductive rights'. But white women have a knack for taking over the conversation and work that black women have been doing for decades without even acknowledging them, as evidenced by the development of the #metoo campaign which was created in 2007 by Tarana Burke, yet it was Burke who was left out of *Time* magazine's Person of the Year cover which was dedicated to 'The Silence Breakers'. Birth and reproductive justice activist, Mars Lord, explains:

> 'White women's experiences are presumed to speak for and represent all women's experiences. They do not. For years black women have been told to put aside their race and focus on gender. This is the agenda of white women so that their issues are the ones heard, and once again black women are erased. "Why do you have to be so aggressive?" "You're bullying me." Words that are thrown incredibly easily at black women. These are just a couple of phrases that are designed to keep black women quiet and to deflect from the questions they are trying to ask, confrontations they hadn't been looking for. The main perpetrators are white men, though black men and white women are not innocent, and it has become the narrative. A black woman standing her ground, saying no, disagreeing with a course of action or frankly standing up for injustice, is aggressive. Once whilst defending a small boy against actual aggressive behaviour from his teacher, I was accused of being angry and aggressive after I asked a question. My tone was quiet and there was nothing accusatory. Being called aggressive was her defence mechanism against me, because who is more likely to be believed, the nice white lady, or the "aggressive" black woman? There is a shifting of blame from the aggressor to the target of the actual aggression.
>
> Microaggressions are something that need to be looked at. Things that are seen as small injustices that should be shaken off are a continual poking of black women throughout each day and week. How then can a black woman manage her anger when anger is assumed to be her default?
>
> Race-based stress has a large part to play in a black woman's actual anger.'

Behind the stereotype of the angry premenstrual woman is the weight of these structural oppressions which we must acknowledge fall far more heavily on the shoulders of black, indigenous women of colour. The anger of women is real, and it exists for very good reasons. PMS only serves to bring our legitimate feelings to the surface and should not be dismissed. Dismissing anger is an extension of suppression and it minimises our experiences so don't shy away from it. You are allowed to be angry. You are allowed to speak up.

Progesterone: The Great Sedater

The second half of your cycle, from ovulation to the start of your period (mid-Summer to the start of Winter), is also known as your luteal phase and is progesterone dominant. Progesterone peaks in the middle of your luteal phase, which would be day 21 in a 28-day cycle, or day 29 in a 36-day cycle. If you haven't arrived in your Autumn before that midpoint then you'll surely find yourself there now. The peak of progesterone often marks the transition day between Summer and Autumn and can feel pretty precarious.

This phase of the menstrual cycle can create such strong reactions in women that they are prescribed medication, and whilst I value how medication can support women who have a harrowing time in their Autumn, my feeling is that cycle awareness should always be used as part of a treatment plan. Whilst I do not want to diminish anyone's experience and need for medication, I have supported women who felt a lot of anger that they were medicated when, retrospectively, they felt that if they'd had this knowledge at the time, they may not have needed drugs.

Progesterone, your pro-gestation hormone, is chiefly responsible for nourishing and maintaining a pregnancy. Whether you want to conceive or not, it is present in your cycle and, as you read in Section One of this book, it has many other ways of supercharging your health beyond breeding.

A reminder that if you're taking a 'progesterone only' form of hormonal birth control, i.e. the mini-pill, the Mirena® IUD, implants, or the Depo-Provera® injection, then you're not receiving all the health-boosting benefits of progesterone, because you're taking progestin not progesterone, and they are very different molecules.

In your luteal phase, where your Autumn lies, progesterone will be slowing you down, making you more cautious and preferring to stay in. It's doing what would be best for you and trying to keep you safe in case you've conceived because it's around this time that implantation will take place if it's going to, at which point the production of progesterone ramps up, as well as human chorionic gonadotrophin (hCG), the hormone that pregnancy tests detect. Not to mention slowing your digestion down so that gut transit time increases, giving your digestive system more time to extract nutrients from your food to potentially nourish a developing embryo. Progesterone is also to blame for the puffiness and bloating you get premenstrually that means you may need jeans that are two sizes larger.

Low Progesterone

Although some of us are sensitive to progesterone in the luteal phase, the imbalance that is most common with progesterone is not producing enough of it, the signs and symptoms of which include:

- Breakthrough bleeding in the second half of your cycle
- Difficulty getting pregnant
- Difficulty staying pregnant
- PMS
- Premenstrual headaches and migraines
- Heavy menstrual flow
- Irregular cycles or more frequent cycles
- Bloating and/or water retention
- Swollen breasts, accompanied by tenderness or pain
- Clumsiness or poor co-ordination
- Itchy or restless legs, particularly at night
- Difficulty sleeping
- Ovarian cysts, breast cysts, or endometrial polyps

It's usually caused by:

- Taking the birth control pill and/or lack of ovulation. If you recall, it's the follicle left behind after ovulation – your corpus luteum – that produces and releases the vast majority of the progesterone you produce (your adrenals also produce a tiny amount), so if you are not ovulating, you're not producing progesterone.

- High cortisol levels brought about by sustained periods of stress.
- A diet lacking in nutrition, or nutritional deficiencies in magnesium, vitamin A, vitamin B6, vitamin C, and zinc (these are all common deficiencies to have after using the pill).
- Low thyroid function (hypothyroidism).
- An insufficient LH surge.
- Ageing.
- Perimenopause and menopause.

Progesterone is commonly tested on day 21 of your cycle, which is fine if you have a 28-day cycle, but if you have a shorter or longer cycle, day 21 will not be the most appropriate time to test progesterone and doing so is a complete waste of time and resources. If your cycle is short/long/irregular, then I recommend BBT charting to establish when you ovulate in order to schedule your blood test at the ideal time; around 7 days after ovulation. You can improve low progesterone by:

- Supporting ovulation.
- Acupuncture and pelvic massage such as ATMAT® (see page 272) can improve blood flow to your ovaries and support progesterone production.
- Seed cycling.
- Hanging out with your mates. Research has shown that enjoying the company of women can raise progesterone.
- Taking supplements such as: Vitex Agnus Castus, Maca, Melatonin, vitamin B6, vitamin D, vitamin C, and vitamin E.
- Taking bioidentical progesterone from ovulation to the start of your period.

Under Pressure

When you're stressed, your body responds by gearing you up to run away or stay and fight, a response coined 'fight or flight', by releasing the stress hormones adrenaline, noradrenaline, and cortisol from your adrenal glands.

Adrenaline and noradrenaline are the first responders to any stressful situation that you find yourself in. Adrenaline makes your heart rate jump up, makes you breathe faster, tenses your muscles and gives you a surge of energy. Noradrenaline diverts blood from the organs that aren't essential when it comes to fighting or fleeing, such as your digestive tract, reproductive system and skin, in order to pump blood to your heart, lungs and muscles (this is why when you lie down after a busy day or stressful journey you'll hear your belly gurgling; it's a sign that blood flow is returning to your gut, and the movement it uses to digest and move food along has been switched back on again, thus producing a gurgle.)

Cortisol is the second responder to the scene, and cortisol secretion is a slower response, taking minutes instead of split seconds. It raises your blood pressure and blood sugar levels and suppresses your immune system. Note that all of these inbuilt mechanisms are about having a quick response to acute situations in order to keep you alive, but the trouble is that, as evolved as we like to think we are, our bodies haven't changed in the last 15,000 years, and we respond to stressful situations like receiving negative feedback at work as if we're about to fight a woolly mammoth, and we're also subject to periods of ongoing stress. When you are under continued stress – let's say you have a commute that is far from enjoyable, a nightmare boss, fertility issues, a relationship problem, postpartum anxiety, or essentially any issue that you stew on for a while – your body keeps releasing stress hormones and can suppress the actions of other hormones which has a massive impact on your health; suppressing your immune system and libido, increasing your blood pressure, impairing digestion, and contributing to acne and obesity. And it's worth noting that your body reacts this way even when you imagine or anticipate something stressful.

But we do need cortisol; when I think of cortisol it's 'I'm a Survivor' by Destiny's Child that pops into my head. Not only is it involved in our fight or flight response, but there are receptors for it on almost every cell in your body, which means it can have a range of different actions depending on the cell it's acting upon, and it therefore plays a role in lots of different functions in the body, such as controlling blood sugar levels and influencing blood pressure, weight control, memory formation. It also helps to reduce inflammation which is good in the short term, but when excessive amounts are secreted over a period of time, its anti-inflammatory action can suppress the immune system. But the amount you secrete should follow a specific pattern over the course of the day. This pattern is known as the cortisol curve and when the cortisol curve is healthy, it starts off high in the morning and should reach its peak within an hour of waking so that you feel alert and ready for your day. Then, as your day continues, it should gradually decline so that by the evening, cortisol secretion is low enough so that you can wind down and relax, and melatonin steps in to make you feel sleepy so that you go to bed and sleep soundly. The high level in the morning that helps you to wake up is known as the cortisol awakening response (CAR) and it's the CAR that establishes your circadian rhythm – the physiological pattern that you go through over the course of 24 hours, often referred to as your body clock, and which also influences the regularity of the menstrual cycle.

But what happens if you don't follow the curve? Just like all your hormones, cortisol can be thrown off and be too high or too low. When it's low in the morning you'll struggle to wake up, but if it's too high you can wake up feeling anxious. If it's higher than it should be in the evening and during the night, you can get a second wind and find it hard to get to bed at a decent hour and/or have disturbed sleep.

When Vanessa came to see me she was in bits. She'd been promoted recently but was beginning to doubt her ability to succeed in her new role because she was so shattered, and she'd heard that acupuncture can help with energy and sleep and wanted to give it a go. She also struggled with PMS and was prone to mood swings and irritability during the week before her period came, which was new for her.

She told me that it was rare for her to wake up feeling rested and rejuvenated in the morning, and because she kept hitting snooze on her alarm, she'd inevitably end up in a coffee-fuelled dash to get to work on time. At 10am she'd finally feel alert enough to concentrate and she'd feel good through till 2pm, at which point she'd crash but a cup of coffee would get her through the rest of the day. She'd typically doze off whilst reading on her tube journey home, but she was frustrated that by the time bedtime rolled around, her mind was racing, and sleep was elusive. I suggested diurnal cortisol testing, in which cortisol is tested at four points in the day, and her results weren't exactly a surprise – they were back to front. Instead of being high in the morning, it was low, and instead of being low in the evening, it was spiking, and we needed to figure out why.

It turned out that although Vanessa loved her new role, she was feeling the pressure to perform and stay on top of things, and that meant that she was prone to checking her emails once she was home and working on things that she hadn't managed to get done in the day. Between the stress this created and the blue-light from her laptop, plus the glass of wine and scrolling on social media that she used to help her wind down and switch off, it was no wonder that she was struggling – everything in her evening routine was stimulating her. I told Vanessa that although acupuncture could really help her, its effects would be short-lived if she didn't make some changes to her daily routine. Thankfully, she was willing to give anything a go if it meant she would feel better. I suggested that Vanessa do the following:

- Use a sunrise alarm clock, and upon waking, immediately open her curtains to let the light in and drink a glass of water.
- Have her morning coffee next to a window, along with some breakfast (which she usually skipped altogether). I recommended that she eat some protein to support her blood sugar and energy, and boiled eggs and toast was what felt doable to her because she could shower while her egg was on.
- Pay attention to her lips over the course of the day so that she could assess if she was dehydrated. She quickly realised that she was because her lips were usually dry, but when she upped her water intake they would plump up.
- Eat a mid-morning snack like apple slices dipped in nut butter or a protein smoothie.
- Eat a decent lunch. She often had soup and a salad in an attempt to be healthy, but this wasn't supporting her energy levels in the afternoon, and I wanted her to eat something more substantial that included some animal protein.
- Before reaching for her mid-afternoon coffee, to take a break from her screen and drink a glass of water, and if she needed some caffeine, to opt for a green tea instead.
- Leave her work at work – no checking emails at home. This one was a tough one but we spoke about the importance of separating her personal and professional life, and setting an example to her team.
- If she used screens in the evening, to take measures to block the blue light they emit and prevent her body from being tricked into thinking it was still daytime. She could choose from using software such as f.lux, wearing blue-light blocking glasses or turning on the 'Blue light filter' setting on her phone.
- To have a hot bath before bedtime with two handfuls of Epsom salts in it, which are rich in magnesium and can help soothe the nervous system and support sleep.

We scheduled her acupuncture sessions for Wednesday evenings, the point in the week when she really struggled and would feel most stressed and did two shorter treatments in the week before her period when she experienced pre-menstrual irritability. Vanessa found the first week hard – she wasn't used to prioritising regular meals and it took a bit of getting used to, but she found that if she ate regularly, had enough protein, and kept herself hydrated then she had lots more energy in the afternoon. The second week was easier and the cumulative effect of her efforts meant she was falling asleep quicker, and in the third week she found that mornings were much easier, but in the fourth week we hit a blip because her colleague went on holiday and her work load increased. This was a temporary problem, but I was concerned that the extra work she planned to do in the evening would undo all her good work, so I suggested that instead of working later, that she get up at 6am instead of 7am and work in the morning. Vanessa was mortified, but knowing it would only be for a week, she decided to give it a go. She was surprised at how well it went but it really demonstrated how far she'd come in the space of a few weeks. Although she was relieved to go back to her regular 7am wake up, the added pressure of that week motivated her to keep up the good work. I treated Vanessa regularly for two months, at which point we reduced her sessions to one treatment at ovulation and one a week later when she entered her Autumn, and two months later her course of treatment ended because her PMS had improved so much.

Adrenal Dysfunction

Caused by:

- Unrelenting emotional and mental stress.
- Food allergies or sensitivities – gluten, sugar, dairy and others.
- Over-exercising, dieting, and disordered eating.
- Notifications (or lack of them) on your mobile.
- Using steroids such as those used to treat allergies and asthma.
- Addison's disease aka adrenal insufficiency, an endocrine disorder in which the adrenal glands don't produce enough hormones to regulate key body processes.

- Congenital adrenal hyperplasia, which refers to a group of rare inherited conditions that affect the adrenal glands, resulting in low levels of cortisol and high levels of androgens.

Signs and symptoms of adrenal dysfunction (you can have both high and low cortisol within a 24-hour period, remember it's all about following the cortisol curve):

- Fatigue and feeling burnt out
- Not feeling rested after sleep
- Relying on caffeine and sugar to function
- Struggling to feel alert in the morning
- Loss of stamina, particularly from 2–5pm
- Feeling tired but wired
- Finding it hard to wind down for bedtime
- Difficulty falling asleep
- Difficulty staying asleep
- Irregular menstrual cycle
- Amenorrhoea (no periods)
- Constantly rushing from one task to the next
- Feeling anxious or nervous
- Easily angered, prone to yelling and/or screaming
- Feeling distracted and not present
- Low/high blood pressure
- Feeling dizzy when you stand up
- Awareness of your heart beating/palpitations even when relaxed
- High blood sugar, insulin resistance, or diabetes
- Low blood sugar between meals
- Decreased fertility
- You catch every cough and cold flying around, and it takes a while for you to recover from illness or to heal a wound
- Asthma/bronchitis/allergies
- Feeling unable to cope and less resilient to stress
- Craving salt
- Sweating excessively

- Nausea, vomiting or diarrhoea (or alternating between loose stools and constipation)
- Muscle weakness and/or muscle and joint pain
- Bruising easily

Plan:

- Ask your doctor to test your cortisol levels in the morning (before 9am), though a diurnal cortisol panel which is taken at four points in the day is far more helpful because it assesses your cortisol curve.
- Find out why your adrenal function has been thrown off.
- Get outside in the daytime to expose yourself to light, and use full spectrum lights when inside.
- Set things up so that you can wind down in the evening and avoid blue light from electronic devices to allow cortisol to decrease and melatonin to increase.
- Stroke a furry friend. Snuggling with pets increases oxytocin and endorphins – calming healing hormones which will dial down stress hormones.
- Work on balancing your blood sugar.
- Lay off caffeine and sugar – your blood sugar could do without the wild ride.
- Watch something funny. Belly laughter is good medicine.
- You can also stimulate the release of oxytocin and endorphins by having an orgasm or by lightly stroking your upper abdomen; close your eyes, take a few relaxing belly breaths, and use your finger tips to lightly stroke downwards from the bottom of your breastbone to your belly button. This feels nice when done through a layer of clothing (particularly if it's got a stretchy quality to it), which means you can do it anywhere, even while you're waiting for the bus.
- Research shows that gardening and reading both lead to decreases in cortisol but gardening outperforms reading. If you don't have a garden or an allotment, find someone who needs help with theirs because generosity can also decrease cortisol levels.

Pregnenolone Steal; are you for Real?

Pregnenolone is made from cholesterol and is the precursor to progesterone, in other words it's what progesterone is made from. Pregnenolone is actually the mother hormone of several hormones: cortisol – a stress hormone, and DHEA, which is converted into oestrogen and testosterone.

There's a theory that because steroid hormones are made from pregnenolone, elevated secretion of cortisol caused by severe stress or a sustained period of stress will result in the pool of pregnenolone being used to create more cortisol, and less being available for other hormones. This has been described as the 'pregnenolone steal' and it's been used to explain how stress can cause diminished production of hormones such as progesterone. But the synthesis of hormone production is far more complicated than that, and most flow charts used to explain how they're made are over-simplified and lead you to believe that there is a single pool of pregnenolone available, but in actual fact the conversion from cholesterol to pregnenolone takes place in different types of cells in the adrenal glands and the different cells are each responsible for the production of specific hormones. Put simply, there is no single reservoir of pregnenolone to be stolen for production of cortisol.

Does that mean that stress doesn't affect hormone production? No, it doesn't, because when your body perceives a threat, it dials down your reproductive function because emergencies and survival always come first. As if that wasn't enough, cortisol does a number on progesterone by blocking progesterone receptors. When hormones are released into the bloodstream we don't want them to affect every cell in our body, only their intended target, so each hormone we release travels around the body, looking for a cell which is receptive to it and has a lock on it that the key, or hormone, fits in to. Cortisol blocks progesterone sites when we are stressed because it has deemed that it is not safe and suitable to conceive, and that responding to what it thinks is a woolly mammoth is a better idea.

If you think that all this chat about stress doesn't apply to you, then I congratulate you, and I also encourage you to *really* observe your reactions to what you experience day to day, because a lot of the time our stress response is so swift and well executed that we don't recognise its presence.

Top Tips to Get the Most out of your Autumn

- Respect where you're at.
- Say 'no' to as much as possible.
- Notice where you peak during the day – that's when to schedule the activities that you can't get away from.
- Leave some wiggle room in your day; you'll be moving slower so give yourself extra time to get to places.
- Stop being a martyr and let others help. Sure, you could do it better and quicker, but maybe you can chill for a minute and let someone else pick up the slack. And if you want them to keep helping (you do, even if they aren't doing it properly) then don't nitpick, encourage them and be thankful. Let them support you.
- Do a big shop in your Summer to give you a head start to eating well in Autumn, which you can top up as you go. Don't ride it out until you've got nothing left in the fridge and you're craving fat, sweet, salty things in your Autumn, because you'll end up with a trolley full of crisps, cheese and Hobnobs. You don't want to be wandering the aisles like a zombie, wondering what the hell you can have for dinner, and end up gorging on pick and mix just so you can survive the journey home.
- Cook ahead. Have some homemade meals ready to go in your freezer so that if you hit a wall of exhaustion, you're sorted.
- Get things out of your system instead of letting them fester or boil over. Go to an 80s dance class, write without restriction, or yell in solitude.
- When you're busy reviewing something, take care not to undo all your good work. Find some softness and space before doing something radical. Pause.
- Towards the end of your Autumn, think about what needs attention in order to feel a sense of completion before your next cycle begins, a bit like finishing things off before you go to bed at night.

Chapter 7

Ch-ch-ch-ch-changes

There are specific times in your life when hormones are apt to go a bit off piste, or when your relationship with your body and your cycle might change. The beauty of The Cycle Strategy is that it isn't fixed; it can be adapted to suit where you're at and it will evolve with you. In this chapter we're going to look at the teen years, the use of hormonal birth control, fertility issues, pregnancy, motherhood, being transgender, as well as how to use the lunar cycle as a replacement for the menstrual cycle if you're not menstruating, or in addition to it.

Girl, You'll Be a Woman Soon

Your first period can be a shock, especially if you haven't been told much, or anything about them. It can also be something that you really want, a desired status – particularly if all your mates have already started theirs. For most people, their first period is accompanied by a mixed bag of emotions, because regardless of whether it was wanted or not, or if the news of it brought celebration or shame, it signifies a change in you, of leaving your childhood and supposedly 'becoming a woman' – whether you wanted to or not.

Although the average age for people to get their first period is 12–13 years, you can fall either side of that average and be younger or older. Puberty is a process, and one of the first signs is the appearance of breast buds, where the breast and nipple area begins to puff out, and the nipples darken and may have little raised dots on them. Two to three years after the development of breast buds, menstruation is likely to start, though this time may be shortened if breast buds don't appear until age 13. Along with changing body shape, boobs appearing, and pubic hair springing out of nowhere, you might notice a whitish fluid on your underwear and in your vagina for up to a year before your period actually starts. This fluid might dry to be a bit yellow on your underwear and can even resemble egg whites in the weeks before your first period arrives. This type of fluid is produced by your cervix; it's a sign that ovulation is about to take place and is a helpful way to predict when your period will arrive – roughly 14 days later – both before your first period starts, and in future cycles.

It's really common for teens to have anovulatory cycles in which no egg is released, and it's 100 per cent normal for it to take several years for you to ovulate regularly. In the first two years of having periods, around half of cycles are ones where ovulation takes place, with this increasing to 75 per cent by five years, and over the following few years 80 per cent of cycles are ovulatory which is considered to be the mature rate. A result of this is that teens frequently have polycystic ovaries, because inside the ovaries their follicles are busy responding to the hormonal cues that are now being chucked around your body and are developing and gearing up for ovulation, but they don't always achieve that. Instead, it's like a series of dress rehearsals, the result of which is a build-up of follicles hanging out on the surface of the ovaries, which become ovarian cysts. Having several cysts (medically referred to as polycystic ovaries) does not mean that you have polycystic ovarian syndrome (PCOS). In fact, because of the prevalence of them during the teen years, to receive a diagnosis of PCOS as a teen you must meet all three of something called the Rotterdam criteria (more on this on page 301). If you have ovarian cysts but they don't cause any issues, your cycle is regular, and you don't have clear signs of androgen excess such as hair growth on your face and body or the results of a blood test, then you probably just need to support your health by eating regular healthy meals, exercising, and getting enough sleep (you can read all about this in Section Three). With time you're likely to start ovulating regularly so unless there is a clear problem, just keep an eye on things and make sure you're limiting your exposure to chemicals which mimic oestrogen such as Bisphenol A (BPA) which is commonly found in plastic food containers and water bottles, as well as in receipts which are printed on thermal paper (see page 266), as not only is BPA linked to early puberty and breast cancer but, until ovulation is a regular event, you're prone to a hormonal imbalance of excess oestrogen which exposure to chemicals such as BPA will exacerbate.

Anovulation

There's an expectation among most medical professionals and the public that when you get a period, that means that you ovulated roughly two weeks before you started to bleed, but when researchers in Norway assessed ovulation in over 3,000 women, they found that only 63.3 per cent had ovulated, despite all of the participants having normal length menstrual cycles. They concluded that anovulation (the lack of ovulation in a cycle) occurs in over a third of normal menstrual cycles.

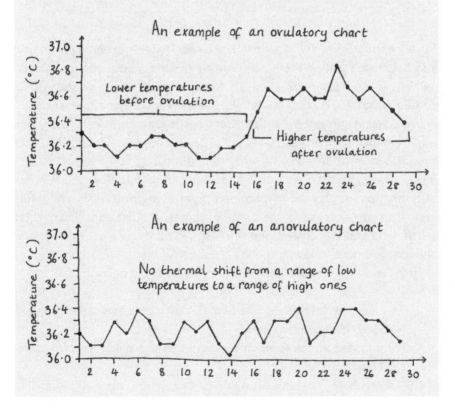

An example of an ovulatory chart

An example of an anovulatory chart

When a cycle is anovulatory, it can result in a shorter or longer cycle, and a lighter or heavier period, and the best way to spot anovulation is by tracking your basal body temperature (BBT) because after ovulation your BBT should rise significantly, resulting in two clear phases; a lower temperature before ovulation, and a higher one afterwards. But if you don't ovulate then your temperature will remain low.

Although it may be stressful if you're trying to conceive, occasional anovulation isn't particularly concerning, but if you start to get them when you haven't previously, or the frequency of them increases (especially if you have several in a row) then it's important to assess why they're happening as they can be a sign of a hormonal imbalance.

In your early years of menstruating, when your body is attempting to ovulate and not always getting there, you're likely to have a hormonal imbalance, and again, this is normal, although there are things you can do to help matters which I'll get on to in a bit. Progesterone is only produced when you ovulate, and its progesterone that keeps oestrogen in check. When you're not ovulating on the regular, you tend to be oestrogen dominant, which can cause heavy periods, PMS, bloating, breast swelling and tenderness, and mood swings. In addition to this, your body isn't used to this sudden influx of hormones yet, and the hormone receptors across your body are highly sensitive while they get in the swing of things, which means you're extra sensitive on a hormonal level, and you may well find this carries through into how you feel emotionally.

In the teenage years, the following are all considered normal:

- An average cycle length of 32 days in the first year of menstruating, but 21 to 45 days is considered typical.
- For it to take several years for you have to have regular ovulatory cycles and because of that you can:
  ○ Experience symptoms of excess oestrogen.
  ○ Have polycystic ovaries but not have PCOS.

If you turn 15 years old and haven't had your first period, your GP should be contacted. There are lots of factors that can delay it, and typically it'll start the day before your appointment, but it's worth investigating to see what might be going on. You should also speak to your GP if you experience menstrual cramps that affect your ability to go to school and do the activities you usually enjoy, and that you have to take painkillers to manage. Period pain is common, but it is not normal, and severe pain can be a sign of a condition called endometriosis (see page 281), which, unfortunately, usually takes years to diagnose and some medical professionals are of the ill-informed opinion that teenagers are too young to have it. This simply isn't true, so if someone tells you that, don't accept it and ask to be referred to a specialist who will hopefully be more clued up on endo. Having painful periods does not necessarily mean that you do have endo, and most cramps usually respond fairly quickly to dietary and lifestyle changes, such as cutting out cow's dairy, supplementing with magnesium, Omega-3 Fatty Acids, and B vitamins, as well as getting adequate sleep and exercise – which will also help with PMS and mood swings too. Addressing the oestrogen dominance that can be behind heavy periods can reduce blood loss, as can supplementing with iron and turmeric and using non-steroidal anti-inflammatory drugs (NSAIDs) such as ibuprofen. You can read more about period problems in Chapter 9, and how to reduce oestrogen in Section Three. If you're concerned about leaking, check out the period-wear companies in the Resources section. They manufacture incredibly absorbent underwear that are designed to catch your blood without needing to use a pad or tampon, though they can also be used as back up if your flow is quite heavy and you want to use them alongside other products.

When it comes to treatments for teen menstruators, acupuncture is incredibly helpful at regulating the cycle, reducing heavy flow, and alleviating pain, but I also love teaching teens how to do castor oil packs (see page 83) and abdominal massage on themselves, because both methods put you in touch with your body. They're also more affordable than seeing a practitioner week after week, and they're techniques that can be used throughout your life. It's never too early to get to know your body and how to care for it, and there's a fabulous opportunity during the teen years to address menstrual problems instead of resorting to unnecessary medication like the pill.

Though you may decide that using hormonal birth control such as the pill is what you want to use to prevent pregnancy (and remembering that it doesn't protect you from sexually transmitted infections), it's not a great way of treating period problems, because it doesn't actually treat them, it just stops them from happening by stopping you from ovulating and getting periods (the episodes of bleeding that you have on the pill are withdrawal bleeds). A common side effect of being on the pill is depression, which nobody ever needs, but particularly not in your teen years when you're figuring the world out and who you are in it. The insights that you have through the process of your menstrual cycle can also point you towards the direction, or directions, that you take in life, and taking the pill can shut down that powerful function. I'm not saying don't take it, but I am asking you to consider all the effects of using it, particularly as it's the hormones of your menstrual cycle that are responsible for your bone density. Not menstruating during your teen years, particularly due to overexercising, can lead to low bone density in your twenties.

Teens and adult menstruators often use the pill as a way to improve the appearance of their skin which is 100 per cent understandable. Having acne is not nice and the presence of it has a huge impact on how you feel about yourself, but there are plenty of other ways to reduce spots. The hormones that are found in dairy produced in cow's milk have been linked to acne, as has consuming sugar and refined carbs such as bread, pasta, rice, and cereals. Whereas limiting all of these types of food has been shown to improve acne, and supplementing with Omega-3 Fatty Acids, vitamin E, zinc, and vitamin A can help too. If you're tempted to take a medication called Accutane® that's used to treat acne, please try other measures first as several studies have demonstrated that it can cause a whole host of nasty side effects, but also long-term damage. You cannot take it during pregnancy as it can cause miscarriage and severe birth defects, which is why the pill is often prescribed alongside it.

Charting your cycle is a great habit to develop; not only will you learn the ins and outs of your particular cycle and how to read your own body, but the American College of Obstetricians and Gynecologists recommend that your menstrual cycle should be considered as your fifth vital sign after body temperature, heart rate, blood pressure, and breathing rate, because it can improve early identification of health issues. It will also help you to establish self-esteem and self-confidence and prove to be a valuable tool in supporting your mental health.

In each cycle you could end up having a fairly long Spring while your body gets used to ovulating and you have cycles that are on the longer side, and this makes sense given that you are in the Spring phase of your life – enjoy it! Young people are faced with tremendous pressure to figure out what they're doing with their lives, and if you're feeling that weight, then use your Spring season to keep things lighthearted and to explore the possibilities that are open to you. Yes, picking the 'right' subjects at school can make a difference when it comes to further education and employment, but they aren't the be all and end all, and this won't be your only chance. Play around with ideas and try a job on for size by contacting professionals within a field to see if you can do some work experience with them; this way you can experiment before you commit to a course of action.

When Desire Emerges

At some point, and most likely in your Springs and Summers, you'll start to experience your sexual desire, and it's important for you to find a way to express it in a way that feels good to you and that's safe, which makes masturbation a fantastic option. It gives you a way to explore your body and experiment with what feels good before you involve anyone else, and also teaches you the valuable lesson that you don't have to rely on someone else for sexual pleasure. Being safe sexually involves using contraception that prevents pregnancy and sexually transmitted infections if you decide to have sex with someone, but safety isn't just about this form of protection – it's also about boundaries and consent.

In our teen years we start to experiment with, and get a sense of our boundaries, and combined with your emerging sexuality, it makes it a good time to get in the habit of letting other people know when you want them to back off. In childhood, girls who are touched by boys and who are clearly uncomfortable with a physical interaction are frequently told by their caregivers that, 'It's okay, he just likes you', which results in us being taught from an early age that we should allow men to touch us even when we don't want them to. In our teens though, there is a chance to address this and to find your voice. Any time you feel uncomfortable because someone gets too close to you or touches you without your permission, let them know that you feel uncomfortable and that it's not okay. You can tell them to stop at any point, including if you've previously said that you wanted to do something, because you can withdraw consent whenever you want to. Doing so doesn't make you a 'prick tease', it means you respect yourself. Boys are typically raised with a sense of entitlement, and told that girls like to play hard to get and that they really want it even if they say that they don't, which means it can be really hard to make it clear to some boys and men that you want them to stop. If you haven't already, get in the habit of giving consent and withdrawing it when you start to feel uncomfortable or change your mind, which you always have the right to do. This applies to when you're being intimate with someone, but also when a person invades your personal space or touches you without your permission.

Your Autumn may prove tricky, as it is for most menstruators of all ages but especially as you learn to regulate your emotions and your brain is changing in structure and function during your teen years (by the way, I'll be 38 when this book is published, and I still haven't figured that one out, so feel free to hit me up with your tips and tricks). Keeping a diary helps you to adjust to becoming a menstruator and will provide clues about what you want for your life, so I suggest taking notes and keeping them somewhere safe. It's up to you what you want to do, but you could let your parents know that you're doing this and explicitly say to them that your diary is for you and that it's private and explain how you'd feel if they read it without your permission. It's important for you to be able to give them boundaries, and if you can do this by calmly instructing them and explaining why this is important to you, then they're more likely to respect your wishes. It also means that the door is open if you do decide that you want to share anything with them and ask for help.

> **Side note for the parents reading this:** Please respect your child's right to privacy, and if they come to you wanting to share their experience of their cycle, be willing to listen. You don't have to have answers; your job is to listen and acknowledge what's going on for them and give them a hug if that's what they want.

Remember:

- Cervical fluid is a sign of health and fertility, and something to be proud of.
- You can get pregnant *before* you get your first period, because ovulation always happens before a period comes.
- Hormonal birth control will not 'regulate your cycles', it prevents you from ovulating and only causes withdrawal bleeds, not real periods.
- It's normal for your cycle to be irregular and it's likely to even out with time.

- There's a lot that you can do to reduce heavy blood loss and painful cramps without resorting to the pill.
- What you eat and drink, eating disorders, lack of sleep, lack of exercise, overexercising, and screen time all influence hormone production and therefore your cycle and your period too.
- Tracking your cycle helps you to understand what's going on with your body and builds self-esteem and body confidence.

I want you to arm yourself with the knowledge in this book, to talk to people that you trust and who care about you. Ask them questions – none of them are silly, I promise you. I hope that you have someone close to you to share your experiences with and to receive guidance from, and most of all I want you to know that your body and mind are strong and beautiful, and that your body is wise, even when you feel broken and confused, so learn to trust what it's telling you.

Hormonal Birth Control

I love birth control that works well for the people using it. That means that it needs to be highly effective as a contraceptive *and* not cause any health issues. And that's why I can't get on board with the pill – because it can cause significant health issues. Sure, its invention was revolutionary, and some people take it without any apparent problems, but it can cause numerous side effects whilst it's being taken, as well as long-term consequences after you come off it. I'm pro-informed choice, but I suspect that most users of hormonal birth control take it without having the kind of conversation that I'd like them to have with their healthcare provider, one in which the side effects and other options are discussed before the prescription pad is reached for. Hormonal birth control is often 'chosen' because of an absence of other options, or the absence of education about other options, but I don't judge you for taking it, especially when it's presented as the be all and end all of women's health issues.

I'm not here to convince you that you shouldn't use hormonal birth control, it's your body and your choice, and I'm 100 per cent behind whatever you feel is appropriate for you, but it is my job to let you know what the negative effects of taking the drugs like the pill can be, because most of the time, it's the benefits which are touted (such as a reduced risk of developing ovarian cancer or endometrial cancer). I've had so many clients over the years who've had significant health issues and they've never considered that the pill could be behind them, and that's what I wish to highlight as much as I can in a very short section. What I describe may not reflect your experience (in which case, great), but it will chime with what a significant number of pill users find. The pill is so ubiquitous that most of the clients that I see who are on the pill don't list it as a form of medication on their medical history. But the birth control pill is a drug and taking it impacts on our mental health, sexuality, behaviour, and relationships. The pill is also an endocrine disruptor that every single one of us is affected by because it's present in the wee of those that take it, and water treatment does not filter it out, which means that we're all exposed to it through our water supply (this is one of several reasons thought to be behind why sperm counts have fallen dramatically in the last 50 years). And there's a lot of people weeing it out, around 80 per cent of us have taken it at some point in our lives, though for 42 per cent of American users, contraception isn't their primary reason for taking it. So why do people take it? A 2011 study carried out by the Guttmacher Institute found that when it comes to pill use:

- 86 per cent of users take it to prevent pregnancy.
- 56 per cent of users also use it for non-contraceptive reasons, 31 per cent of which is because of menstrual pain.
- 9 per cent had never had sex and use it exclusively for non-contraceptive reasons.

And 50 per cent take it to 'regulate' their periods, which is highly problematic because the pill cannot achieve this. When you want your periods to regulate you have to support ovulation, not suppress it, and taking the pill prevents ovulation so you don't get a period when you're on the pill, you have what's known as a withdrawal bleed. Regular menstruation is good for your heart, bone, and breast health, and there's strong evidence showing that a lack of progesterone produced by ovulation is detrimental to our health. One study showed that women with just one nonovulatory cycle a year lost an average of 4 per cent of their spinal bone density, so supporting ovulation is vital.

Hormonal contraception is also routinely prescribed to 'treat' period pain, PMS, PMDD, heavy periods, an absence of periods, PCOS, endo, and adenomyosis, and there are plenty of menstruators who suffer from these debilitating hormonal and reproductive conditions who will experience significant or total relief from hormonal birth control, so that they can actually live their lives, but while the pill can reduce some symptoms, it doesn't actually treat any of these conditions. It simply acts as a band-aid which can unfortunately cause further problems.

A Bitter Pill to Swallow

There are many, many benefits to experiencing the richness of the menstrual cycle, though I appreciate that for some people that can feel a little too rich at times and that they might prefer to dial everything down and 'turn off' their cycle by taking the pill, but at what cost? In her book, *Sweetening the Pill*, which describes the side effects and social consequences of prescribing the pill to millions of women worldwide, Holly Grigg-Spall states; 'when the pill stops the downs, it also stops the ups – it does not differentiate'. The detached, numb state that some users find themselves in has an impact on their ability to participate in and enjoy life. This is particularly relevant during the teen years when we're trying to figure it all out and could do with being tuned into our instincts while we are. Some pill users will find that it doesn't impact on their ambition, motivation, and creativity, but some will experience a decimation of them, and that has huge consequences for every part of life. I went on the pill in my teens when I started having sex. I felt grown up; going to the GP on my own, taking charge of my reproductive health, *being responsible*. I stayed on it for six years and during that time I was depressed and had little desire to have sex. I was numb to a lot of what was going on inside and around me, and whilst I'm sure that it wasn't just the pill that was causing me to feel this way, it was remarkable at how much better I felt when I came off it.

I'm not the only one who experienced a change in mood whilst on it; a study of over one million women in Denmark found that using hormonal contraception, particularly among adolescents and those taking the progestin only pill, was associated with subsequent use of antidepressants and a diagnosis of depression, so can we please stop telling pill users that it doesn't cause depression?

What else does it do? The pill increases your risk of breast, cervical, and liver cancers, and shouldn't be taken if there is a history of breast cancer in your family, or if you smoke because of the increased risk of blood clots. The World Health Organisation classifies it as a known carcinogen alongside tobacco and asbestos. The pill lowers production of cortisol, testosterone, and DHEA. It lowers bone density. It's linked to inflammatory bowel disease such as Crohn's disease. It increases production of a substance called thyroid hormone binding globulin (THBG) which binds to your thyroid hormones and inhibits their actions in the body such as helping you to feel energised, remain at a healthy weight, and have a full head of hair. It also increases production of sex hormone binding globulin (SHBG) – the protein that mops up excess hormones in your system, which is a good thing on the pill but also means that the small amount of testosterone that you do have circulating gets bound up and can't be used, and that impacts on sexual desire. Dr. Claudia Panzer, an endocrinologist and researcher, found that even after four months of not taking the pill, levels of SHBG still remained high when compared to participants who had never taken the pill, and she suggests that long-term research should be carried out to evaluate whether this change could be permanent. Panzer states that, 'it is important for physicians prescribing oral contraceptives to point out to their patient's potential sexual side effects, such as decreased desire, arousal, decreased lubrication and increased sexual pain.' Did yours?

Not only does a decrease in testosterone negatively impact on desire, but because oestrogen also gets bound up by SHBG, it can cause a shrivelling effect on genital tissue and a decrease in lubrication. One study of 22 healthy women found that after three months of being on the pill that:

- The labia minora decreased in thickness.
- The size of the entrance to the vagina decreased.
- Frequency of intercourse decreased.
- Frequency of orgasm decreased.
- Pain during sex increased.

And yes, a study of 22 women is a small one, but I've met so many women over the years whose experiences echoed the findings of this study, and side effects such as these need to be discussed and researched further. Another study found that when on low dose 'oestrogen' pills, 25 per cent of women experienced pain with orgasm (that's twice as many as those taking a higher dose pill or not taking any pill), and one small study found that clitoral volume decreases too. All this makes me wonder, is our focus on suppressing reproductive function at the expense of healthy and enjoyable sexual function? Again, it may not reflect your experience, but if it is, speak to your doctor. Your sexuality matters.

Then we come onto the matter of relationships and how the pill can affect them. When it comes to attraction and desire, pheromones are a crucial component. They're airborne chemical substances that we secrete which are detected by others and can trigger a mating response in them, and are one factor in what makes us feel turned on or turned off by someone. You're genetically programmed to be attracted to the pheromones of someone who is genetically dissimilar to you – nature's way of keeping the gene pool diverse – but studies have found that when you're on the pill, you're more likely to be attracted to the pheromones of someone who has genes that are similar to yours. In this non-ovulating state that's similar to pregnancy (in that you don't have the ebb and flow of a cycle), your body wants to keep you safe – something that would be important in pregnancy and would lead you to seek out the company of people who will protect you, such as members of your 'tribe' who would have similar genes to you, specifically the major histocompatibility complex (MHC) group of genes that help the immune system to recognise foreign substances, including sperm. I've had several clients who were on the pill for the duration of their long-term relationships decide to come off the pill in order to try to conceive, only to find that they were no longer attracted to their other half. So, before you commit to a relationship, or marriage, maybe it would be wise to come off the pill and hang out in your other half's armpit for a bit and see if their natural scent turns you on, or off. Some scientists are of the opinion that there could be a link between couples who share MHC genes which are similar and fertility issues and pregnancy loss, but this is a topic which needs to be researched further before conclusions can be drawn.

Hormonal birth control is either *combined* and is described as having oestrogen and progesterone in it, such as the combined pill, the patch, and NuvaRing®. Or as being *progesterone only*, such as the Mirena® IUD, Depo-Provera® contraceptive injection, and the cute-sounding mini-pill. But when you take these forms of hormonal birth control, you're not taking oestrogen and/or progesterone, you're taking the synthetic versions of them and they are not the same. That means you're not getting all the benefits associated with the form of these hormones that you produce in your body as a result of your menstrual cycle.

Although the Mirena® IUD works primarily by thickening your cervical fluid so that sperm can't penetrate it and reach an egg, and by thinning the lining of your uterus so that a fertilised egg can't implant, it can also suppress ovulation in up to 85 per cent of cycles in the first year of use, with this figure reducing to around 15 per cent of cycles thereafter.

Long-acting reversible contraceptives (LARC) are methods of birth control which provide contraception for an extended period of time, such as injections, implants, and IUDs. While there's clearly no going back from an injection, implants and IUDs can be removed though they leave you reliant on a healthcare professional to take them out, and I'm sad to say that I've had several distressed clients over the years in tears because they've been told they have to wait 6 months to get an appointment to have it taken out (though the appointment to have one inserted was available within a week of them requesting one).

There are also reproductive justice issues around contraception. SisterSong Women of Color Reproductive Justice Collective, an organisation in America, coined the term reproductive justice and define it as; 'the human right to maintain personal bodily autonomy, have children, not have children, and parent the children we have in safe and sustainable communities.' Healthcare providers are often so focused on how effective contraceptive methods are that they fail to take into account their patient's actual needs, and in some cases their perceived need for an individual to use contraception, when they may not want to use it at all. The Reproductive Health Technologies Project, who are now closed as an organisation, worked to advance the ability of every woman to achieve full reproductive freedom, state on their website that:

> 'All people should be able to make decisions about the contraceptive method that is best for them free from coercion and discrimination. However, inequality and disparities in power – across age, race, ethnicity, gender, geography, education, income, sexual orientation, and disability (among other identities) – have often resulted in policies and practices that fail to meet the unique needs of individuals or to respect their dignity and autonomy. Indeed, there are numerous examples of programs that have made birth control, sterilization, or abortion available to low-resourced women, while sacrificing the principles of self-determination and informed and voluntary consent in the name of tackling poverty.'

The Depo-Provera® contraceptive injection is pushed on African-American communities – 9 per cent of white teens versus 18 per cent of black teens. It's also currently used in sex offender rehabilitation centres to decrease the sex drive of offenders, and studies point to a link between using Depo-Provera® and an increased risk of HIV infection which is important, especially when it's pushed in Sub-Saharan Africa, a region with high rates of HIV transmission. Yes, people have a right to access contraception, but that comes with a right to be informed and a right to choose the most appropriate method, and people also have the right to extend their family if they choose to. Population control has long been blamed on women's unwillingness to be responsible and use contraception, but as Grigg-Spall points out, 'pregnancy is made to be the problem and not the poverty itself ... there is no evidence to show that population density causes lack of resources and poverty ... people are purposely kept poor so that developed countries (or at least their corporations) can become richer.' So why aren't we pointing the finger at the multinationals who control the flow of resources? Isn't that what impacts on reproductive choices and access to them?

We are only capable of conceiving for six days in every cycle, whereas men are fertile all the time, so why are we the ones who bear the burden of responsibility with using these drugs and devices? I'm not saying that men should have to take hormonal contraception, because I have concerns about the effects of it too – so far trials have been abandoned because of the unwanted side effects participants experienced; depression, irritability, acne, changes in sexual desire, and a temporary decrease in testicular volume. Yet those same side effects are reported by women all the time and repeatedly ignored and denied (though it's our ovaries that shrink). In fact, if the female pill was researched now, would it even make it through a research trial, or would that be abandoned too?

Post-pill Fertility

If you make an informed choice to use hormonal birth control and the method that you use works well for you – fantastic. But be cautious and considerate of the possible long-term effects. If you're planning on conceiving, come off it before you actually start trying because some people find that they have post-pill amenorrhoea and it takes a while for their periods to return. I often see women in my clinic who've come off the pill to have a baby, but a year or two later their period still hasn't returned so they've been referred for IVF and they've come to me to optimise their chances, and at that point,

I'm usually thinking that if I can work with them for 3–6 months that we'll be able to get their cycle back, because instead of being infertile, they're probably just recovering from being on the pill for a decade or two.

When it comes to fertility, one study found an association between long-term pill use (5–10 years) and a thin uterine lining. This is important because a sub-optimal endometrial thickness has a negative impact on your ability to conceive. If, during a round of IVF, the endometrium doesn't reach the required minimum thickness of 7–8mm, the round is usually called off and all the embryos are frozen so that they can be transferred at a later date.

A Danish study which investigated ovarian reserve in relation to use of oral contraception concluded that using the pill has a negative impact on ovarian volume and AMH – a hormone that's tested to assess fertility – and that practitioners and patients should be aware of the potential for it to affect fertility. But perhaps the most important issue in relation to conceiving after being on the pill is the fact that it reduces your ability to absorb key vitamins and minerals that are essential to fertility and pregnancy (folic acid, vitamins B2, B6, B12, vitamin C and E, and the minerals magnesium, selenium, and zinc), so I recommend giving your body time to adjust and stock up on these key nutrients through diet and supplementation before trying to conceive.

When it comes to birth control, I'm in agreement with naturopath Lara Briden's comment that, 'sixty years of hormonal birth control shows a startling lack of imagination.' And whether you love or loathe hormonal contraception, I hope you'll agree that we need better.

So what are your other options? In the following table you'll find a list of some common methods of birth control, a description of how they work, and their failure rates in terms of their typical use. Perfect use is when a method is always used consistently and correctly, typical use is what happens in real life and, as you can imagine, there's often a discrepancy between the two sets of statistics.

Emergency contraception (EC), aka the morning-after pill (Levonelle®, ellaOne®, Plan B®) can be used to prevent pregnancy after unprotected sex or contraceptive failure such as a condom splitting, but it works by delaying or preventing an egg from being released, so if you've already ovulated it can't be relied upon as it won't prevent a fertilised egg from implanting or disturb it if it already has. Levonelle® and Plan B® must be taken within 72 hours (3 days), and ellaOne® must be taken within 120 hours (5 days). Whereas the copper IUD Paragard®, which can be used as EC and can be

Type	Brand names	Hormones	Works by	Typical use success rate	
Combined pill	• Cilest® • Microgynon® • Rigevidon® • Yasmin® • Ovranette® • Dianette®	Oestrogen and progestin	Supressing ovulation, as well as thinning the lining of the uterus and thickening cervical fluid, making it harder for sperm to enter the uterus and for a fertilised egg to implant.	93%	Missing a pill, vomiting and diarrhoea all make it less effective.
Progestin-only pill (mini-pill)	• Cerazette® • Cerelle® • Noriday® • Norgeston® • Norethindrone® • Ovrette® • Micronor®	Progestin	Thinning the lining of the uterus and thickening cervical fluid. May also suppress ovulation.	93%	Not taking it at the same time every day, missing a pill, vomiting and diarrhoea all make it less effective.
Vaginal ring	• NuvaRing®	Oestrogen and progestin	Supressing ovulation	93%	A flexible transparent ring which you place inside your vagina and leave in place for 3 weeks.
Contraceptive patch	• Evra®	Oestrogen and progestin which are absorbed through the skin and enter the bloodstream.	Supressing ovulation, as well as thinning the lining of the uterus and thickening cervical fluid, making it harder for sperm to enter the uterus and for a fertilised egg to implant.	93%	A 4cm square plastic patch that sticks to the skin. Patches are applied on a weekly basis. Not affected by diarrhoea and vomiting.

Type	Brand names	Hormones	Works by	Typical use success rate	
Implants	• Norplant® • Nexplanon®	Progestin	Prevents ovulation and thickens cervical mucus.	99.9%	Inserted under the skin of the upper arm by a doctor or nurse and can remain in place for up to 3 years.
Injections	• Depo-Provera®	Progestin	Prevents the ovary from releasing an egg.	96%	An injection containing progestin is given every 3 months. Can result in unpredictable bleeding, but periods can also become lighter or stop altogether.
Hormonal Intra-Uterine System (IUS)	• Mirena® • Skyla® • Jaydess®	Progestin	Thinning the lining of the uterus and thickening cervical fluid. May also suppress ovulation, particularly in the first year of use.	99.3%	A small plastic T-shaped device which releases progestin is inserted into the uterus by a doctor or nurse. Can result in unpredictable bleeding initially, but periods may become light or stop altogether. Can be left in place for 3–5 years depending on the brand.
Copper IUD	• Paragard®	None	The copper ions emitted by the copper IUD are toxic to sperm and prevent them from reaching an egg.	99.2%	A small T-shaped piece of plastic and copper is inserted into the uterus by a doctor or nurse, and it can be left in place for up to 10 years. Periods can become longer, heavier, or more painful.
Condoms		None	Prevent sperm from entering the vagina.	87% (male) 79% (female)	Also prevent transmission of STIs.

Method	Description	%		Notes
Diaphragm and cervical caps	Act as a barrier method, preventing sperm from meeting an egg by covering your cervix (entrance to your uterus).	83%	None	Come in different shapes and sizes so it's important to work with a healthcare provider who is accustomed to the various brands in order to find one that's a good fit.
Spermicides	They contain a sperm-killing agent and are usually used alongside other methods such as condoms or the diaphragm.	79%	None	Available as a foam, cream, jelly, film, suppository, or tablet, which is inserted into the vagina prior to sex. Can be messy and irritate the vagina or penis.
Withdrawal	The penis is withdrawn prior to ejaculation.	80%	None	Requires control and trust. Some studies suggest that sperm is present in the fluid that leaks out of the penis prior to ejaculation (pre-cum).
Fertility awareness method	Bodily changes are tracked to identify your fertile window, such as basal body temperature, cervical mucus and cervical position.	85%	None	Penis-in-vagina sex should be avoided or barrier methods used during the fertile window.
Female sterilisation	The fallopian tubes are cut or blocked with rings or clipped, preventing an egg from reaching the uterus.	99.5%	None	Should be considered permanent as an operation to reverse it isn't always successful.
Vasectomy	Simple and quick operation in which the tubes which transport sperm from the testicles to the penis are tied or cut.	99.85%	None	Should be considered permanent as an operation to reverse it isn't always successful.

kept in for long-term contraception, works by impairing sperm and may prevent implantation. It's 99.9 per cent effective if it's inserted by a healthcare professional within 5 days of having sex.

Fertility Challenges

We're raised to believe that all it takes is one sperm to get knocked up and that precautions must be taken in order to prevent pregnancy because all it takes to get knocked up is one eager swimmer. While this is technically true, it's sadly not always so simple.

The intense pain of infertility is traumatic. The ability to reproduce is deeply ingrained in our sense of self, so when it goes awry it affects every single part of your life. It damages your self-esteem and your ability to trust and believe in your body. It's a gaping unseen wound that, even if it heals, always leaves a scar – even after a successful pregnancy.

The effects of infertility play out in the menstrual cycle month after month after month and it can be impossible to enjoy any aspect of it, because even the most positive parts of the cycle can be fraught with tension. The pressure to conceive can decimate the powers associated with each phase, which is why fertility challenges can dismantle a person's identity and self-worth. Conceiving is not a talent for you to master, it is a biological reaction, but when it doesn't happen it impacts on your confidence in other areas of your life.

Spring is the phase of your cycle where you're gearing up for another attempt at trying to conceive, and it's the season that's associated with hope and possibility but allowing yourself to feel this can feel incredibly risky. You may feel that you need to protect yourself from further pain by dialling down your expectations and feelings of positivity. When you're experiencing fertility issues, sex becomes a very serious business. Spontaneity goes out the window along with intimacy and pleasure, but you can use the playful nature of Spring to bring back some connection and fun. The Spring season of the cycle equates to your adolescence, so think back to an activity that you probably did a lot of during your teenage years: Kissing. When was the last time you had a proper smooch and got lost in this oh so important form of intimacy? Kissing helps maintain connection in a relationship, and is the gateway drug to more pleasure, which your relationship is likely lacking in if you're at the point where sex is just about one sperm and one egg.

It's common for people who are intensely focused on trying to conceive to feel robbed of their Summer, and it may only last a few days because as soon as ovulation happens, you enter the two-week wait until you're able to take a pregnancy test. You feel unable to let yourself go and enjoy life lest you do something that inadvertently destroys the embryo that's possibly attempting to nestle itself into your womb (although the reality is that whatever you do now is really unlikely to affect things). If you've been trying for a while then you've probably hit pause on your life which means that there isn't much to enjoy in this phase, especially if how you socialise and whom you socialise with has had to change in order to support your fertility. When you're limiting alcohol intake and going to bed earlier, relationships that have been based on a foundation of drinking bottles of wine go out the window pretty quickly, not to mention that you're likely to find hanging around anyone with kids painful. Infertility can leave you feeling isolated; those around you may have no clue what's going on, and those that do may not get it and make unintended blunders that are hurtful, so you retreat in order to protect yourself. Your Summer is all about connection, but making a baby sex becomes purely functional, a means to an end that increasingly feels like a chore. Connection and communication in a relationship frequently deteriorate, and you can find yourself disappearing into yourself more and more. You might sense an abundance of love with you in the start of your Summer but feel sadness at not being able to pour that love onto a baby.

The second half of the cycle is excruciating when you desperately want to be pregnant and are waiting to see if you are, and the psychological anguish of the two week wait certainly magnifies your experience of your Autumn. Your defences are already fragile and worn away and it's harder to remember all that you've achieved in life because those achievements mean nothing when your womb is empty. Infertility rapidly takes over your identity, and irrational self-blame gives your inner critic a neverending source of fuel, allowing it to run riot all cycle long, so finding ways to create boundaries for it is crucial in order for you to preserve your sense of self. Your experience of PMS may express itself in your attitude towards your partner, particularly if the fertility problem lies with them, because to put it bluntly, and whether it's conscious or sub-conscious, they are failing to get you pregnant. Although men and women share the diagnosis of infertility equally, fertility treatment focuses on the female body, and there may be anger that it's you that has to go through it all.

The arrival of your period serves as a painful and inescapable reminder that your body is betraying you, and its repeated appearance casts a shadow over any feelings of positivity that you have about your body during the sunny seasons of your cycle. The grief and despair of infertility means that the darkness of your Winter can consume you, and it can be hard to feel any sense of purpose in life when the only one that you want to fulfil is having a child. Multiple layers of loss accumulate as your fertility journey lengthens; every egg that doesn't fertilise, the eggs that fertilise but don't implant, the embryos that implant but don't stay, the pregnancy losses, the loss of control, self-esteem, and confidence in your body, the loss of sexual intimacy and spontaneity in your relationship, and the expense of any treatment you undergo. All of which means that when you're experiencing difficulties in conceiving, you do a lot of holding it together in order to get through your day and to preserve your relationship. There's a pressure to think positively, to 'just relax and it'll happen' (as if being told that ever helped anyone to actually relax), and there's usually a limit to how much sadness those around us can handle witnessing, so just as your grief intensifies, you feel that you have to hold it together even more, then you retreat further into yourself and feel a distance between you and the rest of the world that wasn't there before.

When fertility clients come into my treatment room, their sorrow and tears pour out of them as soon as they walk in the door because they know that I value these emotions, and that my clinic is a safe space for them to come out. I hope that you have someone who can simply be there for you, to acknowledge your uncomfortable feelings and experiences without trying to cheer you up (though there are times when that's helpful too) and recommend finding a fertility support group that's local to you, as well as professional support from a practitioner if that's within your budget. Create a safe space for yourself, write and let your tears and thoughts stream out of you, give yourself permission to feel it all because when you allow yourself to be cleared out emotionally in your Winter, you leave space for other feelings during the other seasons.

Working with your cycle can reframe how you experience it and help you to form a more positive relationship with your body. I won't lie to you though, nothing will budge you from the focus of conceiving but practising cycle awareness will make your cycle about more than just conceiving. It allows you to explore and reclaim other parts of yourself, you know, the you before your fertility struggle, the you that you've completely lost sight of.

Moving with your seasons gives you permission to feel all of your emotions, offering a container for them and a way of letting them be, and being aware of your personal rhythm helps you to realise that your hormones are there to serve you in other ways – that there are ways for you to feel the positive effects of them even though they will pale in comparison to your desire for a child.

Tracking your basal body temperature can be immensely helpful for couples trying to conceive and also for the practitioners who support them, but it can also create high levels of anxiety, and instead of being curious and informed by the data on your chart, it becomes something to live by that dictates your every move. Using The Cycle Strategy switches the focus from your temperatures to your experience and gives you a way to care for yourself.

When you're trying to get pregnant, you're likely to investigate every complementary care option that's available to you, and as a practitioner of Chinese medicine and ATMAT® I have a well-founded bias towards these therapies, and I'm pleased to say that a lot of the time the work I do involves being able to celebrate pregnancies and births. But it also involves supporting clients as they work towards accepting that their journey to conceive is ending, and whatever comes after that for them. Please be wary of clinics and practitioners who purport spectacular success rates. Find someone who is knowledgeable and transparent in their approach, someone who's been recommended to you and that you know in your gut you can trust. Infertility treatment, in all its forms, can be exorbitant, so it's crucial that you trust where you're putting your money.

It's also okay to take a break from trying to conceive, really it is. I know that just the idea of losing time can provoke panic but stepping back and away from the continuous rollercoaster of trying to conceive can be hugely beneficial to your mental and physical health, as well as the health of your relationship. It gives you time to remember that you are more than your reproductive capacity, to assess your next steps, and most of the time it feels like a relief to hit pause.

Fertility is yet another taboo topic, but it's even more taboo to speak about the effects of infertility after you've had a baby. The trauma of infertility and pregnancy loss doesn't disappear once a baby is born. It can affect how you view your body in the long-term, and also impact on your ability to allow yourself to experience all the feelings of motherhood, particularly the not-so-nice emotions, such as frustration, depression, and rage, which are intensified by the hormones of the menstrual cycle. Instead of accepting that these feelings are part and parcel of having a child and not beating yourself up about feeling them, you could find yourself feeling intense guilt and place a demand on yourself that it's not okay to feel these emotions, because you're fortunate enough to have a child when so many others don't.

When you really want a baby, your relationship with your reproductive system and your cycle can become a very negative one, but cycle awareness from a non-fertility perspective can help you to claw your way back to a more balanced relationship with your cycle.

Pregnancy

Cycle awareness is fabulous preparation for pregnancy and parenthood, but The Cycle Strategy can also be used during pregnancy and postpartum. Sure, you won't be cycling while you're pregnant (although in some pregnancies, spotting can occur in the first trimester around the time when you would have had your period), instead you'll enter a different cycle and one that takes much longer to move through – something that you may find enjoyable in parts but hard in others.

The first trimester acts as an extended Winter and gives you time to adjust. Even if your pregnancy was planned and wanted, it can still come as a shock, and if you feel anxious or have had a previous loss, it might feel particularly precarious. It's a time when everything slows down, your energy will probably plummet sooner than you expect and you'll fall asleep without a moment's notice (because you're growing a human and a placenta, which both take effort), and your digestion practically grinds to a halt due to the effects of progesterone, the pregnancy hormone that slows digestive transit time so that your body has more opportunity to extract nutrients from the food you eat, which by the way is likely to all come from one food group – beige. In the first trimester, the practicalities of life such as getting on public transport can really wear you down, let alone if you're unfortunate enough to get hit with pregnancy nausea or the extreme form of it, *hyperemesis gravidarum*, in which case resting and retreating is absolutely non-negotiable.

Some of you will transition into the Spring phase of pregnancy as you head into your second trimester, or if you're feeling particularly depleted and challenged by pregnancy or life, you could find yourself remaining in your Winter for another month. You'll know you're entering your Spring because your interest in colourful healthy food returns, you'll want to get up off the sofa and move, and a spark of libido may even surface. Up till now all you could consider was your basic needs of food, water, and sleep, but now you can actually think about people other than you and the child inside you, you're interested in what's going on in the world and you're ready to rejoin it. The Spring season of pregnancy also brings hope and possibility – that this pregnancy has stuck and will work out.

The transition into your Summer at some point in your second trimester may be less pronounced than when you entered Spring but feeling horny again is a sure sign that you're there. Summer is the honeymoon period in pregnancy when your energy and mood improve, and you can still move with ease, so make the most of it. Do the things that you enjoy, go on dates and connect with those that you love, and get the bulk of your pre-baby checklist done so that you can ease up when you enter your Autumn. One potential downside to Summer is that your bump will be more noticeable by now, and everyone feels that they have a right to comment on it, or even touch it – this is the 'feeling too seen' aspect of Summer showing up in the seasons of pregnancy and I suggest that you bat any unwanted hands away.

You'll find yourself transitioning into the Autumn phase of pregnancy around the time you enter your third trimester or at some point during it. Just like the menstrual cycle, every person's experience of pregnancy varies, and the timing of your seasons will depend on how well you've felt throughout your pregnancy and what level of support you've received from others. Perhaps you're slowing down, feeling affected by swings in blood sugar and mood, getting a bit hot and bothered, or feeling utterly wiped out. Listen to your body. If you're feeling irritated and upset, then be mindful that the things that show up now are what you need to address before your baby arrives on the scene, in fact they could even affect how you labour, so don't gloss over them. If you're exhausted, then for goodness sake please rest and focus on nourishing yourself – labouring and entering parenthood when you're already depleted and knackered is hard work.

The Autumn phase of pregnancy is the perfect time to review your life, make some decisions, and start to edit. Sort and organise, give unwanted items away, fill your freezer, get odd jobs done, potter, rest, clear things in you and around you. Have a good old-fashioned sort out and get in the spirit of nesting if that's what you feel like doing (it's okay if you don't feel this urge). If you're unskilled in the art of asking, now is the time to get in the habit. Find your voice and let those around you know what it is you want and need. This might relate to what you need in pregnancy, what you want in labour (a time when even the strongest of women can lose their voice, and the quietest can find theirs), and your wishes for your early days as a family. Lay down the ground rules for your postpartum now so that your loved ones have a chance to adjust their expectations and get in line with what you want.

In the menstrual cycle, you either enter your Winter in the hours or days before you start bleeding – perhaps experiencing a sense of distance from the world – or the physicality of bleeding is what heralds the start of Winter. It's the same with labour; you either find yourself in a time of in between in the days or weeks before it starts or going into labour transports you into the depths of your Winter. And labour is likely to be the Winter of all Winters. It is the ultimate process of letting go and journeying into the depths of yourself, to go through doors you didn't even know were there and that you may rather run from, to let go and allow something that feels bigger than you to take over. But of course, it is you and so labour cannot be bigger than you.

During labour, retreating into a safe dark place is crucial because that's what will allow your hormones to reach optimal levels and enable a smooth and efficient labour, and in the same way masturbation and orgasms can help with period pain, they can provide relief in labour, and along with nipple stimulation, they can encourage contractions too. There are many similarities between menstruation and childbirth, including that no matter what form it takes, childbirth strips you back to your essence and forces you to face yourself – a theme that may feel familiar to you if you're battle worn from dealing with hardcore periods.

After birth you'll be bleeding for a while and, while you are, you're definitely in your Winter, so please act like it. I see too many new parents trying to rush out of the Winter of their postpartum, wincing and hobbling their way down the street when their stitches are still healing, and they should be resting. In the same way adequate rest during your period sets you up for a productive time in your Spring and Summer, resting in your fourth trimester will pay dividends in the coming months and years. It's time you won't get back or get to do again in the same way with any future children, at least not without a serious level of help from others. In the very least aim for a week in bed, and a week around the bed. Pull up the drawbridge and say "no" to visitors, unless of course they are of the super helpful kind that drop food off, hang your laundry up, and do the dishes, but even in those cases a time limit proves useful. When you're deciding who you want to come over, think about who you'd be happy to let see you in your undies and with your boobs out, because regardless of how you plan to feed your baby, it's a helpful marker of who you should have around. Family politics can weigh heavily on this time, but this is your time as a new family, so prioritise yourselves. Do not have people you're not so keen on seeing visit in the first week; your hormones go through a major transition around days 2–5 and most commonly on day 3 or 4, and while some navigate this switch without a hitch (usually when they've had a smooth birth without intervention and a peaceful start to parenting), many of the women I've supported have experienced a teary blip or a major emotional outpouring of some kind – the latter usually being when they've had a full-on birth and/or they've done way too much afterwards, which in actuality needn't be much at all because even the 'little' things like having a shower can be exhausting.

The first three months following birth are referred to as the fourth trimester as it's a time when your baby is going through an enormous transition from womb to world, and you're transitioning too, even if it isn't your first rodeo. Every baby will be different but all of them need time to acclimatise to the outside world, which is very different to the one they've left behind, and your world will have changed too, which means that you also need time to figure things out; how to feed and care for your baby, how to feed and care for yourself, plus all the other influences such as your relationship and professional life. Retreating and giving yourself space to tune into your instincts will help you. The fourth trimester is a time when you're likely to feel permeable and vulnerable. When loved ones and total strangers make unsupportive comments about your baby and your parenting choices, they can pierce you to your very heart and decimate the confidence you've been building as a new mum. When you're considering who to have around you, choose wisely, and above all else, know that the decisions you're making for you and your family are what's best for you. You're doing great, truly you are.

Around the three month mark you'll hopefully be feeling more in the swing of things and getting out of the house will feel easier, a sure sign that you're working your way out of your fourth trimester and your Winter, though to tell you the truth I felt that elements of the fourth trimester remained until the eighteen month mark; some of them were enjoyable and others were hard work, and I suspect that I'm not alone in that. In fact, it wasn't until I started menstruating again that I felt a definite shift.

Breastfeeding and chestfeeding (a term used by some masculine-identified trans people who feed their baby from their chest but prefer not to say breastfeeding) can, but doesn't always, halt ovulation and menstruation, causing postpartum amenorrhoea. But in the absence of breast/chestfeeding you can ovulate as early as three weeks after giving birth so it's worth discussing and making decisions about contraception very early on, even if you have no plans to hop back on the horse so soon. Sex after giving birth can be uncomfortable and painful, even after a caesarean, because it's not just emotional and physical trauma that can cause it, but the low levels of oestrogen that result in vaginal dryness that's common in the postpartum.

If you have PCOS or hypothyroidism, it's important to know that both of these conditions can affect your milk supply when breastfeeding, so I recommend seeking out specialist help from an International Board Certified Lactation Consultant (IBCLC) during pregnancy, in order to prepare for this possibility.

Pregnancy is a liminal state, a time of transition when you're between the place that you used to be, and the place that you're about to enter, and where some people will enjoy this feeling, others will find it deeply unsettling. Not menstruating brings challenges too, because you don't have the moment of release that you're used to having in a cycle, so finding ways to discharge pent up feelings will become important. During pregnancy and postpartum, you can use the lunar cycle in place of your menstrual cycle to provide a way for you to schedule in some down time every month, and to work with the rhythm of a cycle (see page 212).

When Parenting and PMS Collide

Rich and rewarding, oppressive and relentless, parenting presents a whole host of challenges. When you're already struggling to take care of your basic needs, such as staying hydrated, eating regularly, and sleeping sufficiently, how can you tend to the other things that nourish you, like your close relationships, and your personal and professional ambitions? And I haven't even got onto the complexities of what it does to your hormones and how tricky it is to navigate your menstrual cycle when the neverending demands placed upon you feel crushing, but your cycle forces you to reclaim something for yourself and of yourself, the inner seasons once more providing a way for you to explore your identity, desires, and needs.

Spring and Summer are great seasons to parent in. The playful and inquisitive nature of your Spring is a perfect match to hanging out with kids, and the increase in energy and positivity that you hopefully feel in your Summer can make parenting so much easier, so be sure to capitalise on these seasons and schedule in dedicated time that you can enjoy with them. When it comes to supporting their sleep, committing to nappy training, or implementing a new schedule, start these endeavours in your Spring so that you do the bulk of the work when you're feeling up to the challenge. Trying to get your kid to sleep through the night when you're having a hard time in your Autumn is not going to work out well.

In raising a human, you are doing the biggest job out there, but it's one where you don't necessarily benefit from seeing and celebrating the results of your constant hard work, either because you're so entrenched in the tasks at hand that you can't see the wood for the trees, or because you're not working with others who can acknowledge what you're doing and reflect back how they see you to you. Spring and Summer can also be frustrating if you want to do work other than parenting but aren't able to in the way that you used to, but a lack of time can be highly motivating, and you'll likely surprise yourself with just how much you can get done. But despite it being the 21st century, it's our willingness to set our ambition aside as mothers that's expected and rewarded by society, and your return to work may be met with negativity. Even in writing this book I have been told that I can't have it all i.e. be a mother and commit to such an intense project, but nobody has told my boyfriend that *he* can't have it all.

Most mums I know are desperate for time out, period, but particularly so during the Autumn and Winter phases of the cycle when premenstrual irritability and depression make you want to abandon ship. The overwhelming need to walk away and to retreat is often impossible when your children are young, and you can't even poo on your own, they're highly attuned to any attempt at separating and spending time apart, but for the sake of your sanity, it's vital that you do. Remember, *whatever bothers you in your Autumn is there all cycle long,* but in the first half of your cycle oestrogen camouflages what's going on, so it isn't revealed until you hit your premenstruum. The combined effect of the heavy mental load experienced by mums, and the tendency for them to be doing the bulk of unpaid work in a household in terms of chores and practical and emotional caregiving, usually results in a tempestuous time in your Autumn, even if all the thoughts and feelings you experience remain inside you. Keep track of what sets you into a fiery rage or a downward spiral of tears and depression and make plans to change matters. Not sure what it is that you need to do? I'll hazard a guess that it involves doing less for other people and doing more for yourself.

If you suspect that you're depressed, you're not alone; 1 in 5 women have maternal mental health issues, and it's no surprise given the lack of support available to us. We weren't meant to do it alone and it really does take a whole village to raise a child, mainly because the parents need help staying sane. When you have a child there's a tremendous shift within yourself and in your close relationships. You're likely to be getting bugger all sleep so you can say hello to unstable blood sugar and mood, inflammation, and food cravings, and you're less likely to be eating the healthy, nutrient-dense diet that you prioritised during pregnancy and more likely to be surviving on crappy carbs, sugar, and caffeine, which results in more inflammation and unstable blood sugar. With the combination of massive psychological and physiological changes in the year after childbirth, lack of support and sub-optimal self-care it's no wonder that so many of us experience mental health issues. If you've experienced a mental health issue in the past then there's a 50 per cent chance of it returning in the postpartum, and having a child can trigger premenstrual dysphoric disorder (PMDD, the extreme form of PMS), which means it's essential that you form a support team and develop a care plan before you have your baby.

Postpartum Thyroiditis

A hormonal imbalance that can result in postnatal depression is postpartum thyroiditis, where the thyroid gland at the base of your neck becomes inflamed in the year after giving birth. It can be a tricky condition to recognise as the signs and symptoms of it are usually attributed to the reality of life with a newborn, but 1 in 18 new mothers develop it. There are two phases of postpartum thyroiditis, in the first phase the thyroid is overactive, and in the second, it's underactive, though you can have postpartum thyroiditis and only experience one phase – 43 per cent of cases present with only hypothyroidism.

The phases of postpartum thyroiditis are:

- One to four months after giving birth, symptoms that are similar to hyperthyroidism appear, such as; anxiety, irritability, fast heart rate, palpitations, rapid weight loss, fatigue, insomnia, tremors, and sensitivity to heat. These symptoms typically last for 1–3 months, and the second phase may then develop.
- As thyroid function diminishes, symptoms of hypothyroidism arrive on the scene, like; exhaustion, depression, weight gain, hair loss, constipation, aches and pains, trouble concentrating, low desire for sex, and a tendency to feel cold. These symptoms typically occur 4–8 months after giving birth and last for 9–12 months.

The effects of postpartum thyroiditis can really mess with your life and adjusting to motherhood is hard enough without your hormones screwing you over too. Although most doctors say that it will resolve itself with time (most cases do within a year), I don't think that's good enough – not only is it dismissive of women's experiences, but it can rob them of a crucial bonding period with their baby. And women who develop postpartum thyroiditis have a 25–30 per cent chance of developing permanent hypothyroidism within the following 5–10 years. That means that the year following childbirth provides a window of opportunity in which the risk of developing permanent hypothyroidism can be assessed, and flags up those who need to be assessed regularly over the subsequent years.

If you or someone in your family has a history of autoimmune or thyroid disease, or if you have type 1 diabetes, then you should have your blood tested in pregnancy for thyroid hormones and antibodies because you're at an increased risk of developing postpartum thyroiditis, and of those who test positive for thyroid antibodies in the third trimester of pregnancy, 80 per cent will go on to develop postpartum thyroiditis. If you feel there's more to how you feel than the stress of having a newborn, please speak to your GP about testing your thyroid, especially if you've been diagnosed with postpartum depression, because it may be that instead of being prescribed an antidepressant what you need is some thyroid medication and support (and remember, just testing TSH isn't enough and, even with full thyroid testing, hypothyroidism is frequently subclinical so you can have just about every sign and symptom of it, but your lab tests will still appear as normal in which case a diagnosis may have to be made according to your signs and symptoms as opposed to the results of a blood test, see page 290). We've got to stop accepting 'well you've got a kid so of course you feel that way' as a good enough answer.

When you have a child, your job is to love them, feed them, and keep them warm. To ensure that you're focused on doing this and nothing else, your brain undergoes a transformation during pregnancy; it shrinks slightly and restructures itself. That, as well as having low levels of hormones in the postpartum means that your days of multitasking are long gone, and the simple act of remembering to make a phone call is problematic. Simple tasks become overwhelming and stressful, and you can enter a state of hypervigilance that's impossible to switch off from, leaving you feeling tired but wired. When you're stressed the adrenal hormone, cortisol, takes over in order to survive the crisis, but motherhood can end up being a constant crisis, and your adrenal glands can have a hard time keeping up with the sustained stress. They work best when you eat regularly and get good quality, uninterrupted sleep, which I know you're managing with ease now that you're a mum, right? Left untreated this can lead to weight gain around your middle, fatigue, and depression – just what you need. You can help your adrenals by staying hydrated and eating regularly, and do not limit food intake or skip meals in a bid to lose weight because you'll end up with low blood sugar, be moody AF, and you'll trigger the secretion of cortisol which then shuts down fatburning in order to preserve fuel, so it won't even help you to lose weight.

Signs of adrenal dysfunction include; struggling to get out of bed in the morning; feeling shattered in the afternoon; craving sugar, fat, and salt; decreased immunity; depression; low sexual desire; feeling light-headed or dizzy, especially when moving from lying or sitting to standing; brain fog and poor memory; irritability; decreased ability to handle stress; trouble falling asleep or waking up feeling wired in the middle of the night (because low cortisol affects how you regulate your blood sugar level in the night, and low blood sugar can trigger you into waking up to refuel); and increased PMS and symptoms of perimenopause.

Perimenopause and Menopause

Menopause itself only lasts for one day because you reach it after a year of having no periods. What most of us think of as menopause is actually perimenopause – the period of time that precedes it during which symptoms such as changes in menstrual pattern and flow, hot flushes, night sweats, insomnia, fatigue, and PMS can appear.

Ninety-five per cent of us will experience menopause at some point between 44 and 56 years of age, with the average age being 50 years old. Genetics and whether you smoke or not can impact how early you make the transition, and there's a dose-related response of smoking and early menopause. In other words, the more you smoke the earlier it can happen. Premature menopause – when it occurs before the age of forty – occurs in around 2 per cent of women and there appears to be an inherited risk, so if there's a history of early menopause in your family, it's wise to bear this in mind when making decisions about having your own family.

As eggs start to run low and as their quality diminishes, follicular development is impaired, resulting in a decline in fertility and the appearance of irregular cycles. To begin with, your pituitary gland works harder to pull follicles out of your ovaries by pumping out more follicle stimulating hormone (FSH) in an effort to stimulate them, which shortens the first phase of your cycle, and creates more frequent cycles. This is your body's way of creating chances for you to conceive before you stop ovulating, and it's the irregular (usually shorter) cycles that commonly start in your 40s and even in your 30s that mark the beginning of the perimenopause – although your menstrual cycle may not actually cease for another ten years.

If you recall from Chapter 1, thousands of follicles undergo a natural process of atresia (dying off) in every cycle so by the time perimenopause rolls around the number of follicles we have left has greatly declined, which means that the cells on the follicles which are responsible for manufacturing hormones has also lessened, resulting in a decrease in ovarian hormone production. This causes an increase in anovulatory cycles that tend to be on the long side and you'll start to go several months without a period. In the absence of regular ovulation and a functioning corpus luteum to produce progesterone, oestrogen is no longer kept in check and begins to run riot if it hasn't already and symptoms of oestrogen dominance appear, such as heavier and/or longer periods, PMS, tender breasts, bloating, headaches, and water retention. Without the calming effects of progesterone on your nervous system, you could be feeling agitated and anxious, and your ability to sleep soundly plummets, which means you're exhausted and find yourself in a vicious cycle of low mood and shit sleep.

With time, oestrogen levels begin to fall too, and symptoms of oestrogen deficiency appear, such as vaginal dryness, painful sex (that's if you're even interested), a leaky or over-active bladder that's also prone to infections, hot flushes, night sweats, trouble sleeping, poor memory, and generally feeling the ageing process. You're probably getting palpitations even when you're feeling relaxed and waking up in the middle of the night to find that you're drenched in sweat and need to change your bed linen too. Most of my clients find that these symptoms are immediately exacerbated by drinking a glass of wine or eating rich, spicy food, so be wary of foods and drinks that are heating in nature and lean towards a diet that's cooling and nourishing (think lean and green).

This may sound like a reasonably predictable linear process, but while the overall hormonal sequence might sound clear and sequential, the daily reality can feel like you're on a rollercoaster and you most likely are. Take a look at the diagram opposite and you'll see that far from having a predictable ebb and flow of hormones in every cycle, in perimenopause they fluctuate wildly.

This is all probably sounding pretty shit so it's worth bearing in mind that menopause is not a condition, it is a life event and plenty of people have a positive experience of it. It is a time when you truly come into your own power, but for some, the process of getting there will be rocky. The more

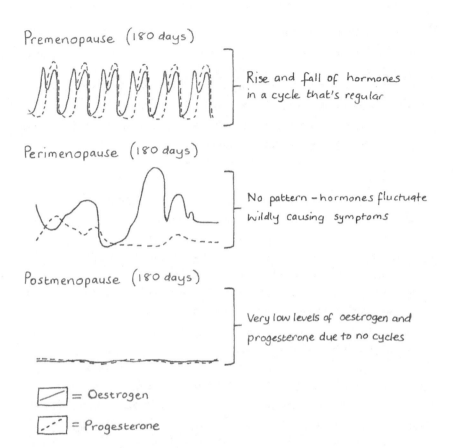

Premenopause (180 days)

Rise and fall of hormones in a cycle that's regular

Perimenopause (180 days)

No pattern – hormones fluctuate wildly causing symptoms

Postmenopause (180 days)

Very low levels of oestrogen and progesterone due to no cycles

= Oestrogen

= Progesterone

you work with your menstrual cycle in the years that lead to menopause, the easier your psychological transition will be. Anything that's unresolved in your life will loom large now and you can no longer stick your head in the sand. Without oestrogen to gloss over the not-so-nice side of life, you'll view your life and your relationships through a different lens. Oestrogen makes us care about others, so when it starts to wane, our tolerance for putting up with people and their bullshit goes with it, and you could find yourself acknowledging all the times that you cared for others instead of yourself and feel bitter and resentful of how your own needs have been abandoned and ignored. This is why it's so important to work with the menstrual cycle early on in life; each cycle refines you towards menopause and helps to develop self-awareness and kindness towards yourself – including developing healthy boundaries and maintaining a balance between caring for others and ourselves.

During perimenopause, PMS can start earlier and hit harder than it used to, and your experience of the Autumn season of your cycle will be confounded by the fact that you're also in the Autumn phase of your life, and this powerful double whammy will heighten the powers and pitfalls associated with your Autumn. Autumn is all about editing in order to focus on what's important, particularly relevant when – whether consciously or sub-consciously – you'll have an awareness that the Winter phase of your life is around the corner, and that brings about a sense of urgency which may be about having a child or pushing for what matters in your professional life.

As you head towards the Winter season of your life, you'll step further into your inner wisdom and feel surer of yourself, but this phase of life is associated with the metal element in Chinese medicine, so it's important to watch out for hardening and becoming brittle both in body and mind, and to work at maintaining flexibility.

While oestrogen and testosterone are high in relation to other hormones, sexual desire can hit a lifetime peak, then as oestrogen declines, particularly after menopause, genito-urinary issues can get in the way of having a good time. Less oestrogen causes vaginal atrophy in which the vaginal walls thin and dry and there is a reduction in the rate of production and volume of arousal fluid, making penetrative sex uncomfortable and painful. Itching, irritation and burning can all occur even in the absence of sexual activity, and because the collagen that keeps your skin elastic and supple is oestrogen-dependent, as oestrogen declines so does your ability to hold your wee. Unfortunately, urinary leakage isn't the only bladder symptom that can emerge; an overactive bladder and urinary tract infections are more prevalent too.

In my clinic the most common uterine problem that I treat perimenopausal clients for is abnormal uterine bleeding – bleeding that occurs outside of the normal menstrual cycle that isn't caused by a disease. It can take the form of light continued spotting or be a very heavy flow that seems like it'll never stop and may feature lots of clots that can be large in size. Abnormal uterine bleeding is yet another symptom of oestrogen dominance so it's vital that you reduce oestrogen by making dietary changes, limiting exposure to oestrogen mimickers in the environment such as BPA in plastic is also key, and improving the pathways in the body which allow you to excrete oestrogen. Chinese medicine and/or ATMAT® can work wonders in situations like this to reduce heavy bleeding and prevent anaemia, a common complication which can cause further blood loss, as well as treating the underlying cause. I really wish that these treatments were available through the NHS, because I don't doubt that they would save thousands of people from having unnecessary hysterectomies, a surgical procedure in which the uterus is removed, sometimes in addition to the cervix, fallopian tubes, and ovaries.

Hysterectomy

Though there are menstruators who suffer so much that they're desperate for their uterus to be taken out and who have found having a hysterectomy to be a very positive decision, every person I've spoken to about having a hysterectomy would prefer to keep their uterus as long as their troubling symptoms could be resolved. There's still a tendency for medical professionals to believe that you've got no need for a uterus now that you're over the hill, and that it's only going to cause problems, so why not just whip it out and be done with it? But in my experience, this can cause psychological trauma, particularly when it's a solution that is forced instead of chosen, and when it doesn't address the root of the problem; oestrogen dominance. Now is the time in life to really look at what's going on with oestrogen because, in excess, it can cause plenty of other troublesome symptoms and increases your risk of developing oestrogen-receptor cancers.

Hysterectomy increases your long-term risk of vaginal prolapse and urinary incontinence, but it can become an appropriate course of action when all other treatment options have been exhausted, or if cancer has been detected. But remember that it does not treat endometriosis and will only be helpful in a select number of cases of it. Regardless of age, when the ovaries are removed in addition to the uterus, it instigates an immediate menopause which is referred to as surgical menopause. The loss of ovarian hormones due to menopause is linked to a decline in cardiovascular health and the advancement of conditions such as osteoporosis, dementia, Alzheimer's, and some cancers, and even after natural menopause, research has shown that the ovaries continue to produce hormones that benefit your health, which means that it's a good idea to hang onto your ovaries unless there's a clear medical reason to take them out.

If you've had a hysterectomy but managed to keep your ovaries, then you'll still experience a menstrual cycle, just one that doesn't involve having a period. That means that you can still get PMS and feel a sense of relief as your hormone levels wane when your period would have started, and that you'll also still benefit from experiencing the four inner seasons. Once you begin to experience bouts of amenorrhoea where your period doesn't show up for several months at a time, and you feel that your body is moving beyond its cycling years, you can use the lunar cycle as a way of bringing in a cyclical way of living, and to create scheduled periods for rest and rejuvenation (see page 212).

When oestrogen levels start to fall, the uterus and breasts shrink in size, but prior to that, from 35–45 years of age, women are prone to weight gain more than any other time in their lives, meaning that by the time we hit our perimenopause, most of us are carrying excess weight, and that's a problem because not only does our risk for diabetes and cardiovascular disease jump up at menopause, but carrying excess weight is yet another risk factor for oestrogen dominance because fat cells make their own oestrogen. If you're trying to lose weight, don't limit your intake of healthy fats – you need them to manufacture hormones, and to break down excess stored fat and lose it. They also reduce inflammation and are crucial when it comes to nerve function – which means they promote brain health and your ability to remember where you put that thingamybob.

If you notice that your memory has become abysmal and it feels as if there's a fog clouding your brain, declining oestrogen could be to blame but it could also be the influence of your thyroid. In fact, menstrual irregularities, heavy periods, amenorrhoea, and weight gain are also all signs of perimenopause *and* of hypothyroidism, a condition which increases with age and is more common in women than in men. Up to 45 per cent of the thyroid glands of women over sixty shows signs of hypothyroidism, and up to 20 per cent of women over sixty have subclinical hypothyroidism – that's to say that it isn't detected by clinical tests – so it's worth assessing your thyroid function if these appear in addition to other signs and symptoms associated with the condition, and particularly if you are trying to conceive whilst dancing with perimenopause, because there is an increased risk of miscarriage in those with hypothyroidism (it often takes several miscarriages for it to be picked up).

Your likelihood of having depression does increase in perimenopause, perhaps in response to symptoms such as interrupted sleep and hot flashes, as well as facing adversity in life, and a history of PMS does appear to be a strong predictor of perimenopausal depression – I suspect because the same issues that cause tension in every cycle still remain and are intensified by hormonal fluctuations. But it's important to bear in mind that the Harvard Study of Moods and Cycles found that 83 per cent of women experience no mood changes.

There are a whole host of herbs and supplements that can be invaluable during perimenopause and post-menopause, as can the use of bioidentical hormones and hormone replacement therapy (HRT). Bioidentical hormones can reduce bothersome symptoms such as perimenopausal insomnia and hot flushes. They're hormones which have the same chemical structure as the ones you produce naturally in your body but are derived from an ingredient in Mexican yams – the same source for many a hormonal treatment, including the all singing, all dancing birth control pill. They're prescribed in the form of a cream or lozenge by licensed practitioners, and as they're 100 per cent identical to the hormones you manufacture in your body; they replicate the same effects and benefits.

Discussing the pros and cons of HRT goes well beyond the scope of this book, but here are some key points to consider:

- Despite oestrogen being prescribed for women since the seventies, it wasn't tested on women in clinical trials until 1991. Instead, it was tested on men.
- There are more than 50 types of HRT.
- HRT tends to focus on putting more oestrogen into the body, but perimenopausal symptoms are often a consequence of oestrogen dominance, so question if putting more oestrogen in the body is a good idea. What about using progesterone and androgens such as DHEA and testosterone instead of, or in addition to oestrogen?
- I strongly recommend doing the DUTCH test – an incredibly comprehensive hormone test, see page 237 for more information – prior to starting any HRT or bioidentical hormone treatment because it provides

an unparalleled amount of information about your hormones and how you metabolise them, which will help you and your doctor to figure out what the best options are specifically for you.

- Whether you use bioidentical hormones, HRT, herbs, or vitamins, it really is about finding the right approach and the right dosage, which is why I recommend working with a qualified professional who specialises in menopause.
- One troubling symptom is enough to severely impact your life, and all of the aforementioned methods can make a massive difference to this stage of life, but it's vital that you don't just take HRT, and that stress, diet, and sleep are addressed.

Having high cortisol levels impairs cognitive function and memory, and increases symptoms such as hot flushes, depression, and anxiety. Given how distressing these symptoms are, reducing stress is going to be key when it comes to having healthy cortisol levels, and after decades of caring for others and ending up at the bottom of the list of priorities, it's high time that you took care of yourself. Thankfully, declining oestrogen is going to help you to achieve that, because self-care is no longer open to discussion, it is a must. If you haven't done so already, get really clear about what it is that you want in your life as you transition into the next phase. Make some decisions, even if they're just based on what you don't want because some judicious pruning will make space for the new.

Exercise can work wonders for stress levels, but if you do exercise and you're not coping well with stress, try exercising less and easing up on the intensity of your workouts because they can exacerbate stress hormone imbalances. If your resilience to stress is strong then embrace HIIT workouts as they improve insulin sensitivity, aid weight loss, improve growth hormone levels for building muscle, and increase bone density. Your need for calories is much less than it used to be, and it's better that you get your nutrition from vegetables, healthy fats, and protein, though that doesn't mean that you need to avoid carbs entirely, just don't let them be the majority of your plate and go for complex carbs, not crappy ones.

There's a final push to sort your shit out in perimenopause that working with your cycle can help you to achieve; a sense of urgency to do the inner work required of you before you cross over into your wise years, where you move into a larger consciousness and set the world to rights.

Post-menopause is associated with an improvement in emotional wellbeing, I suspect because we feel more certain of ourselves and our place in the world, stop caring about other people so much, and especially what they think of us. Thanks to the baby boomers and the fact that we're living a lot longer than we used to, there are now more post-menopausal women on the planet than there has ever been; that's a hell of a lot of powerful women and we need their voices in positions of authority.

Not Everyone who Menstruates is a Woman

Periods can be uncomfortable and painful, but if you're trans, non-binary, or intersex, then they can bring the added challenge of gender dysphoria – the distress a person experiences as a result of the sex and gender they were assigned at birth. As trans male model Kenny Jones points out, 'periods make you hyperaware of the parts of your body that don't necessarily feel like "you", it was like my body was saying "by the way, in case you forgot, you're still a biological woman" and I noticed I would get really anxious – my body seemed to know it was about to go through something I didn't like.'

> **Transgender people** are those whose gender identity does not match the sex they were assigned at birth.
>
> **Non-binary** is a way of describing people whose gender identity can't be defined within a male and female gender binary.
>
> **Intersex** is a general term which describes a variety of conditions in which a person is born with reproductive and/or sexual anatomy which doesn't fit the typical definitions of female or male.
>
> **Cis-gender** refers to people whose gender identity matches their assigned sex at birth.

There's an assumption that I frequently run into on social media platforms (usually when someone can't accept that there are people who menstruate who don't identify as female), and that's when they state that if someone doesn't want their period, that they should just take testosterone and stop it. Unfortunately, it's not that simple. Although some people who take testosterone (T) will find that their periods stop soon after they start taking it, it won't work that way for everyone, and as Cass Bliss, aka The Period Prince, a non-binary and trans period activist and artist explains, not everyone will want to take T, and even if they do, they might not have access to it or be able to afford it if it's not available to them through their healthcare system or medical insurance. In terms of how taking T has affected their cycle ('their' is Cass's preferred pronoun), so far Cass's experience has not been great, as they explained in their article for *Seventeen*: 'Before I started testosterone, I had a moderate 3–5-day cycle that came with few side effects. But after 3–4 months on hormones, my period became extremely irregular, lasted up to two weeks, and caused the worse cramps I've ever experienced in my life. This continued for the six months I was on testosterone and hasn't slowed down since I had to stop hormones due to financial and insurance issues.'

For people who take T and find that it does stop their periods, they may still experience menstrual symptoms. Kenny started his medical transition when he was 16 by taking hormone blockers which, after a few months of a gradual diminishing amount of blood loss, eventually stopped his periods. He then switched to taking T when he was 18 and found that he started to experience some pain and spotting for a while. He hasn't bled since he was 19, but at 24 he still occasionally experiences subtle period symptoms such as cramps, bloating and emotional changes.

Cass's website Bleeding While Trans features incredibly helpful reviews of period products and how they measure up for non-female menstruators, in terms of the issues that come up with using particular products, as well as how gendered product packaging is, and how actively companies are affirming a space for all people with periods. They explain that although companies who manufacture period underwear may promote a product that's described as a 'boy short' as being one suitable for all genders, some of them are clearly designed for cis-women to wear and don't take into account the fact that trans menstruators really don't want their butt cheeks peeking out of their underwear. But there are companies like Lunapads and Pyramid Seven who have period boxers that are designed specifically with the needs of menstruators who don't identify as women in mind, and the language and photos on their websites reflect the brands' gender inclusivity.

Cass points out that although having to engage with your genitals to insert a tampon or menstrual cup can result in further dysphoria, using a cup has an advantage in that it can be worn for up to 12 hours which makes using a public toilet a safer prospect. Though Cass explains that: 'The major downside to cups over pads and tampons is that they do require a direct interaction with your menstrual blood when you slide the cup in or pull it out. For me, the discomfort of a cup is far easier to deal with than the panic I used to experience changing my tampon 3–4 times a day in a men's bathroom.'

Self-care during your period is non-negotiable, not just in terms of your physical and mental health but in terms of your personal safety. The risk of physical violence is a very real one to anyone who doesn't conform to the genders that we're assigned at birth, but that risk skyrockets when you're menstruating. Managing your flow in a gendered public bathroom can be fraught with danger because of the very real risk of being outed, and if you're prone to your breasts/chest becoming swollen and/or tender then wearing a chest binder can be so uncomfortable that it's not possible to wear one, which is Cass's experience; 'my boobs would swell which is particularly frustrating as a trans person, it got so bad that I couldn't wear a binder and that meant I would be misgendered a lot'.

Retreating in your Autumn and Winter may be even more necessary for you than it is for cis-women, and keeping track of your cycle can help to plan for when you might want to lay low. Kenny finds that if he misses a couple of days of T (he currently applies a gel every day), his body starts to feel like he's going to come on his period and he prefers to take some time off:

'If I miss a couple of days of T then I start sinking in to myself and don't want to be social. I know that I need a day off to chill and do nothing so I'll reschedule things if I can and try to go with how I feel. There's no point fighting my own body, it only causes me more harm, and I notice that when I sink into myself, that's when I'm most creative. I hated having my period and dealing with it was one of the hardest things I've had to accept about my body, but dramatic times like that are when you can find out who you are and I found peace with it. As much as I wanted to avoid it, I needed to learn about my body so I could take care of myself, and the more I push against it the worse it was. Accepting that I was going to have to live with it was the best decision I've ever made.'

Cass is contacted by a lot of people who don't want to get their period and are considering transitioning medically in order to stop them. As well as cautioning them that they may not get the results they want in the timeframe they imagine, Cass tells them: 'The fact that an organ in your body has the ability to shed its lining every once in a while does not determine who you are as a person, or how the world should recognise you ... Your period does not define who you are.'

Sisters of the Moon

The lunar cycle is 29.5 days in length – strikingly similar to the so-called average menstrual cycle of 28 days, and there's an increasing amount of chatter over social media around synchronising our menstrual cycles with the moon. However, from the research available to us – in this case, the analysis of 7.5 million menstrual cycles by the menstrual app *Clue* – there appears to be no correlation between the two. Even so, there are menstruators who find that their experience of their menstrual cycle is intensified by the phases of the lunar cycle, and who find that charting the two cycles concurrently is both helpful and profound.

Working with the lunar cycle is particularly advantageous during phases of life when periods cease; in bouts of amenorrhoea, using hormonal birth control, pregnancy, breastfeeding, during perimenopause when cycles become less frequent, and post-menopause when you've stopped bleeding. The lunar cycle is also a wonderful tool if you've had a hysterectomy or if you're a transwoman who wants to work with a cycle. Michaela, a post-menopausal client of mine, was relieved that her heavy periods had finally come to an end but found that she felt at sea without the presence of her menstrual cycle, 'even though I always had horrifically heavy periods and I was glad to see the back of them, I miss having a cycle because I took great care of myself in my Winter and knew how to play to my strengths in the other phases. When my cycle stopped I was feeling ungrounded but using the moon's cycle has made me feel anchored and allowed me to experience a rhythm again. It makes me stop and take a breath, to pay attention to my energy, my desires and needs.'

In each phase of the lunar cycle, there are qualities and actions which mirror those of the seasons of the menstrual cycle, as Sarah Gottesdiener, an artist, designer and writer who creates and publishes the cult classic workbooks *Many Moons*, explains:

'*During the New Moon we set intentions, during the Waxing phase we take practical steps to move forward, during the Full Moon we celebrate, affirm, aim even higher; during the Waning Moon we release, work through blocks, and get rid of that which is no longer serving us; and the Dark Moon is a time for finality. While the Moon is from New to Full, the focus is on growing, building, and protecting. While the Moon changes from Full to Dark, our work centres on releasing and letting go.*'

If you aren't menstruating and want to work with the moon, these are how the seasons of the menstrual cycle correspond to the phases of the lunar cycle:

- Menstruation/Winter is the time of the New Moon.
- Pre-ovulation/Spring is during the Waxing Moon.
- Ovulation/Summer is the time of the Full Moon.
- Premenstruum/Autumn is during the Waning Moon.
- The Dark Moon is the void time before and at the start of Winter.

Sarah has generously allowed me to use her words from *Many Moons* to describe the phases of the lunar cycle here:

New Moon (menstruation, Winter)

This is the time from when the moon can't be seen and appears completely dark, to its first sliver of a smile. The glimmering hint of possibilities is shown to us, igniting hope and imparting new beginnings. It's a wonderful time to set new intentions, for beginning new projects, for interviewing for jobs, and for allowing new opportunities to unfold. It's this phase of the lunar cycle that's perfect for career advancement, creative endeavours, and for love and romance. Plant the seeds of hope, faith, and optimism. Gather resources, schedule meetings, strategise, and formulate your ideas.

Waxing Moon (pre-ovulation, Spring)

As the Moon continues to grow it reaches its first quarter, where exactly half of what's visible to us is illuminated. If the time during the New Moon was about planting seeds and gestating in hope and optimism, the Waxing period is about putting the pedal to the metal and bringing your work out into the world. You're surrounded by resources, so begin building what you wish to see, hear, and touch around you. This period is good for attraction, amplified success, and fertility. Build structures, better habits, network, and launch your new project during this time.

Full Moon (ovulation, Summer)
The Moon is now at her fullest and the entire sunlit part of the Moon is facing us, while the shadowed portion is entirely hidden from view. Reach for what you want, draw down the energy of the Moon and sit with her. Give thanks and pay attention to your instincts. Think about what would transpire in your life if absolutely nothing could go wrong; if everything you wanted was in front of you, just waiting for you to choose it. Gather with others if you are energetically inclined to, throw a dinner party or invite loved ones over for a craft night. Create a supportive Moon circle where you can all share your intentions and send them out into the universe, amplified. The Full Moon is a great time to draw in energy and reconnect to what it is that you want to see happen in your life.

Waning Moon (premenstruum, Autumn)
The Moon is now waning and journeying from Full to New. This phase is about getting things in order that are not in order; paperwork, doctor's appointments, closets. Creating space to bring in new opportunities, thought patterns, and positive people and experiences that will help you. But first you yourself need to get moving and make space for the new! This is the time to do so. Energetically you might feel tired or low. Recognise the importance of quietude. Spend more time resting or sleeping, more time listening. This is a wonderful time to go inward and connect with your intuition – ask your intuition questions and listen for the answers. It's ok to say goodbye and write the letter you will never send. Forgiving yourself and others, as well as making amends internally are opportune exercises at this time. The Waning Moon favours releasing yourself from any pulls to other people, places, and the past, to close the door on what no longer serves us.

Dark Moon (the hours and days before and at the start of Winter):
The Dark Moon is when the last slivers of the Waning Moon have gone, and the Moon is in darkness. The two or three days of void time before she appears

again. It is the time to practice concentrated rest. Take a long bath, lay down and close your eyes. Focus on being quiet and sleeping more. Our culture does not often allow us to prioritise rest. Yet now is the time we need it more than ever. Can you give yourself one or two days of committed rest and relaxation during the Dark Moon time?

Paying attention to the phases of the lunar cycle and living in tune with them allows non-menstruators to benefit from the containers created by cyclic living, the most beneficial of which is often time dedicated to rest and rejuvenation.

SECTION THREE

TREAT YO'SELF

Let's get down to business and talk about actually sorting your cycle out. There are lots of things that you can do to improve your periods and support your reproductive health, on your own and with the support of a qualified practitioner, but before we get on to them, I want to make it clear that the act of tracking your cycle is an incredible act of self-care in itself, and you'll see massive improvements solely being aware of and working with your cycle.

The world of wellness can be confusing and overwhelming. There's lots of conflicting research as well as trends that come and go, so my aim with this is to give you the information you need to make decisions about your health. Try things out and see how they feel; it is 100 per cent okay to cherry pick your way through this section and see what will work for you right now, and what won't. When it comes to making changes, here are my recommendations:

- **Make one change at a time and take your time**
  If you try to do several things all at once, it'll be a shock to your nervous system and result in you feeling stressed, which is exactly what we're trying to avoid. Slow gradual change is usually more long-lasting than a sudden one.
- **Start by adding a behaviour in**
  There's a tendency to focus on what you shouldn't do, but I find it's easier to start to make a change by adding in a behaviour rather than getting rid of one, then once you're on a roll and feeling some positive benefits, you can work on something that you want to limit or cut out.
- **Start small by chunking things up**
  When you have a large long-term goal it can feel overwhelming, so breaking it up into smaller goals feels entirely more manageable. Newbie runners don't start off training for a marathon by running 26.2 miles, they start with a couch to 10k programme. How can you use a similar approach to achieve your goals?

- **Make a plan that will stick**
  When it comes to making a successful change, the devil really is in the details, so get out some pen and paper and come up with a plan that leaves you feeling motivated and prepared. What do you want to change? What are the positive outcomes if you succeed? What are the negatives if you don't make this change? What time of day will you do it? What could get in the way of achieving your goal and what do you need to get in place in order to prevent this from happening? Put your plan somewhere visible so that you continue to be inspired by it.

- **Involve a buddy**
  Sharing your plans with a friend, colleague, or family member will give you someone to be accountable to so you're more likely to follow through with them, and – even better – they might join in.

- **Ask for support**
  You don't have to do it alone. There are a whole host of support groups out there (you could even start your own), and loved ones are often very willing to help if you let them know what's going on and accept their help. Qualified practitioners can help you get off to a good start and use techniques to enhance your efforts. If you don't feel that working with a practitioner is within your budget, check out local colleges and universities to see if they have student clinics, where student practitioners gain clinical experience under the direction and supervision of their teachers. Student clinics and community projects are a significantly cheaper option.

- **Do a Jerry**
  Consistency in our daily actions is what leads to success, and my favourite tool to achieve this is to use a method that comedian Jerry Seinfeld uses to keep him motivated to write jokes every day, and it's this: Get a wall calendar that has a whole year on one page and hang it somewhere where you're forced to look at it, and every day that you carry out your intended behaviour – not skipping breakfast, walking a mile, taking a nutritional supplement – you take a red marker and put a big red X over that day, and after a few days a series of crosses start to form a chain, and the longer it gets the better it feels, and the harder it will be to break it. The key is to not break the chain.

Chapter 8

Self-care

Caring for myself is not self-indulgence, it is self-preservation, and that is an act of political warfare.
– Audre Lorde

Self-care is a loaded phrase these days, or should I say; hashtag. The line between indulgence and self-care is a blurred and debated one, but what you'll find in this chapter is self-care at a fundamental level:

- Staying hydrated.
- Eating well, and I don't just mean what you eat, it's how you eat too.
- Optimising your digestion.
- Getting decent sleep.
- Avoiding hormone disruptors in your food and environment.

No Guts, No Glory

When I meet with a new client and we go over the issues that they have with their reproductive health, my next path of enquiry is to find out what's going on with their gut, because, as you're about to read, healthy digestion makes for a happy life, but it's a tricky topic because not everyone wants to go there. When I ask what a client's digestion is like, the most common answer is, 'It's fine.' with punctuation that suggests that's the end of the sentence *and* the topic. But we have to go there, because without optimal digestion, you will struggle to achieve hormonal health, no matter what you eat.

When your gut is in great shape it extracts and uses the nutrients in the food you eat, your immune system will be strong, and you're able to detoxify and eliminate waste with ease. When your gut is struggling it can cause digestive upsets such as constipation, loose stools, bloating, and gas, but digestive complaints are only the beginning. When your digestive function is compromised it can also cause hormonal imbalances, skin conditions, recurrent infections, depression and other mental health conditions.

Eating diets that are traditional such as the Mediterranean and Japanese diets is linked to lower rates of depression when compared to the average Western diet, which tends to be high in calories but low in nutrients, and there are a few reasons why there's such a strong link between depression and diet. Let's talk about serotonin first; serotonin is a wonderful molecule within the body that you may have heard of, it functions as a neurotransmitter and as a hormone. It's implicated in just about every type of behaviour such as appetite, sleep, and mood. There's a link between low levels of serotonin and depression and obesity, and selective serotonin reuptake inhibitors (SSRIs) are commonly prescribed for depression. Now, here's where it gets interesting; 95 per cent of serotonin is manufactured in the cells of the digestive tract, so if you want to feel good in yourself and maintain a healthy weight, it's essential that you improve your diet and digestion. Depression can also be due to chronic inflammation in the body. There are a whole host of reasons why people suffer from depression, including traumatic life events, but it's thought that at least 30 per cent of all cases of depression feature an elevated presence of C-reactive protein and cytokines – inflammatory markers which appear in the bloodstreams of people who are depressed but are otherwise healthy. Care to hazard a guess at where this inflammation starts? Yup, the gut.

Generation Inflammation

Inflammation in the body is a good thing in certain circumstances, such as if we've been wounded or come into contact with an infectious illness. Your body deals with potential threats to it all day long and when it detects a hazard, an inflammatory response is initiated that causes an increase in temperature, redness, swelling, and pain, all of which are the immune system's way of limiting the effects of harmful substances and pathogens that find their way into the body. But we don't want inflammation to take hold in the body because persistent low-grade inflammation causes food intolerances, eczema, brain fog, weight gain, fatigue, depression, anxiety, insomnia, migraines, and fibromyalgia (a chronic health condition which features widespread pain, a heightened pain response, and profound fatigue). Inflammation is also important to address if you have period pain, PMS, PCOS, fibroids, endometriosis, adenomyosis, and breast tenderness or cysts.

Poor sleep can cause inflammation, as can a diet that's full of inflammatory foods and drinks. Sugar, alcohol, processed foods, and beige foods like pasta and bread can all cause inflammation, and while supplements such as probiotics, turmeric, resveratrol, Omega-3 Fatty Acids, liposomal glutathione, N-Acetyl Cysteine, and bioflavonoids like green tea and grapeseed extract can all help to reduce inflammation, there's no point in taking them without addressing your dietary exposure to the substances that cause the inflammation in the first place. Following an anti-inflammatory diet that avoids common culprits will help most people, but if you want to go the whole hog, and especially if you suspect that you have food intolerances and sensitivities, consider an elimination diet.

Set Things Straight: Eliminate

No current food sensitivity test is as accurate as the elimination diet. It's an affordable way of assessing food sensitivities and it puts you in touch with your body – something that a pricey blood test won't do. Admittedly, it can be challenging and takes commitment, so it's worth really planning for it way in advance by planning and preparing your meals, and of course starting it at the ideal time in your menstrual cycle; your Spring.

The autoimmune paleo protocol is what I recommend following. In the first phase the foods that most commonly cause problems are eliminated, including: grains, dairy, sugar, alcohol, nuts, seeds, and nightshade vegetables (aubergine, tomato, bell peppers, and white potatoes). To be thorough, they should be excluded for at least three weeks before moving to the second phase of reintroducing them one at a time, in which you eat each one for four days by consuming approximately three servings per day, or less if they cause a big reaction, then you remove it again and see if how you react resolves before moving on to the next food. This approach means three weeks of restricted eating, but around three months of careful eating in total. Gentle reintroduction allows you to keep track of how you feel after eating these foods again and if they cause a negative reaction such as pain, headaches, digestive issues, skin issues, nasal congestion, fatigue, brain fog, weight gain, mood changes, this lets you know what you need to exclude on a more permanent basis. It's hard work to begin with, but fascinating. I've managed to do this once, and being someone who only gets one or two headaches a year (usually of the adult variety), I was astounded at the headaches I got once I brought dairy back in, not to mention the sneezing and abundance of snot coming out of my nose. Prior to eliminating them, I was largely unaware of the effect they had on me, which is why I suggest doing the protocol once in a while, as our dietary sensitivities can change throughout our lifetime. I also really recommend doing it if you have a condition like endometriosis, interstitial cystitis, pelvic pain, and vulvodynia. If you have a history of disordered eating then I don't recommend doing an elimination diet as you could find that the restrictive element triggers you. If you have a condition called leaky gut then consider if an elimination diet could end up being a depressing venture for you if you discover that you react to a lot of foods, or if you'll find it empowering while you work on healing your gut.

Leaky Gut

The surface area of the lining of your gut is gigantic; it's the size of a tennis court and it's highly permeable so that you can maximise your ability to absorb nutrients. It also has to protect you from contaminants and pathogens, and one way it does this is by distinguishing whether a substance is friend or foe before it allows it to penetrate the intestinal wall and enter the bloodstream. There are tight junctions between the intestinal cells in order to achieve this; a bit like having a tightly-guarded narrow door to a nightclub – everyone outside wants in but the people at the door decide who comes in, and who doesn't. Stress, infections, toxins, and age can make the tight cell junctions that form your intestinal wall break apart, causing a condition called leaky gut in which undigested food, bacteria and toxins permeate the lining of the small intestine and enter the bloodstream, triggering the immune system and causing inflammation. It's like the security team getting a bit slack and leaving the door wide open, and then someone leaves the emergency exit open too, and before you know it, the club's full of troublemakers.

In some people inflammatory foods such as gluten and dairy cause a leaky gut, but other potential causes include; trans fats that are found in fried foods, sugar and artificial sweeteners, alcohol, processed oils such as canola, corn, sunflower, and margarine, emotional and/or physical stress (including intense exercise and dehydration), not chewing enough, candida overgrowth, a condition called small intestinal bacterial overgrowth (SIBO) which can cause IBS, intestinal parasites, exposure to environmental toxins such as pesticides and BPA, and the use of some medications such as ibuprofen and antibiotics. Signs and symptoms of a leaky gut include:

- Digestive issues such as bloating, gas, diarrhoea, irritable bowel syndrome (IBS), inflammatory bowel diseases (Crohn's, ulcerative colitis).
- Food allergies or intolerances.
- Mental health issues such as depression, anxiety, ADD or ADHD.
- Hormonal imbalances like PMS and PCOS.
- Seasonal allergies or asthma.
- Skin complaints like acne or eczema.
- Diagnosis of an autoimmune disease.
- Diagnosis of candida overgrowth.
- Diagnosis of chronic fatigue or fibromyalgia.

Following an elimination diet in which you remove foods that commonly cause a leaky gut gives your digestive system time to heal. It's a great way of assessing if you have any food sensitivities, even in the absence of any troubling symptoms, and following an anti-inflammatory diet will benefit most of us in some way. But there's one more dietary-related intolerance that you should know about, and that's histamine intolerance.

Histamine Intolerance

You've probably heard of histamine – it's the chemical produced when you have allergies and it causes an immediate inflammatory response. Taking an anti-histamine drug like Piriton® or Benedryl® provides relief because it dials down the inflammatory response created by histamine by reducing histamine's action. But if your body doesn't break down histamine properly, you can develop a condition called histamine intolerance in which eating foods which are rich in histamine or which cause a release of histamine results in an annoying bunch of symptoms, including:

- Headaches and migraines
- Nasal congestion and sneezing
- Flushing and sweating

- Difficulty breathing
- Dizziness or vertigo
- Anxiety
- Insomnia
- Brain fog
- Hypertension
- Abdominal cramps
- Nausea and vomiting
- Fatigue
- Swelling
- Breast tenderness
- Period pain

It's a hard condition to spot because its symptoms are varied, and not many people know about it. I had symptoms of it for ten years before I learned about histamine intolerance and the penny finally dropped – and I work in the field and have been treated by plenty of practitioners in that time. It's also a frustrating condition because, as you'll see shortly, loads of food and drinks that are meant to be really healthy for you actually cause symptoms, which is incredibly frustrating when you're putting a lot of money and effort into improving your diet. Histamine rich foods which can cause a reaction include:

- Fermented food and drink such as wine, champagne, beer, kombucha (a fermented tea which has a slight fizziness to it), kefir (a fermented drink traditionally made with milk which has the consistency of a drinkable yoghurt), sauerkraut, sourdough, sour cream, buttermilk, yoghurt, soy sauce.
- Bone broth.
- Vinegar (apple cider vinegar, wine vinegar, pickles, mayonnaise).
- Cured meats (bacon, pepperoni, salami, prosciutto).
- Dried fruit (apricots, figs, prunes, raisins).
- Most citrus fruits.
- Some vegetables (aubergine, avocado, spinach, tomatoes).
- Some nuts (cashews, walnuts).
- Smoked fish and some species of fish (mackerel, tuna, sardines, anchovies).
- Aged cheese.

Histamine-releasing foods include:

- Alcohol
- Bananas
- Chocolate
- Cow's milk
- Papaya
- Pineapple
- Shellfish
- Strawberries
- Tomatoes

High histamine levels can be caused by allergies, SIBO, leaky gut, and deficiency of an enzyme called diamine oxidase (DAO) which helps to break histamine down. Low DAO can be caused by gluten intolerance, leaky gut, SIBO, Crohn's disease, ulcerative colitis, inflammatory bowel disease, and some types of medication such as NSAIDs, antidepressants, and anti-histamines. And alcohol, energy drinks, and black and green teas can all block the action of DAO so that it's harder for your body to break histamine down.

Oestrogen stimulates the production of histamine and also suppresses the action of DAO, which means symptoms of histamine intolerance often get worse at the points in the cycle where oestrogen is high in relation to progesterone; at ovulation and just before menstruation. It doesn't help that histamine also stimulates the production of oestrogen which results in more histamine production – a truly vicious cycle.

You can test for histamine intolerance by following an elimination diet which prioritises the food and drink listed above and then reintroducing them to see how you respond to them. Your doctor can also test your blood for histamine levels and for DAO, though blood testing should be done when you've been eating histamine-rich and histamine producing foods, not after you've eliminated them. As well as avoiding foods that trigger it, supplements such as magnesium, vitamin B6, SAMe, quercetin, and DAO can be used to treat it, and supporting regular ovulation is important because progesterone stimulates production of DAO, which is why symptoms often improve as progesterone levels increase after ovulation. Due to the high amount of progesterone that's produced in pregnancy, which stimulates

DAO production, symptoms often get better or disappear entirely during pregnancy and then reappear afterwards.

Once you've figured out what foods don't agree with you, you can get to work on repairing your gut and rebalancing your microbiome – the helpful microorganisms in your body.

Only 10 per cent Human

You harbour a vast array of bacteria, fungi, viruses, and other microbes. There's over 100 trillion microorganisms living in and on your body and they outnumber your own cells ten to one. They might sound like they're a force to battle and destroy but your particular population of microbes – your microbiome – is hugely beneficial to you. Not only do they make up the bulk of your immune system, but 99 per cent of metabolic functions in the body are carried out by bacterial DNA, and your microbiome has its own endocrine system – it produces and secretes every single hormone in the body, as well as responding to the hormones produced by our own cells and regulating them. There's even a set of bacteria in the gut called the oestrobolome and when the oestrobolome is out of balance your body reabsorbs oestrogen that was meant to be excreted via your intestines and poo, and it ends up being recirculated in your bloodstream instead, which leads to oestrogen dominance (see page 235).

Needless to say, when your microbiome is out of whack, it causes pandemonium in the body. Antibiotic exposure during your mum's labour with you or at any other point in your life, being born by caesarean, not being breastfed, eating processed foods, and a lack of diversity in your diet all negatively influence the health of your microbiome and how diverse it is, and the more diverse it is the better.

Getting the Microbiome off to the Right Start

If you're pregnant, please consider how you can help your kid's microbiome get off to the best start, because the health of your vaginal microbiome in pregnancy, as well as what happens during labour, birth, and immediately afterwards are what determine your baby's microbiome for life. There are numerous ways of supporting your child's microbiome, even if you have a caesarean birth and decide to feed your baby formula. These include:

- Before and during pregnancy; don't use anti-bacterial washes and hand sanitisers, avoid unnecessary antibiotics, improve gut function, and eat sweet potatoes and squash (and fermented foods if they agree with you).
- Avoid antibiotics in labour because your baby will also receive a small dose and they are associated with an increase in infant gut microbiome dysfunction. So many women are given them prophylactically 12–24 hours after their waters break ('prolonged' rupture of membranes) or when they have an epidural and develop a fever, which can be a sign of infection which would warrant the use of antibiotics. But simply having an epidural can also cause your temperature to spike. Thankfully there are some NHS trusts who are sensible enough to want there to be two clinical indicators of an infection before administering antibiotics.
- A vaginal birth is preferable to a caesarean birth because as your baby moves through your birth canal and comes out of the vagina it comes into contact with your vaginal and faecal bacteria. This is hugely beneficial because it's these bacteria which colonise your baby's gut, rather than the bacteria in the hospital environment. Cleaning the perineum, or heaven forbid, applying anti-microbial products to them, can interfere with this crucial exposure.
- If you have a caesarean birth, there are ways in which you can protect and 'seed' your baby's microbiome, including:
  - Tell your obstetrician that you only consent to antibiotics being administered *after* your baby has been born. Whilst a caesarean is surgery which absolutely necessitates the use of antibiotics to prevent infection, there is no reason why they can't be given to you immediately after your baby comes out so that your baby isn't exposed to them.
  - Use a vaginal swab to 'seed' your baby's microbiome by taking a piece of sterile gauze which has been soaked in sterile saline, folding it up concertina-style into a tampon shape and inserting it into your

vagina. Leave it in place for an hour, remove just prior to surgery, and store it in a sterile container. Then, immediately after your baby has been born, the midwife caring for your baby should apply the swab to your baby's mouth, followed by their face and the rest of their body so that they are coated in your bacteria. In my experience of being at hundreds of births, most in-labour caesareans aren't actually emergencies and there is usually plenty of time before going into theatre to do this, but if you have a true emergency caesarean in which you really wouldn't have time to do it, this process can be carried out afterwards.

- Babies born at home and who are exclusively breastfed have the most beneficial gut microbiome. If, for whatever reason, you don't breastfeed, consider giving your baby a probiotic which includes *Bifidobacterium infantis*, a key bacterium that's present in breastmilk and which dominates the gut microbiome of babies who are breastfed, but thanks to generations of formula feeding, caesarean births and use of antibiotics, has diminished greatly. It's worth giving to your baby even if you breastfeed because people in developed countries have significantly less *B. infantis* than those in developing countries, and it's passed down through generations, which means if you weren't breastfed and the chain of inheritance was broken, then you won't have it to pass on to your child.

- After birth, your baby's microbiome continues to be colonised, so lots of skin-to-skin contact and naked time together is beneficial (and is also a great way to keep people you don't want around away), as is not washing them. Seriously, they do not need to be cleaned. Wait at least a week before bathing your baby and when you do, don't use anything other than plain old brilliant water.

- Let your kids eat dirt – something they seem genetically programmed to do. In the past we wouldn't have scrubbed our vegetables so scrupulously, and we would have benefitted from the bugs that coated them, but these days we don't eat 'dirty' food and nor do we get dirty like we used to. There are more microorganisms in a teaspoon of dirt than there are people on the planet, so let your kid eat some.

The great news is that your microbiome responds quickly to lifestyle changes, sometimes in as little as four days, so if you want to improve yours, do the following:

- Eat a wide variety of different unprocessed foods.
- Make fermented foods like sauerkraut and kimchi and eat a spoonful of them every day (unless you're histamine intolerant that is).
- Up your intake of foods which are rich in prebiotics – types of dietary fibre such as sweet potato, carrots, and squash, which feed the good bacteria in your gut.

Antibiotics

Antibiotics can save lives, but they are overused and antibiotic resistance is a very real concern. Just one round of antibiotics has the potential to wipe out an entire species of your gut bacteria, and antimicrobial products such as hand sanitisers not only disrupt your hormones and are linked to fertility issues, but they also encourage antibiotic resistance. It's far better to actually wash your hands with soap and water, or just let go of the need to be overly clean (unless of course you work in a field where hygiene is paramount), because over 95 per cent of bacteria are harmless to humans, and many are helpful. Be mindful that livestock are routinely given antibiotics to prevent infections that they're at risk of catching due to the squalid 'living' conditions that they're kept in, so buy organic meat where possible, or from a source where you know about the meat's provenance.

A diet made up of processed foods that's filled with sugar and alcohol and absent in fibre messes with your gut's microbiome, but a diet high in vegetables and fibre helps your gut flora to flourish. Probiotics feed your gut bacteria, support weight loss, and reduce inflammation. Lack of sleep and stress both damage your microbiome, but fermented foods like sourdough bread, sauerkraut, and kimchi, and fermented drinks such as kefir and kombucha (which are available in health food shops but are easily made at home too, *see* Resources) encourage the growth of helpful bacteria – though if you have a histamine intolerance they could trigger your symptoms.

If you absolutely need to take antibiotics, take them, but be sure to help your gut bacteria rebalance afterwards. Antibiotics are usually prescribed for urinary tract infections (UTIs) but this isn't advisable as the most common risk factor for developing recurrent UTIs is the use of broad-spectrum antibiotics which are used to treat infections such as recurrent UTIs. But there are some simple remedies which you can keep in your cupboard to treat UTIs:

- Drinking homemade lemon barley water drastically reduces symptoms within 24 hours and resolves them entirely soon after. You can make it by taking 150g of pearl barley and rinsing it until the water runs clear, then place in a saucepan along with the zest of two lemons, 1 tbsp of grated ginger, and 2.5 pints of water. Bring to the boil and turn down to a gentle simmer for ten minutes. Remove from the heat, strain and save the liquid, then add the juice of the two lemons (and 4 tbsp of honey, optional). Set aside to cool and drink at room temperature throughout your day.
- D-Mannose, the active ingredient in cranberries and other types of fruit such as apples, peaches, oranges and blueberries, can be taken as a supplement and is preferable to store-bought cranberry juice, which contains a lot of sugar that aggravates UTIs.
- If you get recurrent UTIs, evaluate the health of your microbiome, particularly if you've been taking antibiotics which have killed off the beneficial bacteria as well as the bad. Your bladder has its own community of microorganisms, but it's important to address your gut microbiome as when it comes to location-specific communities in your microbiome, such as the bladder, it's your gut microbiome which acts as central command.

SIBO: When Bacteria Go Wild

Your bacteria are fabulous, they're an integral part of you, but they need to know their place. Most of them are meant to hang out in your large intestine and colon, but when they head on up to your small intestine, or the ones that should be in your small intestine overgrow, they start to feed on the undigested food transiting through your small intestine and cause a condition called small intestinal bacterial overgrowth (SIBO). Causes of SIBO include:

- The presence of an infection.
- An underactive thyroid.
- Physical obstructions such as scarring from surgeries or Crohn's disease.

- Damage to the nerves and muscles in the gut.
- The use of antibiotics and steroids.
- A decrease in the amount of stomach acid, due to: the ageing process, the presence of a bacterium called Helicobacter pylori in the stomach, diluting them by drinking too much fluid alongside meals, and the use of drugs used to treat heartburn such as; antacids (Rennies® and Pepto-Bismol®), histamine receptor (H2) blockers which increase the risk of SIBO by up to 17 per cent, and proton-pump inhibitors like lansoprazole, omeprazole, and esomeprazole which raise SIBO risk by 53 per cent.
- Some experts believe there to be an association between the use of oral contraceptives and the incidence of SIBO (fingers crossed for some research on this).
- A diet that's full of sugar, carbs and booze – their favourite meal! When they feed on these delicious substances, they cause them to ferment, a process which creates hydrogen, which, in turn, feeds microbes in your small intestine called archaea. As archaea gobble up hydrogen, they produce methane, which means that with SIBO you can have an excess of both hydrogen and methane in your digestive tract, leaving you with a hell of a lot of gas. Bloating, burping, and farting are all symptoms of SIBO, as are:
  - Diarrhoea
  - Constipation
  - Abdominal pain
  - Food intolerances such as gluten, lactose, casein, fructose
  - Histamine intolerance
  - Leaky gut
  - Diagnosis of IBS or inflammatory bowel disease
  - Vitamin and mineral deficiencies
  - Fat malabsorption
  - Reacting negatively to probiotics which contain *Lactobacillus* or *Bifidobacterium* (because they increase your bacteria and exacerbate the problem)

If you've got IBS, then there's a strong chance that you have SIBO, as it's been found in 80 per cent of IBS cases and is thought to be a cause of it. The best way to test for SIBO is by doing a breath test where you fast for 12 hours, eat some sugar and then breathe into a small balloon every 15 minutes for 3 hours, so that your breath can be tested for hydrogen and methane. Your urine can also be tested but won't provide information about which gas is the problem. Treatment involves starving the bacteria of their preferred foods such as alcohol and sugar, then using antibiotics or herbal antimicrobials such as berberine to kill the bacteria off (the latter clearly being the preferred route because antibiotics don't discriminate and wipe out more than is necessary). After that you can carefully begin to restore the good bacteria by eating fermented foods and using a SIBO-friendly probiotic such as those that are soil-based.

Detox Like A Pro

The aim with oestrogen is to use it and lose it, and your liver is in charge of getting rid of it. When the liver can't do its thing, you end up with excess oestrogen in your bloodstream and that leads to PMS, heavy periods, bloating, water retention, menstrual migraines, and puts you at greater risk of developing breast cancer. To do its job well, your liver doesn't need an extreme spring clean once a year, it needs year-round support. Liver detoxification takes place continually in your body and it's how your body takes oestrogen that's no longer needed and gets rid of it. It does this in two phases; during the first it breaks oestrogen down into smaller units called metabolites, and in the second it changes the metabolites from fat-loving molecules into water-soluble ones. Steroid hormones such as oestrogen are fat-loving and don't dissolve in water so they can't pass easily into your urine, so various enzymes convert them into water-soluble metabolites which can then enter your urine and bile so that they can be excreted. The trouble is, there are different pathways that the oestrogen metabolites can go down. Some are healthy and some are associated with heavy periods, tender breasts, PMS, and hormone-dependent cancers, so it's important to encourage the healthy pathways. That's the short and extremely simplified version of oestrogen detoxification. Here's the more detailed picture of each phase:

Phase 1: Preparation
In this phase your liver does the prep work that's needed in order for you to then get rid of oestrogen by breaking oestrogen down into smaller units. It takes oestradiol and oestrone (the two main forms of oestrogen in your body) and converts them into one of three oestrogen metabolites: 2OH, 4OH,

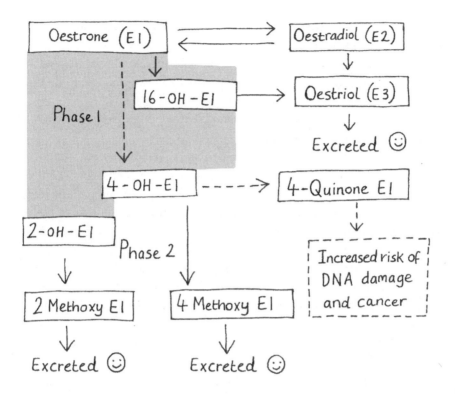

and 16OH. But let's just call them routes 2, 4, and 16. Of these metabolite pathways, route 2 is the safer route. Route 4 *can* be okay, but it has a pitchfork in it, and it's only an okay route if it goes down the right pathway; if it goes down the pathway in which an enzyme called quinone converts it, then your risk for oestrogen-based cancers goes up. Route 16 is the pathway to avoid because it's associated with heavy periods, clots, tender breasts, and an increased risk of oestrogen-based cancers such as breast cancer – it's the pathway that makes things grow; the lining of your womb, your boobs, and cancerous cells.

Phase 1 is inhibited by nutritional deficiency, low protein intake, drinking alcohol, heavy metal build-up, and using medications like paracetamol, and you can support the 2OH pathway and encourage phase 1 detox by eating cruciferous vegetables like broccoli, kale and cauliflower which contain diindolyl-methane (DIM). DIM promotes healthy oestrogen detoxification by reducing the formation of the 4OH and 16OH metabolites and increasing the 2OH metabolites, and it can be taken as a supplement. Other supplements which can support this phase include; liposomal glutathione, N-Acetyl Cysteine, and resveratrol.

At the end of phase 1, you're left with phase 1 metabolites which you now need to get rid of before they recirculate and give you grief, and to do that a reaction needs to take place.

Phase 2: Addition (methylation)
Next up comes the phase where the oestrogen metabolites from phase 1 are added to. Prior to this phase oestrogen is fat-soluble, so think about if you were to fill a bathtub up with water, pour oil into it, and then pull the plug – what happens? The water goes out but the oil clings to the side of the tub and won't go down the drain. In phase 2, the oestrogen metabolites gain a water-loving molecule which makes them water-soluble, and therefore able to leave the body via your urine, bile and intestines. During methylation they gain a methyl group of atoms and go from being 2OH and 4OH into 2Methoxy and 4Methoxy, the change in name reflecting that they are now water-soluble.

Dr. Carrie Jones uses the bathtub analogy to explain phases 1 and 2 of liver detoxification: water filling up the bathtub is phase 1, and the ability of your body to get it out is phase 2. In order to reduce symptoms of oestrogen dominance and reduce your risk of developing oestrogen dominant cancers, both pathways need to be working optimally – the right water should be filling your tub up *and* your drain should be able to get rid of it.

When phase 2 isn't working as well as it could, oestrogen metabolites can't leave the body and the 4OH metabolite goes down the not-so-great quinone enzyme pathway, potentially increasing your cancer risk. Genetic factors can impair this process so genetic testing of these markers can help you to understand how you methylate your hormones, and exposure to chemicals in your diet, personal care products, and environment can all limit your liver's ability to do its job well. Sulphur-rich foods such as eggs, garlic, onions, leeks, mushrooms and cruciferous vegetables, as well as supplements like S-adenosylmethionine (SAMe), magnesium, and methylated B vitamins can support the methylation process, and staying hydrated will clearly help you to excrete the metabolites. Limiting exposure to environmental chemicals in your food, personal care products, and home and workplace is important because they impact on your liver's ability to do its job well.

Oestrogen isn't all bad though; it's actually a really great hormone that's responsible for over 400 processes in the body and which comes with lots of health benefits such as protecting your heart, brain, and bones, improving mood, keeping your vagina moist, and making the lining of your uterus plump up every month in preparation for pregnancy. You just don't want it lurking around your body. We all need to consider how we detox oestrogen because we're all exposed to it through the food we eat and in the environment, and even more so if you get symptoms of excess oestrogen, which you're more prone to having if you're in your teens, are perimenopausal, or if you have endometriosis.

Excess Oestrogen

Symptoms of excess oestrogen can show up when it's high in relation to progesterone so it's important to evaluate what's going on with both hormones. Remember, it's progesterone that keeps oestrogen in check, so not ovulating regularly or not producing enough progesterone after ovulation can result in excess oestrogen.

> **Note:** You can have low levels of oestrogen, but if it's high in relation to progesterone, you can still have signs of excess oestrogen, so it's all about the relationship between the two hormones.

Signs and symptoms of excess oestrogen include:

- Heavy menstrual bleeding
- Breast tenderness
- Cysts
- PMS
- Painful periods
- Endometriosis
- Fibroids
- Menstrual migraines

- Mood swings and irritability
- Moodiness and meltdowns
- Depression
- Weepiness
- Mid-cycle pain
- Brain fog
- Weight gain around the middle
- Bloating, puffiness or water retention
- Abnormal smear tests

Oestrogen imbalance can be caused by:

- Anovulatory cycles (common during teen years and perimenopause)
- PCOS
- Impaired oestrogen detoxification
- Poor diet
- Histamine intolerance
- Gut issues like constipation
- High levels of cortisol competing for and blocking progesterone receptors
- Environmental toxins such as BPA and phthalates that are commonly found in plastics, which mimic oestrogen and interfere with its action in the body
- Alcohol consumption
- Weight gain and obesity (because fat cells produce excess oestrogen)
- Diabetes
- Some autoimmune conditions

You can address oestrogen imbalance by:

- Supporting liver detoxification and improving gut function.
- Increasing your intake of dietary fibre to support oestrogen detoxification via your colon (and poo).
- Increasing your water intake to support oestrogen detoxification via your wee.
- Getting some decent shut-eye. There's a relationship between a disruption to the circadian rhythm and the incidence of breast and colo-rectal cancer,

which is thought to be because of reduced melatonin secretion and an increase in light exposure at night.
- Reducing alcohol intake.
- Exercising, particularly types which are high intensity and make you sweat.
- Losing excess weight.
- Eating broccoli sprouts. You can sprout them at home in three days which makes them a very affordable way of supporting your health. They contain the highest concentrations of glucoraphanin and sulforaphane which encourage oestrogen metabolites that are going down the unhealthy quinone 4OH route to head back to the start of the pathway so that it has a chance of going down a better route. Sulforaphane also has anti-oxidant, antimicrobial, anticancer, anti-inflammatory, and anti-diabetic properties, and can help to protect against cardiovascular and neurodegenerative diseases – bring on the broccoli sprouts!
- Using supplements such as Calcium D-glucarate, iodine (which makes oestrogen receptors less sensitive), vitamin D, N-Acetyl Cysteine (NAC), and resveratol.

If you want to know what's going on with oestrogen in your body (which we all do), DUTCH testing offers the most accurate and comprehensive insights into your oestrogen levels and which pathways your metabolites are going down.

Go DUTCH

DUTCH is an acronym that stands for Dried Urine Test for Comprehensive Hormones. It's a simple but incredibly comprehensive method of testing your hormones, as well as showing how you process and metabolise them. The collection is easy; all you have to do is wee on a series of pieces of filter paper over the course of your day and/or your menstrual cycle, depending on which specific test you do, send them to Precision Analytical (the lab who created the test) for testing, and your results are sent to your healthcare provider so that they can explain them to you and come up with a suitable treatment plan.

The level of detailed information that you get from DUTCH testing is unparalleled and you get a heck of a lot more information than you would from a sample of blood or saliva. It doesn't just look at what your hormone levels are, it looks at your hormone metabolites and the pathways that they're going down, which is particularly relevant when you want to understand how you are processing and excreting oestrogen, and also when assessing androgens such as testosterone, because it's possible to have a 'normal' testosterone level but experience symptoms of high testosterone such as acne, thinning scalp hair, and an increase in facial and body hair (all symptoms of PCOS) because of how testosterone is being metabolised.

It gives an accurate representation with what's going on with cortisol and cortisone (the deactivated form of cortisol). By testing cortisol and cortisone at four points throughout the day, your cortisol curve – which should be higher in the morning and lower as the day goes on – can be assessed to see if you follow a healthy curve or vary from it, which is really important when it comes to understanding fatigue, anxiety, stress, depression, libido, and problems with sleep. It also assesses melatonin levels, which is important not just in assessing sleep issues, but because melatonin is an antioxidant and optimal levels of it are associated with a reduced risk of breast cancer.

You can use the DUTCH test prior to starting bioidentical hormones or HRT to understand how you will metabolise them, as well as assessing their effect once you start taking them. The DUTCH test doesn't assess thyroid hormones because urine tests for them aren't as adequate as comprehensive blood tests are, but some of the markers that it does test can give clues about thyroid function. Recently they added organic acids to the test – markers for neurotransmitters which help to understand mood and sleep issues.

The DUTCH test can help you get to the bottom of why you're struggling with:

- Mood swings, depression, anxiety
- PMS
- Low sexual desire

- Irregular menstrual cycles
- Fertility issues
- Fatigue
- Insomnia
- Symptoms of perimenopause

The DUTCH test is paid for privately (though some insurance companies will reimburse you) so it is a financial investment, but it truly speeds up the diagnosis process and enables the most appropriate treatment plan to be developed, saving you time and money that's potentially wasted exploring different avenues before arriving at an answer and a solution.

You can find a healthcare provider who uses the DUTCH test through their website www.dutchtest.com

It's Time to Give a Crap About your Crap

Oestrogen, along with other hormones and toxins, is also excreted through your bile – a fluid secreted by your liver – and then enters your intestines, enabling oestrogen to leave your body via poo. This wonderful process gets mucked up when the bacteria in your gut are imbalanced – from inflammation, use of antibiotics, and a poor diet – as well as when you're constipated, and instead of oestrogen exiting your body, it gets reabsorbed and recirculates, leaving you with symptoms of excess oestrogen; not good.

Think about how smoothly food exits your body. Do you poo regularly or are you backed up? Healthy elimination means having at least one satisfying and complete bowel movement per day, that's a four on the Bristol stool chart (like a sausage or snake, smooth and soft). Constipation is improved by increasing your intake of water and fibre (that means veggies), and by movement, either by moving all of your body or using manual therapies such as abdominal massage. It's no wonder that so many of us are constipated – we're sat down all day, dehydrated, and our diets lack sufficient fibre. And that's before we add in being scared to poo in the workplace.

The take home message here is that you cannot expect to have balanced hormones when your gut and liver are struggling.

Food as Medicine

Some people do well with diets that are meticulous, but most don't so I'm going to avoid being overly prescriptive. Start off with adding things into your diet such as vegetables, protein, and healthy fats (such as avocado, nuts and seeds, oily fish, olives and olive oil), then work on removing the not-so-good stuff, like processed foods and sugar. There are hundreds of diets and methods out there and I'll be mentioning a few of them, but what I want you to remember is that you know your body best and that by being mindful of what you eat and how you feel afterwards, you're in a great position to assess what works for you and what doesn't.

It can be hard to talk about diet. Most of us feel judged, and eating can be emotional, so before we get into the specifics of particular types of food, take a moment to recall what mealtimes were like in your family when you were growing up and what food story you've been left with. Here are some common scenarios:

- Food was scarce and you either shoved food down your throat because you feared that someone else would take it, so now you eat hurriedly and barely chew, or you feel guilty about taking more than you feel is yours.
- Food was abundant, but mealtimes were tough because you could feel the tension between your parents, and that made you feel tense, so you ate a lot to try and quash your own feelings or felt so tense that there's no way you could eat – a pattern that's remained into adulthood.
- Your mum (or dad) took it personally if you didn't eat everything they put on your plate, as if you were refusing their love somehow, so you got used to overeating and overriding your instinct about what you want to eat, and how much.
- Family members made comments about how much or how little you ate, perhaps in relation to your body type and weight, so now you still feel conscious about your intake of calories and fat.

- Food was restricted in some way if you were 'bad' and provided if you were 'good'. This one is a biggie and incredibly common. We really need to stop punishing and rewarding our kids with food.
- Your family encouraged you to get involved with preparing and cooking meals, and mealtimes were a relaxed affair where you connected with loved ones and enjoyed your food and time together.

It's easy to get caught up in what you should and shouldn't eat, but it's important that we consider where we eat, who we eat with, and how we eat. Here are my recommendations:

- Eat somewhere that's conducive to digestion i.e. away from your desk and any screens, and not while you're running for the bus.
- Hit pause before you start eating. Take three slow, deep breaths to help your nervous system move away from *fight or flight* and into *rest and digest*. If taking a moment to give thanks, or to say a prayer of some kind feels right, do that too. You're more likely to eat your meal mindfully if you slow down before that first forkful.
- Eat till 80 per cent full. Your brain needs up to 20 minutes to catch up with your stomach and receive the signal that you're full. Eating slowly is not only beneficial to digestion but gives your brain and stomach a chance to communicate before you overeat.
- Chew your food. Forty times per bite of hard food is optimal according to the research but that can feel like a ridiculous amount if you usually only manage two chews per bite of food, so start with ten and see how you get on. Chewing your food properly means you'll extract more nutrients from your food, helps to maintain a healthy weight, prevents digestive upsets, and it's good for the health of your teeth and jaw too.
- Put your utensils down between bites to help you slow down and be present so that you chew and really enjoy your food.
- Eat protein and veg first and see if you have room for all those carbs you thought you needed to feel satisfied.

Before I get into the juicy topic of what to eat and what not to eat (though I prefer to frame it as foods to lean towards and away from), let's start with some overall aims for you to always come back to. Your diet should be:

- Enjoyable to eat
- Nutritionally rich and diverse
- Providing you with enough fuel to feel energised throughout your day
- Helping you to maintain an appropriate weight
- Supporting the health of your microbiome
- Keeping your blood sugar levels in check
- Targeting any specific health issues that you have

What to Actually Eat

Breakfast
Eat breakfast within an hour of waking and don't you dare skip it – you can't expect to balance your hormones if you do. When clients tell me that they don't have time to make or eat breakfast before they leave the house, I ask them to evaluate how much time they devote to getting the outside of their body ready by washing, dressing, and doing their hair and make-up, versus how much time they spend taking care of their insides.

Cereal does not count as breakfast, and neither does toast with jam. Your breakfast must always include protein and healthy fat in order to sort your blood sugar out first thing in the morning, and this is even more relevant if you have PCOS or your periods are MIA. Eggs are a breakfast favourite of mine, not least because they're so quick to cook. Scramble them and serve on top of some toast or a tortilla with some avocado on the side, or fill an omelette with some pre-cooked veg. If you're really pressed for time then boil some eggs and store them in the fridge or make a vegetable frittata the night before so that it's ready to go the following morning (and the one after). Oats, quinoa, millet, and amaranth can all be used with plant-based milks such as oat and almond to make porridge and topped with fruit, nut butters, and a sprinkling of seeds. But in all honesty, I'd love it if we got rid of our very Western idea of what constitutes breakfast. I quite like to have some cooked salmon with cooked greens and rice or quinoa for mine, all of which can be cooked in advance and reheated quickly in a pan. If you're really not a breakfast person, have protein smoothies and make sure that you're not eating your dinner too late (eating earlier in the evening often stimulates your need to eat in the morning). Any carbs should be complex, such as whole grains and starchy veg, and caffeine should be consumed alongside or after eating breakfast, not before.

Regular meals

Three satisfying square meals a day and no snacks does work well for most people, but if you're prone to low blood sugar or have hypothalamic amenorrhoea (see page 287), then you probably need to eat more frequently than that, perhaps eating every 2.5–3 hours. Whatever camp you're in, just don't skip a meal because your blood sugar levels will suffer. And bear in mind that you are not a cow – you don't have four stomachs to deal with all-day-long grazing, so don't nibble continuously.

Feeling Hangry?

You're not alone. So many of my clients are prone to feeling hungry and angry as a result of unstable blood sugar levels (and probably lightheaded, forgetful, and anxious too), and it's often symptomatic of our busy lifestyles. We're always trying to get things done and often prioritise other people and tasks over our need to eat regularly, or we're so caught up in what we're doing that we don't even realise we're hungry, and this plays havoc with our hormones.

Your blood sugar level is the amount of glucose that you have in your blood, and it's in constant flux. There are two imbalances of blood sugar that we're concerned with. The first is low blood sugar, or hypoglycaemia. Hypoglycaemia can leave you feeling grumpy, irritable, nauseous, sweaty, and ravenous to the point of panic. When your blood sugar is low you crave sugar and carbs because they're a quick-fix solution to the problem, but they also go on to cause blood sugar crashes that cause more instability and cravings. A little bit of hunger before you eat is okay but riding it out and getting hypoglycaemic just because it's two hours till lunch isn't. If you are prone to hypoglycaemia, then it's really important that you eat regularly enough to stave it off and that you eat protein at every meal.

Habits that lead to hypoglycaemia include:

- Eating breakfast hours after waking or skipping it altogether
- Surviving on caffeine and sugar to get through the day
- Grazing your way through the day
- Suppressing your appetite with caffeine and cigarettes
- Exercising a lot without replenishing calories

When you eat something sugary, whether that's a sweet treat, a croissant, some pasta, or some fruit with a high sugar content, your blood sugar level goes up and your body responds by releasing insulin. Insulin's job is to allow the cells in your body to let sugar (glucose) in so that it can either be used as fuel or stored as body fat. By doing this it keeps your blood sugar balanced, but consistently high levels of insulin can lead to insulin resistance, a condition in which your body doesn't respond as well to insulin. It's caused by obesity, surviving on carbs, sugar, and processed foods, and lack of exercise. There may be no signs of insulin resistance initially, but as the effects of it progress, signs and symptoms include:

- Feeling tired all the time, particularly after eating meals
- Feeling hungry
- Gaining weight easily and having a hard time losing it, especially weight around your middle
- Difficulty concentrating
- High blood pressure
- High cholesterol levels
- Eating sweets doesn't relieve your craving for them

High levels of insulin are a big problem because they set off a chain reaction with your other hormones. Cortisol (the stress hormone) goes up which is a problem because cortisol and progesterone compete for the same hormone receptors, but cortisol pips progesterone to the post, which can lead to progesterone deficiency and oestrogen dominance. There are also insulin receptors on your ovaries and excess oestrogen makes them produce more testosterone than oestrogen which can interfere with ovarian function and cause irregular or absent menstrual cycles, and an increase in body hair and acne (all indicators of PCOS, a condition with a strong link to insulin resistance). High levels of testosterone can also come about because excess insulin decreases sex hormone binding globulin (SHBG) – the protein that binds up testosterone so it's not all available at once – so that more testosterone is in the bloodstream. Insulin resistance can lead to weight gain (which also contributes to PCOS) and it can develop into diabetes, so treating it is incredibly important.

Taste the Rainbow

Eat 8–10 servings of vegetables and – to a lesser extent – fruit per day, making sure that you consume a variety of colours.

Vegetables

If you only make one change to your diet, let it be putting vegetables front and centre in every meal you eat. Vegetables are packed full of a massively diverse range of nutrients that help to prevent and treat most of the diseases that we get. They're also a rich source of fibre and help to keep your bowel movements regular and easy. They're great for you – stack 'em up so that they take up half of each plate of food that you eat. There are two types of veg; non-starchy, and starchy. Non-starchy vegetables are rich in vitamins and minerals, fibre, and water, and they have a low glycaemic index, which means you can go wild and eat loads of them. Non-starchy veg includes:

- Raw and cooked leafy greens. Mix it up, there's more to greens than a sad serving of iceberg lettuce.
- Cruciferous veg such as broccoli, cauliflower, brussel sprouts, bok choy, cabbage, collard greens, kale, rocket, watercress, and radishes are associated with reduced inflammation, and because they're high in fibre they can regulate blood sugar, promote weight loss, and help reduce oestrogen excess. If you find they give you gas, experiment with different

cooking techniques and make sure you chew them properly. And if you have a thyroid condition, be sure to eat them cooked as eating them raw can cause your intestines to release goitrogens which increases your need for iodine and can damage the thyroid gland.

- Cucumbers, celery, carrot, green beans and mushrooms.
- Sprouts such as alfalfa, broccoli, and mung bean. Grow your own at home.
- Garlic, onions and artichokes.
- Aubergines and peppers (though these can cause an inflammatory response in some people).

Starchy vegetables are a great source of carbohydrates, so they tend to be more filling than their non-starchy companions, but they can also have a higher glycaemic index which means you should have smaller amounts of them. That being said, they're a far better source of carbs than those that come from grains such as bread and pasta. Starchy veg includes:

- Sweet potato (my favourite superfood)
- White potato
- Squash (including butternut, acorn, spaghetti, and pumpkin)
- Parsnips
- Plantain
- Corn (though as a highly genetically modified crop, it's not one to go wild with and best if you can stick to non-GMO)
- Beetroot

Fruit

Fruits are full of nutrients and fibre and are a healthy source of carbo-hydrates, but they also contain substantial amounts of natural sugars so it's better to eat more veg than fruit. Eat fruits which have lower sugar content, and pair them with some protein and fat in order to balance their effect on your body. Fruits with a lower sugar content include:

- Berries: blackberries, blueberries, cranberries, raspberries, strawberries
- Grapefruit
- Lemons

- Limes
- Olives (yep, technically they're a fruit)
- Avocado (also a fruit)
- Peaches
- Papaya

Fruits with the highest sugar content include:

- Mangoes
- Bananas
- Pineapple
- Grapes
- Figs
- Dates
- Cherries
- Pomegranate
- Kiwis

Buy Organic

I'm a big believer in buying the best food that your budget allows, and I find it eternally frustrating that foods with low nutritional value are so cheap. When you're considering what organic foods to splurge your hard-earned money on, prioritise the *Dirty Dozen*, a list of the most pesticide-laden foods that's produced every year by the Environmental Working Group (EWG). It changes slightly every year but commonly features strawberries, spinach, peaches, nectarines, cherries, and apples. The EWG also produce a *Clean Fifteen* list of the fruit and veg that tends to have the lowest amount of pesticides on them, or in other words, produce that needn't be organic unless your budget allows for it (*see* Resources for their website).

One particular time in life when eating organic is best is when you're preparing to conceive or are already pregnant. We know that pesticides from food are present in the umbilical cord blood of newborns (along with plenty of other chemical nasties), so it's crucial that exposure to pesticides and other chemical nasties is limited when babies are in utero.

Make Friends with Fat

Fat isn't the evil ingredient that we've been led to believe it is. It's been blamed for obesity and cardiovascular problems for decades, yet evidence shows that it's crucial for your health. Your brain is made predominantly of fat, and you need fat to build cell membranes and to protect the sheaths that coat your nerve cells. Fat is a key source of energy which also helps you to feel full and regulate your blood sugar and hormones. When fat is removed from foods or it's absent from a meal, you end up eating more in order to reach the point where you feel full because fat helps you to feel satiated, and because of this, an absence of fat can contribute towards obesity – not to mention the fact that low-fat foods are pumped full of sugar and salt to compensate for the flavour that's lost when fat is removed. Fat also enables you to absorb some vitamins and minerals.

Monosaturated fats are liquid at room temperature, they only have one bond (mono) and they're really good for your health. Extra virgin olive oil, avocado oil, seed oils, nut oils, and coconut oil are all good examples of healthy monosaturated oils, and the latest research shows that contrary to popular belief, olive oil does remain stable when you're cooking at higher temperatures and is therefore safe to cook with. Eggs, olives, and avocados are other sources of monosaturated fat.

Polyunsaturated fats can be healthy but aren't always. Polyunsaturated fats in the form of vegetable oils such as sunflower, corn, and canola are usually heavily processed; the heat, chemicals and light that they're exposed to during processing damages their delicate bonds and makes them harmful. They're also high in Omega-6 Fatty Acids which increase inflammation in the body, so you really want to be limiting them as much as possible or cutting them out altogether. Healthy Omega-6 Fatty Acids come from nuts and seeds, and unrefined seed oils such as sesame, walnut seed, and evening primrose oils. Omega-3 Fatty Acids – the kind of healthy fat that comes from oily fish and nuts and seeds and which most of us are deficient in – are really beneficial as they help to reduce inflammation, period pain, fluid retention, PMS, acne, insulin sensitivity, depression, anxiety, and improve your skin, hair, and nails. Omega-3 Fatty Acids, and fat in general, are vital during the preconception period, pregnancy, and postpartum, as they're crucial for a growing baby's development.

Saturated fats are the kind of fats found in butter and other dairy produce, eggs, meat, and coconut oil. They're a hot topic because how good they are for you is debatable. I think it's fair to say that they do have health benefits but that they shouldn't be overused, and how good they are for you will largely come down to the quality of the products that you have access to, such as organic butter from grass-fed cows.

The one type of fat to totally stay clear of is trans fats. They're the type that are found in fried and greasy foods and appear as 'hydrogenated fat' or 'partially hydrogenated oils' on food labels, and are associated with heart disease, high cholesterol, obesity, as well as encouraging oestrogen to go down the pathways which increase your cancer risk.

Cholesterol-rich foods such as egg yolks contain the essential nutrient choline which you really want to consume during pregnancy because a deficiency in it is associated with neural tube defects. Remember that 60 per cent of the human brain is fat – your baby needs you to eat fat, and no, you won't pile on the pregnancy pounds by eating it. The Department of Health recommend eating oily fish two to three times per week, and you can also take an Omega-3 Fatty Acids supplement, but be warned, some people find that it makes them burp, and burping Omega-3 Fatty Acids is not pleasant. Your reaction will vary across brands; I find that BioCare Mega EPA doesn't make me burp at all, and I like that they regularly test their Omega-3 Fatty Acids for contamination (fish in the sea accumulate toxins and mercury that you want to avoid ingesting). If you're vegetarian or vegan then you can take Omega-3 Fatty Acids that's derived from algae instead of taking fish oil.

Oestrogen, progesterone, DHEA (the 'mother' hormone that other hormones are derived from), cortisol, and testosterone are all made from cholesterol from dietary fat, which means that your intake of fat is essential for hormone production and function. If you've got a hormonal issue such as low libido, PMS, or amenorrhoea, take a minute to look at how much fat you're getting in your diet. Every meal you eat should include a serving of healthy fat. One serving is roughly 1–2 tbsps of oil, half an avocado, or a shot glass of nuts and seeds.

Sources of healthy fats include:

- Avocados
- Olives

- Eggs
- Nuts and seeds
- Fatty cold-water fish such as salmon
- Fatty, grass-fed meat
- Use olive oil, flaxseed oil, walnut oil, and avocado oil in dressings and to drizzle over meals
- I also love to keep the fat that floats to the top of homemade bone broth when you refrigerate it and use it for sautéing

Pulses

Pulses include: beans, chickpeas, lentils and peas. They are plant-based sources of protein which are an excellent source of fibre and resistant starch – starch which helps to feed the healthy bacteria in your gut and is associated with weight loss, improved blood sugar control, insulin sensitivity and digestive health. They're also rich in vitamins and minerals, help you to feel full, and eating them is associated with lowered cholesterol levels, improved gut function, and an overall reduction of the risk of chronic disease. Many people avoid legumes though because they find that eating them makes them fart, but staying clear of legumes is a shame because they're an easy way to resolve common gut complaints such as constipation.

If you find eating beans makes you gassy, try methods such as soaking, sprouting or fermenting as they can help to reduce their gassy effect as well as increasing their nutritional value. People who fart a lot after eating them are likely to have a diet which is low in dietary fibre and/or lack the beneficial bacteria needed to process them but, for most people, eating small amounts of pulses on a daily basis has been shown to result in a return to normal levels of farting within two to three weeks of increased consumption. This is likely because eating pulses regularly enables your gut to produce the helpful bacteria that you need to digest them, whereas infrequent consumption means your gut is never ready to handle them and will result in an increase in gas. If you want to include more pulses in your diet, start with a small amount (even a spoonful) every day so that you can acclimatise to them gradually. If you know or suspect you have IBS or SIBO, or if you're particularly sensitive to pulses, then consider working with a nutritionist who can give you specific recommendations as some diets used to treat gut dysfunction recommend avoiding or limiting pulses.

Eggs

Eggs have got to be the healthiest fast food out there, they're a nutritional powerhouse and they're a wonderful source of protein. When I'm working with a client who could do with upping their protein intake – which is most of the people I support – eggs are my favourite recommendation, but you've got to eat the yolk to benefit from their nutritional value. If you're of the belief that eating egg yolks raises your cholesterol and increases your risk of having a heart attack, know that for 75 per cent of the population, dietary cholesterol has very little impact on blood cholesterol. The remaining 25 per cent are referred to as *hyper-responders*, and dietary cholesterol will modestly increase both their LDL ('bad' cholesterol) and HDL ('good' cholesterol), but it doesn't affect the ratio of the two, or increase the incidence of heart disease. Buy organic and free-range if you're able to or keep your own chooks.

Meat and fish

Protein provides the building blocks for all the structures in your body, is a major source of energy, and it keeps your blood sugar steady. Meat and fish are good sources of protein and can also provide important vitamins, minerals, and Omega-3 Fatty Acids – but this varies depending on the quality of the produce and how they're cooked.

You are what you eat, but you're also what you eat ate, and that's definitely the case when it comes to meat and fish. Livestock are routinely given low-dose antibiotics to prevent infection from the appalling conditions they're usually kept in, and 80 per cent of antibiotics that are sold are used on them. They're also frequently pumped full of growth hormones, which means that by eating them, you're increasing your exposure to hormones too, so it's better to eat organic poultry and meat – especially if you're eating their organs or using their bones to make broth. Organic produce can end up eating up most of your salary, but there are less popular nutrient-dense cuts which are delicious and more affordable.

Larger fish have higher levels of mercury in them and are the ones to be wary of such as tuna, marlin, swordfish, grouper, king mackerel, and shark. Fish that are generally lower in mercury include sardines, anchovies, wild Alaska salmon, sockeye salmon, crab, Atlantic mackerel, Atlantic pollock, shrimp, crawfish, and mussels.

Mackerel, sardines and salmon are all great sources of Omega-3 Fatty Acids but opt for wild salmon where possible because farmed salmon are given antibiotics and are frequently dyed orangey-pink, whereas wild salmon are naturally pink, and won't have the antibiotics and chemicals that farmed salmon do.

Carbohydrates

Simple carbohydrates such as natural and refined sugars, pasta, and white bread can all cause your blood sugar to spike quickly, whereas complex carbs such as brown rice, quinoa, legumes, pulses, and starchy root vegetables give a slow release of energy that helps to balance your blood sugar. Most of us could do with eating less carbs and eating more vegetables, but carbs do not have to be excluded. In fact, depriving your body of carbs can make your body think that food is scarce and it will slam the brakes on ovulation rather than waste energy on it. So, complex carbs are better, simple ones less so. Wondering just how much complex carbs to eat? A small fist size is plenty for most people if they're eating sufficient protein and loading up on non-starchy veg too.

Water

Always start your day with water. It'll rehydrate you and help you to wake up, as well as encouraging your bowels to get going before you have to leave home. Most people could do with increasing their water intake but just how much to have gets confusing, so I recommend paying attention to your thirst, and also to your lips because they show signs of dehydration quickly. When you reach for your lip balm, consider if you're dehydrated, and if you feel tired during the day, drink some water before you resort to caffeine and sugar because dehydration also manifests as fatigue. Once you start upping your water intake you'll probably notice that you feel thirstier than you used to. This is normal and is a sign that your body likes you drinking more water. Remember that you do get a lot of water from vegetables (which you're eating more of, right?) as well as soups and other non-caffeinated beverages. If you have a tendency to feel cold, then drink tepid or hot water and herbal teas. Avoid drinking water from the fridge and using ice. Cold water is a shock to the body and is said to dampen your digestive fire in Chinese medicine. Room temperature is much better – save your ice for a gin and tonic instead. And don't flood your stomach while you're eating as it can weaken your digestive juices. Try to drink water 30–60 minutes before a meal instead.

What to Avoid

Food keeps us alive and many people on the planet have limited access to foods, even in developed countries, and it's increasingly common for people to develop orthorexia in which you become obsessed with eating 'healthy' foods and avoiding those that aren't, often to the point where meals are skipped entirely if something 'healthy' isn't available. So when it comes to diet, I really caution against becoming brittle in your mind about what's good for you and what isn't. There's a balance to aim for between recognising what foods don't work for you at the moment and ending up feeling fearful of food. It is there to be enjoyed after all.

Deadly white powder

No, not cocaine. I'm talking about a highly addictive substance that rats prefer to cocaine – sugar. Our DNA makes us primed to go for foods that give us a lot of energy, because in our hunter-gatherer past it was important that we took up the limited opportunities that we had to benefit from foods that delivered a high amount of energy, but sugar-rich food back then was berries, not a snickers bar or a tub of salted caramel ice cream.

There are lots of snazzy forms of sugar available to us, including 'natural' sugars, such as:

- Agave syrup
- Brown rice syrup
- Coconut sugar
- Corn syrup
- Dextrose
- Galactose
- Glucose
- Honey
- Lactose
- Maltose
- Maple syrup
- Molasses
- Saccharose
- Sucrose

You really want to avoid them as much as you can because the more you eat the more you crave. They disrupt your microbiome; cause inflammation, obesity, blood sugar imbalances, and mid-afternoon dips in energy; damage your adrenal gland; and affect your stress response. When we're talking about sugar, I mean the white stuff and the brown stuff, as well as carbohydrates such as bread, cereal, rice and pasta – all of which get broken down into glucose (sugar) – even the wholemeal variety.

Once they're broken down, your pancreas pumps out a hormone called insulin. Insulin regulates the amount of sugar in your bloodstream by signalling to the body's cells that they should pick up the glucose in your blood and store it. How sensitive you are to insulin determines how effective your body is at using carbs, and for the majority of people, the more sensitive you are, the better, because your body only needs to secrete a small amount of insulin to get the job done. When insulin sensitivity is poor, you produce a lot of insulin, and the body doesn't respond to it as it should, causing you to become insulin resistant which puts you at risk for becoming obese and developing type 2 diabetes. Excess insulin production can also impair ovulation and is associated with PCOS.

You can improve insulin sensitivity by getting more sleep, exercising, consuming more fibre, losing excess weight, reducing stress, and *reducing your sugar intake.*

Got milk?
Dairy is a divisive topic. In the West we're brought up being told that we need to consume lots of calcium, that milk is an excellent and healthy source of it, and that drinking it will help to prevent our fracture risk. Yet there's no medical evidence that humans need to consume milk from animals. If you exercise regularly and have a healthy diet with lots of leafy greens in it then you're likely to get all the calcium you need without needing to eat dairy, and a 12-year study of over 70,000 women conducted by Harvard found that consuming dairy does not reduce fracture risk. Health agencies have been lowering their recommended daily allowances of calcium through diet and are promoting exercise to improve bone density instead.

When I'm helping a client to assess if they want to experiment with cutting out dairy, here's what I explain:

- The majority of cow's milk contains a hell of a lot of synthetic hormones which are given to them to sustain milk production such as oestrogen, testosterone, progesterone, cortisol, and insulin. Consuming these hormones via the dairy in your diet can disrupt your hormones.
- On average, dairy cows receive two antibiotic treatments annually, one to prevent and one to treat mastitis (an inflammation of the udder), and evidence of antibiotic use in food animals resulting in antibiotic-resistant infections in humans has existed for decades.
- When clients want to consume cow's milk, I prefer them to stick with full fat in limited amounts. Low-fat and fat-free milk don't help with weight loss, and they may contribute to weight gain as well as reducing ovarian function. When fat is removed from milk it also reduces the absorption and use of fat-soluble vitamins A and D which are required for bone health, and it makes calcium more likely to go into the soft tissue of the body instead of your bones.
- Dairy triggers inflammation in some people, probably because of a protein that tends to be present in cow dairy called A1 casein, whereas dairy with A2 casein is better tolerated by most people. A2 dairy comes from some breeds of cow such as Jersey, as well as dairy that comes from sheep and goats (if you're anything like me you'll be relieved to hear that cheeses that are A2 include feta, halloumi, manchego, pecorino, ricotta, roquefort, and of course goat's cheese).

If you're going to have cow dairy, look for produce which is full fat, grass-fed and as hormone-free as you can get it.

Gluten: The enemy of the 21st century

Gluten intolerance is not a food allergy, it's an autoimmune reaction that can cause depression, fatigue and weight gain. If you have gluten intolerance then you aren't able to digest the protein part that's in many types of grain, and when you eat it the lining of your intestines recognise it as a foreign substance and an immune response is stimulated in order to take care of it. It's this response that causes inflammation, damages the lining of your intestines, and causes digestive upsets such as bloating, cramping, diarrhoea, constipation, and gas, as well as feeling tired. This constant immune response leads to depletion and the inability to absorb vitamins and minerals from your food, causing even more deficiencies and tiredness. I really recommend trying a gluten-free diet if you have endometriosis as it can dramatically reduce the pain that's typically associated with endo. When it comes to Hashimoto's thyroiditis, 51.48 per cent of people with Hashimoto's test positive for gluten specific inflammatory antibodies, and 15.98 per cent test positive for the inflammatory antibodies linked to celiac disease, so if you have Hashimoto's, then go wheat free for 6–12 months and see how you get on.

Be aware that, for most of us, wheat is the primary source of prebiotics in our diet and prebiotics are the compounds in food which cause growth or activity of beneficial microorganisms. When we cut wheat out we significantly reduce our intake of prebiotics and therefore see a reduction in our number of probiotics – the living microorganisms which populate our gut – which were being fed by the wheat, and that means the unhealthy bacteria in our gut that the probiotics were previously keeping in check can multiply, which results in an unhealthy microbiome and inflammation. To avoid this, increase your intake of other prebiotics before you cut wheat out, and you may want to use a supplement which has both prebiotics and probiotics in it. Prebiotic foods include:

- Onions
- Chicory
- Garlic
- Asparagus
- Jerusalem artichokes
- Cruciferous vegetables
- Raw honey
- Resistant starch (which is found in rice and potatoes that have been cooked and cooled, and green bananas as well as other food sources)

Some people find they can tolerate sourdough bread and pizzas, but if you have a histamine intolerance like me, then sourdough could trigger your symptoms because it's fermented.

Molecular Mimicry

Your immune system's ability to recognise harmful molecules isn't flawless. If a molecule's shape looks similar enough to a known offender, the immune system will attack it, and this is what can happen with gluten and dairy. Fifty per cent of people who are sensitive to gluten will unfortunately experience molecular mimicry with a protein that's found in some dairy called casein and will react to it as well as gluten, so if you're planning on eliminating gluten, you might wanna go the whole hog (or cow) and cut out dairy too.

Alcohol

Alcohol messes with your hormones by increasing oestrogen and contributing to oestrogen dominance. Limit it as much as you can but if you do have some, be sure to drink after you've eaten, and drink plenty of water alongside your booze of choice. Alcohol is also high in sugar and some forms of it more than others, so opt for a glass of wine over a rum and coke. Although red wine does contain resveratrol, a compound that's highly anti-inflammatory and a powerful antioxidant, the amount in one glass of wine is insignificant. And no, that doesn't mean you should drink a whole bottle instead.

Types of Diet

I'm of the opinion that no one diet is best, because not only are we all different, but a diet that works well for you in your twenties won't necessarily suit you in your forties or sixties. Listed below are the diets that come up frequently in my practice and the potential issues that they can result in so that you can evaluate if a particular diet is supporting your hormonal and reproductive health, or harming them.

Veganism and vegetarianism

There are vegans and vegetarians who eat lots of nutrient-dense plant-based meals who are mindful that they get enough protein, healthy fats, and important minerals such as copper and zinc in their diets. And then there are the vegetarians whose diets are like the one I had as a teenager and are based around cheese. Clearly, the former is the healthier version, but even with careful consideration of dietary intake, some vegetarians and vegans will struggle to consume enough protein, healthy fats, and vitamins and minerals.

Over the years, close examination of my vegetarian clients' food diaries has, in the majority of cases, revealed an absence of protein until their evening meal, and this is of concern because not only does it leave you open to blood sugar instability but if you're not getting enough protein then you may not have enough amino acids to make sufficient thyroid hormones. Good news though, eating more plant-based foods means that the level of oestrogen in your blood could be 15 to 20 per cent lower than your meat-eating mates.

When I work with a client who's deficient and particularly if their periods have stopped or they're planning to conceive, then I always explore the possibility of introducing some animal protein into their diet. If your choice not to eat meat is an ethical one, you may not be willing to eat meat and that's fair enough, but in my practice, clients are usually vegan or veggie because that's how they were raised or they're doing it to be 'healthy', and these are the clients who are usually up for adding some chicken broth to their soups and sauces, or eating some meat, and find that they respond quickly and positively to it. It's not that being a vegetarian is bad, but when it comes to hormonal health, a vegetarian or vegan diet can come at a cost.

Ketogenic diet

The aim with a ketogenic diet is to eat a diet that's low in carbohydrates and high in healthy fats so that the body goes into a metabolic state called ketosis. By changing the dietary source of energy from sugar (through carbs) to fat, the body is forced to convert its fat stores into energy and as such, it's known for causing rapid loss of body fat in some instances as well as an increase in mental acuity. But it can also result in menstrual irregularities, tiredness, and an increase in cortisol production (a stress hormone) which can go on to cause inflammation and weight gain, so it's important to weigh up if it's actually working for you.

Intermittent fasting

The practice of intermittent fasting, which involves abstaining from eating for 16–24 hours at a time, perhaps once or twice a week, is associated with weight loss, improved blood sugar metabolism, and a reduced risk of diabetes – in men. In women, however, depriving ourselves of regular meals can be catastrophic because our bodies perceive our little experiment as a time of starvation, and it goes into survival mode, slamming the brakes on the menstrual cycle because that's a waste of energy when times are lean, and activating your stress response, because guess what – starving yourself is stressful for the body.

Time restricted feeding, in which there's a 12-hour period where you eat, and a 12-hour window where you don't, is a different kettle of fish. Practically it means eating your evening meal a few hours before you go to bed and not eating while you're asleep but making sure that you can eat breakfast at a suitable time in the morning. If you like to eat your breakfast at 7.30am, you just need to be done eating your evening meal by 7.30pm. As a dietary approach, I think it's one of the healthiest eating behaviours that we can adopt, but that doesn't mean that you have to do it every single night, and it is not appropriate if you have a history of disordered eating, if you're prone to low blood sugar, if you have hypothalamic amenorrhoea, or if you're pregnant. Got it?

Paleo Diet

A paleo diet is very on trend, and I love that it's based on some excellent principles; eating whole unprocessed real food and healthy fats, lots of veggies, aiming to eat produce that's organic, local, and grass-fed, and eliminating inflammatory foods like gluten, dairy, and soy. But, it's a low-carb diet and not everyone handles low-carb well, and in the same way the ketogenic diet can trigger a stress response, so can the paleo diet. Carbs aren't the devil, it's just about moderation and leaning towards healthier sources of them. The paleo diet also excludes legumes, which isn't necessary for everyone and may be an important source of plant-based protein for those who like to limit or exclude animal protein.

If you Don't Snooze, you Lose

Women experience sleep differently to men and it's the onset of menstruation that stimulates the main differences in sleep between the sexes. As oestrogen and progesterone begin their cyclic ebb and flow, they regulate sleep-wake cycle regulation, and as you transition through each phase of your life, you're increasingly likely to experience a sleep disorder. By the time we reach our perimenopausal and postmenopausal years, 53 per cent of us will be having poor quality sleep; trouble falling asleep, staying asleep, and getting enough sleep. Night sweats, needing to wee, and restless leg syndrome all impact on our ability to get a solid night of sleep, and then there are the years of interrupted sleep we get when we become parents and the hypervigilance that some mums are unable to switch off from, even though they're desperate to get some shut-eye.

Not enough decent sleep increases your appetite, upsets your blood sugar balance, and reduces your ability to burn fat, thanks to an increase in production of ghrelin which stimulates your appetite, and lowered levels of leptin, a hormone which tells your brain that you have energy and inhibits hunger. And when I say not enough sleep, I mean one night of crap sleep can have that effect. It also makes you crave carbs and sugar that you can't process as well, triggers inflammation, lowers your immunity, makes you more prone to obesity, diabetes, autoimmune and cardiovascular disease, increases your cancer risk, and makes you less resilient to stress, moody as hell, and tired AF.

Sleep is critical. When I treat someone who has sleep issues, no matter what other health issues they've got going on, improving their sleep is at the top of my list of treatment aims because without sufficient good-quality sleep all our other results will be limited. My aims are for clients to:

- Fall asleep easily within half an hour of winding down and getting into bed.
- Be horizontal by 10pm at the latest.
- Sleep soundly for 7–9 hours (less than that is associated with a whole host of negative health outcomes).
- Be free of night sweats and dreams which are disturbing or exhausting.
- Wake up feeling refreshed and restored in the morning.

Elevated cortisol in the evenings can make falling asleep just about impossible, so it's worth looking at what is stressing you out, and you might have to rethink that 7pm spin class that you love. Sure, it's great exercise and all that sweating helps you to excrete oestrogen, but what is it telling your adrenal glands? That you've got something scary to cycle away from – your body thinks that your instructor barking at you through a microphone and you pedalling and sweating away means that what's actually going on is that a sabretooth tiger is after you, so it ramps up cortisol secretion and despite you being absolutely beat by the time you wobble home and into bed, sleep eludes you.

Another key hormone when it comes to sleep is melatonin – the dracula of hormones because it only comes out in the night. Melatonin is secreted by the pineal gland in your head, during the day it's inactive, but when the sun goes down and it becomes dark, the pineal gland gets going and begins to produce melatonin which is then secreted in to your blood and it tells your body that it's time to hit the hay. Melatonin levels stay high throughout the night, and then when morning rolls around melatonin levels drop to almost nothing, which is why it's generally easier to feel alert in the mornings during the Summer months, because we are exposed to sunlight earlier than in the Winter. If you're someone who struggles to get going in the morning, open your curtains and let light in as soon as you wake – let your pineal gland know that it's time to get going. If mornings are a struggle for you, it could be that your cortisol awakening response isn't optimal, leaving you feeling groggy and reliant on caffeine.

Your body likes to keep to a schedule; eating, exercising, waking, and sleeping at set times per day all let your body know what's coming up next, and means that your pineal gland will know when to start secreting melatonin and it'll release it at the same time every day, which is important because melatonin initiates the sleep cycle hours before you actually fall asleep. Being asleep by 10pm results in optimal production of melatonin and using screens in the evening can dramatically delay production of this sleep-inducing hormone. Some medications may suppress melatonin production if they're taken in the evening, such as beta-blockers and NSAIDs, so speak to your GP about adjusting the time at which you take them if you feel they could be impacting on sleep.

Melatonin also has an influence on the menstrual cycle. Although as a species we breed all year long, compared to mammals who breed seasonally, there are seasonal fluctuations in conception rates in northern countries, as well as in IVF success rates, suggesting that light exposure and melatonin exert an influence on our reproductive function. Some research also suggests that there's a link between melatonin and ovulation, cycle regularity, and progesterone production in the second half of the cycle. It's thought that melatonin may also play a role in menopausal transition, with the age-related disruption of circadian rhythm leading to an irregular cycle and amenorrhoea, and also because a drop in core body temperature accompanies the onset of sleep and is strongly linked to melatonin secretion, but in post-menopausal women this drop is lessened. One study found that supplementing with melatonin can improve quality of sleep and period pain within 2–3 menstrual cycles and out-performs meloxicam, an NSAID.

Most of the clients I treat who have hypothalamic amenorrhoea (where they stop getting their periods, see page 287) have trouble sleeping. They usually fall asleep without issue, but then wake up feeling really alert in the middle of the night, and as well as using acupuncture to improve things, I always recommend a snack that's got protein and fat in it before bed. Here's why – unless you're prone to sleepwalking and raiding the fridge in your sleep, you don't eat overnight and so your body has to compensate for this if you're hypoglycaemic in order to keep your blood sugar stable. It achieves this by secreting cortisol, which stimulates your brain and tells it that you'd better wake up and eat something. You can improve your sleep by:

- Exposing yourself to bright light during the daytime and by getting outside as much as possible.
- Keep your room cool and well ventilated.
- Ensure your room is dark at night. Blackout blinds can really help to block out streetlights.
- Replace stimulating LED lightbulbs with incandescent bulbs which emit a softer light.
- Don't consume caffeine after 2pm.
- Reduce fluid intake in the evenings if your bladder wakes you up in the night (and see an acupuncturist if you still have to get up to pee).
- Avoid eating within three hours of bedtime.
- Avoid alcohol and sugar before bed as it disrupts ability to sleep well.
- Eat enough protein and fat during the day so that your blood sugar is balanced, and if you're prone to wake ups because of low blood sugar, have a snack before bed that has protein and fat in it.
- Avoid napping during the daytime.
- Exercise does improve sleep, but sleep is more important than working out, so sleep should be your priority.

- If stimulating evening workouts are preventing you from winding down, replace them with calming ones such as restorative yoga.
- Consider using supplements such as magnesium, B vitamins, 5-HTP, and melatonin.
- Listen to a guided meditation or have a hot bath before bed.
- Using essential oils such as lavender, frankincense, vetiver, ylang ylang, cedarwood and chamomile.
- Stock up on sleepy-time teas such as chamomile and valerian.
- Don't use stimulating electronic screens before bed.

Baby, Don't Keep the Blue Light on

Once upon a time, not too long ago, we used to finish work and switch off. If we took work home with us, it was either in the form of paperwork or it was a problem that we thought about and maybe discussed with a loved one once we were home. We'd eat at a fairly regular hour, listen to music or the radio, and can you believe it – even talk to each other and have sex! Then came an exciting new development: a magical box called a television. Ooooohh, let's just sit down with a cuppa on the sofa and watch something instead of being intimate and relieving our stress levels. Next up came mobile phones that took a ridiculously long time to write a very short text on, and the ringtones and novel vibrating alerts would snap us into a state of alert and caused our stress hormones to spike and cause anxiety. Then came the advent of our favourite addiction; smartphones. And that's when things got really fucked up.

You know when you're in a dark room with someone and they're on their smartphone and their face is lit up with a creepy blue light? That blue light screws with your hormones in a very big way, and it's not just emitted by your phone, it comes from e-readers, laptops, tablets and televisions too – anything with a digital screen. In fact, blue light is technically everywhere, it's even emitted by the sun, which is why the sky looks blue. Your sleep-wake cycle is regulated by exposure to light, and until very recently in our evolutionary history it was only the sun that supplied us with light, then the use of lightbulbs and electronic devices started exposing us to blue light in the evening, instructing your body that despite it being 11pm, it's actually time to be alert and awake. This is why the use of screens in the evening disrupts your ability to fall asleep and sleep soundly.

Exposure to blue light in the evening and at night increases alertness, lowers your production of melatonin by 55 per cent, delays your production of melatonin (which means you take longer to fall asleep), reduces the amount and timing of REM sleep (that's the restorative phase of sleep in which the parts of your brain responsible for learning and making or retaining memories are activated), and reduces alertness upon waking in the morning.

Mobile device use is also associated with a decline in production of thyroid hormones TSH, T3, and T4, and you only have to be on your phone for a couple of hours a day to experience that decline, which is important given that average usage varies from 2–5 hours a day. How many hours are you clocking up on your phone?

Here's what you can do to help:

- Turn your phone off for portions of the day (71 per cent of Britons never do this). Tuck it away in a drawer and focus on what's in front of you, or at least have it on silent and set not to vibrate.
- Keep your devices away from your body – in a bag or corner – and out of your bedroom.
- Stop using devices two hours before you go to bed (a third of Britons check their phones right before going to bed).
- Failing that, invest in some glasses which block blue-light (such as TrueDark) and wear them in the evening when you're using electronic devices to prevent disruption to your circadian rhythms. They can help to stimulate production of melatonin, so consider using them if you have any sleep issue, regardless of screen use.
- Install f.lux on your computers and devices. It's software which adjusts your screen's colour temperature to match the time of day.
- Read an actual book, instead of one on your e-reader.
- Swap fluorescent and LED lightbulbs for incandescent bulbs that produce less blue light.
- If you really need to use a nightlight – if you have a baby who needs to be fed in the night or you have to get up to wee – then use a red bulb as they are least likely to disrupt your circadian rhythm and suppress melatonin production.
- Use candles instead of bulbs in the darker months of the year.

Endocrine Disruptors

Endocrine disruptors are everywhere and they aren't good. They're synthetic substances which disrupt your hormones and they're found in plastics, pesticides, flame retardants, chemicals, and water systems. You're probably breathing them, drinking them, eating them, putting them on your skin, cleaning your kitchen with them, and putting them inside your vagina. They're even found in ovarian follicles and the umbilical cords of newborns.

They are similar in structure to the hormones that you produce in your body such as oestrogen and are referred to as hormone mimickers, as they mimic them and bind to hormone receptor sites. Hormones work as a lock and key system (see page 29) – hormonal glands release hormones which travel around your body in your bloodstream until they reach their intended target, at which point they bind to it and cause a reaction. Each of these hormones has a different shape, and in the same way a key will only work in the lock that it fits in to, so each hormone will only go into the receptor site that it's intended for and have an effect in the places that it's needed. Endocrine disruptors are little buggers because they can cause an increase or decrease in hormone levels in three different ways:

1) Fitting in the lock convincingly enough to trick the body into thinking it's a naturally produced hormone. The mimicker can cause a signal that's stronger than one produced by your natural hormone, which can cause an overproduction or underproduction of hormones, such as excess oestrogen or an underactive thyroid, or cause a signal at the wrong time.
2) Fitting in the lock but they can't turn it, so no reaction takes place, but they plug up the hole and prevent your natural hormones from binding and turning the lock, so the normal hormone signalling fails.
3) They can also interfere with the way natural hormones and receptors are made.

Clinical evidence of the effects of exposure to endocrine disruptors is limited, but vast amounts of research on animals has shown that they may cause:

- Female reproductive health issues, including early onset of puberty and menstruation, fertility issues, and early menopause.

- Increases in breast, ovarian, and prostate cancers.
- Increases in immune and autoimmune diseases, as well as some neurological diseases.
- Reductions in male fertility and a decline in the number of males born.
- Abnormalities in male reproductive organs.

Common endocrine disruptors include:

- **Bisphenol A (BPA)** is found in a lot of plastics and in countless products that we all use on a daily basis: food containers, water bottles, baby bottles, thermal paper used to print receipts, the lining of aluminium cans, milk containers, optical lenses, dental sealants, water storage tanks and water pipes. And as a result of its production around 100 tons of BPA is released into the environment every year, so it's been found in dust particles and drinking water, all of which means we have to limit our exposure to it as much as possible. It's linked to early puberty, breast cancer, and infertility.
- **Phthalates.** Think of this guy as the compound used to make plastic soft. It's in food packaging which is hard to avoid these days but do your best and opt to use glass containers to store food instead of cling film and plastic Tupperware®, and any plastic Tupperware® that you do use should be kept out of the dishwasher, freezer, and microwaves because hot and cold temperatures cause phthalates to be released. They're also found in Styrofoam™ cups, baby toys, PVC, vinyl flooring, shower curtains, shampoo, hairspray, perfume, and nail polish. Phthalates have been linked to problems with ovulation and fertility, obesity, type 2 diabetes, and cancer.
- **Pesticides** commonly used on fruit and vegetable crops, as well as in your garden, are known endocrine disruptors that can also cause cancer. They'll also be present in any meat or dairy products you eat if the animals consumed feed that was laden with them.
- **Surfactants** in cleansing products. Commonly labelled as sulphate, anything that foams contains surfactants, such as facial wash, shower gel, and shampoo. They work by stripping oil away and therefore can cause initial dryness, followed by an overproduction of sebum (the oily substance produced by the glands in your skin which keeps it nourished

and moisturised) because the drying out nature of surfactants makes your body thinks it needs to produce more sebum.

- **Parabens.** Found in shampoos, soaps and shower gels, toothpaste, cosmetics and many other personal care products.
- **Dioxins** are known as persistent organic pollutants (POPs) because they take a long time to break down once they're released into the environment. They form as a result of waste incineration (including backyard burning) and burning fuels such as wood, coal, and oil, and the chlorine bleaching of pulp and paper. They're highly toxic and can cause cancer, reproductive and developmental problems, and damage to the immune system as well as screwing with your hormones. You can find them in bleached products such as coffee filters and tampons.
- **Solvents** in nail polish and nail polish remover.

The list of sources can feel overwhelming, but I find it encouraging and motivating that one study found that using products without phthalates, parabens and phenol brought down levels of substances by 20–45 per cent in just three days. You can reduce your exposure by working on a couple of things at a time, starting with the products that you use most frequently and/ or liberally such as the products you use to wash or moisturise with every day. Here are my top tips for limiting your exposure to them:

- Eat organic where possible, especially meat and dairy products, and the fruit and vegetables on the EWG's list of the *Dirty Dozen* – to avoid the produce with the highest levels of pesticides (*see* Resources).
- See how your personal care products measure up by looking them up on the EWG's Skin Deep database or on *Think Dirty*, an app which allows you to scan the barcode of cosmetics and personal care products as you shop and identify cleaner options (*see* Resources), and start by replacing those that you use most frequently or liberally such as body wash or moisturiser.
- Store food and drink in glass or stainless steel containers.
- Avoid canned food and drinks as cans are usually lined with BPA (though some companies like Biona use BPA free cans).
- Buy food in glass jars instead of cans.
- Don't reheat or freeze food in plastic.

- Keep water bottles out of the sunshine as the heat can cause BPA to leach out into the water.
- Filter the water that you drink.
- Stop using hormonal birth control, which by its very nature is an endocrine disruptor.
- Don't take receipts printed on thermal paper unless you really need them or have them emailed to you instead and if your job requires you to handle receipts, consider wearing gloves.
- Don't use plastic lids on your take away coffee unless you have to as the heat from your coffee can cause any BPA in it to leach out.
- Don't use hand sanitiser or antimicrobial washes.
- Avoid having your clothes dry cleaned or the use of dryer sheets.
- Use natural household cleaning products and laundry detergent.
- Use unbleached products; coffee filters, tampons, toilet paper. The environmental protection agency (EPA) have determined that just using bleached coffee filters can result in a lifetime exposure to dioxin that exceeds acceptable risks.
- When carpeting your home, avoid synthetic carpets and be sure to air your home afterwards as the solvents in the glue used to hold them in place are also hormone disruptors.
- Fill your home and workplace with houseplants which cleanse the air and pump it full of oxygen (*see* Resources for the NASA clean air study which details suitable plants).

Think Twice About What you Put in your Vagina

Just like all your other orifices, your vagina is lined with a mucosal layer and anything that comes into contact with it can disrupt it and your vaginal microbiome. Yep, your vagina has its very own bacterial community too.

Your vagina is highly permeable, readily absorbing chemicals through its mucus membrane. Tampons, laundry detergent, chlorine from swimming pools, intimate cleansers (which you have no need for FYI), spermicides, penises, and lubricants – even natural ones – can all affect the balance of your vagina's microbiome, as can smoking, and when the five main strains found in there end up being in a lower proportion compared to the other minor strains, you can end up with yeast infections and bacterial vaginosis.

In recent years coconut oil has been touted as an excellent natural lubricant, but it's antimicrobial and can therefore disrupt your vaginal microbiome.

Now that you've got a general sense of how you can improve your hormonal and reproductive health (not to mention your digestion!), let's take a look at specific issues and conditions, why they happen, and what you can do to sort them out.

Chapter 9

When things fall apart

If a woman's uterus is out of balance, so is she.
– Don Elijio Panti, the great Maya Shaman of Belize

Before we get into the nitty gritty of what can go wrong with your hormones and your reproductive system, let's take a moment to clarify what a healthy and normal period and menstrual cycle looks like. Please bear in mind that the almighty caveat to this is that you should consider what's normal for you. What's most significant is when you notice something changing, i.e. if your period used to come every 29 days and lasted for five days, but now it comes every 23 days and you bleed noticeably more or less than you used to, that's a significant change and is worth investigating and treating.

- Although 28 days is stated as the average length of a menstrual cycle, only 12.4 per cent of cycles are 28 days long, and a cycle length of 21–35 days is considered normal, though as a practitioner who does a lot of fertility work, I feel there's an optimal range within that of 26–32 days, and that anything outside of that warrants treatment.
- A period usually lasts 2–7 days. For me the optimal is around 5 days as a period that's shorter or longer can be a sign of an imbalance.
- Premenstrual spotting should turn into your period within 24 hours of it starting. Spotting for longer before your period is due can indicate a progesterone deficiency which is also referred to as a luteal phase defect.
- Your period flow should feel steady and be neither light nor heavy.
- Although the colour of your menstrual blood and whether it contains clots is largely insignificant in Western medicine, practitioners of Chinese medicine will use the colour of your flow and information about clots to aid their diagnosis.

- When it comes to cramps, mild cramping in your lower abdomen during your period which doesn't require the use of painkillers and that doesn't interfere with your ability to live your life is reasonable, anything more painful than that or that involves other areas of your body such as your back, hips, or thighs, isn't okay.
- Your cervical fluid should be noticeable as you head towards ovulation, getting increasingly wet and slippery, and ideally resembles egg whites for at least a day.
- Variations in appetite, energy, mood, sexual desire, and interest in social activity are all 100 per cent normal (as they are for all human beings, regardless of the menstrual cycle or not).

99 Problems, and your Period is the Main One

If you already suspect that you've got something untoward going on, or as you read this chapter you begin to think, 'Yes, that's me!', then please, please, please seek out appropriate help from your GP and/or a qualified alternative health practitioner. Too often we accept that menstrual symptoms are our lot in life and it's time that we changed that. Women are in a disadvantaged position when it comes to healthcare; research shows that hospital staff take women's pain less seriously, spend less time with female patients, and are inclined to write off physical pain as 'just emotional' and 'all in the mind', even when physical tests show that their pain is real. As such, women are more likely to be prescribed sedatives or psychotropic drugs than pain-relieving drugs which is of course what they really need. This gender disparity is even greater if you're a person of colour.

My biggest recommendation is that you become an advocate for yourself and get a healthcare team who listen to you and work with you to develop an appropriate treatment plan. Most conditions can be managed, improved, or resolved with nutritional support, manual therapies like women's health physiotherapy and the Arvigo Techniques of Maya Abdominal Therapy® (ATMAT), and Chinese medicine techniques such as acupuncture and herbs. There's also a whole host of straightforward things that you can do by yourself which you'll find in this section of the book. Will you need to do all of what I suggest and spend a significant amount of your salary on seeing a practitioner forever? No, but committing to treatment for a short period of time to help you get going with things is a worthwhile investment, I promise you. Many practitioners offer sliding scale payment options, and lower cost community practices are increasingly common and are a great way of keeping treatments like acupuncture accessible and affordable. Always work with a qualified and licensed practitioner, and ideally one who has been recommended to you by someone that you trust. You can find a list of places to find practitioners in the Resources section, along with educational resources. I've suggested supplements for you to explore, but I always recommend working with a naturopath who can look at your health and lifestyle and make the most appropriate suggestions for you.

Some conditions respond very quickly to the recommendations I'm giving you, and others take a while. It takes several months for an immature follicle to make it all the way to ovulation, so sometimes you won't see the results of what you start to do now until the follicles beginning to develop now mature, so if you want to try a technique out, commit to it for at least 3 months before you start to assess if it's helped or not.

ATMAT®

The Arvigo Techniques of Maya Abdominal Therapy® (ATMAT) are founded on the ancient Maya technique of abdominal massage. Practitioners primarily use massage to improve the flow of blood, lymph, nerve, and energy through the pelvis, relieve menstrual cycle issues, improve reproductive and digestive function, and gently encourage organs that have shifted position – such as a tilted or prolapsed uterus – back into an optimal position. During a session with a practitioner they will teach you how to perform the massage on yourself so that you can use it as a form of self-care, and five minutes a day is all you need to feel the benefits of it. I love that it's not the kind of treatment where you're reliant upon having a treatment week after week. Instead, you might see your practitioner once or twice a month for continued support and treatments, but if you're diligent with your self-care massage then you may not even need to see them again. ATMAT® is incredibly healing when you're experiencing fertility challenges, and after a pregnancy loss or traumatic birth, it's a great way to get to know your body, and it gives you a ridiculously simple but highly effective way of caring for your body for the rest of your life.

Premenstrual Syndrome (PMS) and Premenstrual Dysphoric Disorder (PMDD)

I'm guessing that either you or someone you know struggles with PMS, but despite it being the most commonly talked about menstrual disorder, the medical community are still debating what premenstrual syndrome actually is and whether it even exists at all, let alone actually figuring out what causes it and how to treat it. We commonly use *PMSing* as a term to describe how we feel and act before our periods start, but PMS also refers to a dazzling array of physical signs and symptoms. There are supposedly over 150 different signs and symptoms which can appear in the second half of the menstrual cycle and have been attributed to PMS, including:

- Acne
- Anxiety
- Bloating
- Bowel changes such as constipation and diarrhoea
- Breast tenderness
- Changes in appetite and sexual desire
- Clumsiness
- Cravings for sweet and salty foods
- Crying
- Depression
- Difficulty concentrating
- Disinterest
- Fatigue
- Headaches
- Irritability
- Joint pain
- Insomnia
- Migraines
- Muscular pain
- Nausea and vomiting
- Social withdrawal
- Suicidal thoughts
- Weight gain

With a list that long, it's likely that every single one of us experiences at least one symptom of PMS, so it won't surprise you when I tell you that research studies have found that as many as 90 per cent of us have PMS, but that doesn't mean that most of us are in tears in the toilet or punching pillows with rage, because statistics like this also include the physical symptoms associated with this time of the month. But a 2014 study investigating the incidence of depressive symptoms premenstrually found that depressive symptoms were not associated with concentrations of reproductive hormones, and a review of the scientific literature on PMS that was conducted in 2012 concluded that the studies analysed 'failed to provide clear evidence in support of the existence of a specific premenstrual negative mood syndrome in the general population' – so what is this PMS that we all talk about? It's entirely reasonable to expect that hormonal changes in the cycle will create the appearance of one symptom or another, and as you've read in the previous chapters, my take on a lot of the physical, emotional, and behavioural variations that we experience throughout the menstrual cycle, is that they are healthy, normal, and even beneficial. But from my training, my own experiences and certainly those of the women I've treated, I know that these symptoms can be challenging, uncomfortable and in some cases, debilitating. In some instances, there will be an underlying hormonal imbalance that can cause or contribute to PMS, including diminishing hormone levels just before a period starts, but when it comes to the mood changes experienced by some of the people who have menstrual cycles, I suspect that our hormones are simply revealing something that's going on all the time but which oestrogen glosses over in the first half of the cycle.

At What Point Does PMS Become a Disorder?

In 2013 the Diagnostic and Statistical Manual of Mental Disorders (DSM-5) made waves by including premenstrual dysphoric disorder (PMDD) as an official diagnosis – the first and only diagnosis related to the menstrual cycle. PMDD is an extreme form of PMS and its symptoms can include depression, extreme irritability, anxiety, suicidal thoughts, feeling overwhelmed, panic attacks, and bouts of crying. Menstruators who have PMDD often describe themselves as living a Jekyll and Hyde life; their extreme symptoms appear premenstrually and respite from them finally comes when their period starts. They can then feel pretty good up to ovulation. Because of the on/off feeling great then feeling fucking awful cyclical nature of these symptoms, PMDD is commonly misdiagnosed as rapid-cycling bipolar disorder.

To receive a diagnosis of PMDD, you must experience at least five of the following eleven signs and symptoms (and one of the first four must be present):

1) Marked changes in mood swings or increased sensitivity.
2) Marked irritability or anger or increased personal conflicts.
3) Marked depressed mood, feelings of hopelessness or self-deprecating thoughts.
4) Marked anxiety and tension, feeling on edge.
5) Decreased interest in usual activities.
6) Difficulty concentrating.
7) Lethargy and marked lack of energy.
8) Marked change in appetite (e.g., over-eating or specific food cravings).
9) Excessive sleepiness and/or insomnia.
10) Feeling overwhelmed or out of control.
11) Physical symptoms (e.g., breast tenderness or swelling, joint or muscle pain, a sensation of 'bloating' and weight gain).

They must occur specifically in the week before your period starts, improve once it begins and become minimal or resolve entirely in the week after your period, have featured in most of your menstrual cycles for the past year, and be severe enough to affect your work, education, social activities, or relationships with others.

In most menstrual cycles, I definitely experience at least one of the first four symptoms, and of the whole list, I can have anything from 5 to all of them. But although I meet the diagnostic criteria and they can affect my personal and professional life and my relationships, I don't consider myself to have PMDD, largely because my symptoms perhaps lack the severity that warrants the diagnosis, but also because I rail against the idea of being labelled as having a mental illness when I know from tracking my cycle that what I experience is down to my tendency to hold my emotions in instead of simply stating my needs to those around me (which by the way, they'd be only too happy to oblige in – if only I'd just let them know). But that's my experience and understanding, and other people's will be different, so let's get back to your experience; how do you differentiate between what's normal and healthy, and what constitutes an illness?

I think you're the best judge of your menstrual cycle and whether your experience of your Autumn is a disorder that needs to be treated. It's estimated that 3–8 per cent of menstruators suffer from PMDD, and those that have it really do suffer. PMDD is often triggered or aggravated following a pregnancy, miscarriage, and perimenopause, and it's associated with an increased risk of postnatal depression and suicide.

PMDD is believed to be a genetic disorder and studies have demonstrated that individuals with PMDD have a variation in their oestrogen receptor alpha (OSR1) gene, are more likely to be sensitive to the effects of oestrogen and progesterone across the menstrual cycle, and that their cells respond differently to exposure to these hormones. But this testing has been carried out as part of medical research studies, and you're unlikely to be tested for it in order to receive a diagnosis.

PMDD can also occur alongside other mental health conditions such as depression, anxiety, and bipolar disorder, exacerbating them premenstrually. This is referred to as premenstrual magnification and can also affect other physical conditions such as digestive disorders.

The classification of this severe form of PMS as a psychiatric disorder is not without debate. Some argue that it medicalises a perfectly natural physiological process, labels us as hormonal liabilities, and serves to benefit the profits of the pharmaceutical industry, because while there are plenty of menstruators who have benefitted from receiving a diagnosis, for each condition or syndrome listed, there will be at least one large pharmaceutical company benefitting from the new inclusion, so we have to question who does it serve; us, or the drug companies? While we do need to be wary, I also believe that there's a very real need for those with PMDD to receive help, and sometimes that needs to be in the form of medication which of course requires a diagnosis. Selective serotonin reuptake inhibitors (SSRIs) such as fluoxetine (Prozac® or Sarafem®), sertraline (Zoloft®), and paroxetine (Paxil®) can be prescribed to alleviate the psychological symptoms of PMS and PMDD, and as symptom relief can be felt in 1–2 days they don't have to be taken throughout the whole of your cycle. Instead, they're taken when symptoms begin and discontinued once you come on your period. Careful tracking of your cycle will help you to establish when your symptoms typically start and end, so that you can get a sense of when you might need to time the use of SSRIs as well as bringing in other strategies that work for you.

Plan for PMS and PMDD:

- If you're doing the bulk of the caregiving or chores in your workplace or home, or if you're not expressing the things that bother you, address this imbalance and find a way to say the words that you swallow time and time again.
- Get really good at saying *no, I prefer not to,* and *let me get back to you about that.*
- Eat regularly and do not skip meals in your luteal phase. Keep your blood sugar balanced by eating plenty of protein and healthy fats.
- Cut out food that causes inflammation in the body (see page 220).
- If you have symptoms of low oestrogen (see page 106), or excess oestrogen (see page 235) and/or low progesterone (see page 159), follow the relevant guidelines.
- Experiment with exercise and rest in your premenstruum and see what helps you.
- Consider using supplements such as magnesium, B vitamins, Omega-3 Fatty Acids, and *Agnus castus* (vitex).
- Question if histamine intolerance (see page 223) could be contributing to or causing PMS/PMDD.
- Speak to your GP if you think that you might have PMDD and ask to be referred for mental health support.

Menstrual Cramps (Dysmenorrhoea)

As many as 84 per cent of us have primary dysmenorrhoea – period pain that isn't caused by another condition such as endometriosis or fibroids – and while a small amount of mild lower abdominal cramping is deemed as normal, it shouldn't be to the degree that you have to stop what you're doing or use pain relief. Most of us are socialised into believing that because period pain is common, it's normal. It isn't. We're not badly designed, we're not being punished for Eve's original sin in the Garden of Eden, and it's not your lot in life to put up with it, so if you're in the 50 per cent who describe their period pain as severe, please don't suffer in silence.

WTF does it happen? Towards the end of your cycle, just before your period begins, the lining of your womb begins to break down and as it does it releases prostaglandins which make it contract and limit blood loss during your period. Period pain occurs when you release too many prostaglandins and most menstruators who experience severe cramping have an increased secretion of them. Prostaglandins are algesic substances, which means that they prime the nervous system for pain and heighten the pain response, resulting in painful contractions *and* an increase in pain signalling to the brain. And if that wasn't enough they're to blame for the nausea, vomiting and period poops that can accompany your period. Nice one.

Some menstruators have stronger and abnormal uterine contractions which result in an increase in intrauterine pressure and an impaired ability to deliver oxygen to the contracting muscles, creating more pain. These contractions have been measured as being as strong as the contractions experienced towards the end of labour, and as someone who used to have extreme period pain and who's given birth, I can tell you that I'd take labour over that kind of period pain any day of the week.

Pharmacologic help can be given in the form of non-steroidal anti-inflammatories (NSAIDs) such as ibuprofen and naproxen, but research shows that heat therapy in the form of a hot water bottle, heat pad, or hot bath can be just as effective.

The pill is frequently offered as first line treatment for period pain, but there are plenty of other ways to treat it without resorting to suppressing your entire reproductive system – remember, the pill works by preventing ovulation, and it's ovulation that results in the production of progesterone which is an important hormone when it comes to your health, and it can also cause a whole host of unpleasant side effects.

If you're planning on having a kid, I strongly recommend getting your period pain under control before you start trying to conceive because, from a Chinese medicine point of view, the syndromes that are behind period pain can also be involved in fertility challenges and complications in pregnancy and birth. There's a fantastic opportunity before you conceive to get everything sorted, which will pay off in terms of less period pain but also when it comes to conceiving and labouring with ease.

Pain is not normal. Pain is your body asking for help, and painkillers, which are often 100 per cent necessary, silence those screams. I get that the whole point of them is to do that, but can you take them and still listen to what your body is asking for instead of ignoring its requests?

When you see your GP about period pain they will carry out a pelvic examination to assess if any abnormalities can be felt, but that's usually about it and in most cases, they'll conclude that there's nothing to suggest an abnormality, and suggest stronger painkillers and/or hormonal birth control. If, in reading about endometriosis and adenomyosis in the following sections, you start to think that they could account for the pain you experience, insist that your doctor refer you for further investigation. It takes an average of 7.5 years for endometriosis to be diagnosed, and sometimes as many as 12, and that is not acceptable.

Plan for menstrual cramps:

- Get resting or get moving. Weekly exercise throughout your cycle is associated with an improvement in pain, but what about exercising when you're actually bleeding? I find that some clients will find that their menstrual related symptoms (period pain, mood swings, headaches etc.) improve when they exercise during their period, because movement helps to get their energy moving and relieve the blockages that cause these issues according to Chinese medicine. Whereas if they're deficient, they are exhausted by exercise during their period and possibly after it's finished too, so nourishing activities like eating well and resting suit them better (yes, rest is an activity, we just don't see it as such because we value growth and movement).
- Smoking, both actively and passively, is related to menstrual pain so ditch that habit.
- Reduce inflammation by cutting out or limiting your intake of sugar, alcohol, and dairy, particularly in the second half of your cycle. I know it's a big ask to do this, so if you're going to focus on cutting one out, make dairy the priority. My clients find that it can make an almost immediate difference, with them noticing an improvement within 1–3 cycles.
- Cut out nightshades; white potatoes, aubergine, peppers and tomatoes have pro-inflammatory properties in those that are sensitive to them. The best way to find out if you are is by excluding them from your diet for a few weeks, see how you feel, and then reintroduce them and see how you react.
- Consider if you have histamine intolerance (see page 223).
- Magnesium can be taken with food throughout your cycle. Magnesium glycinate is easily absorbed and doesn't result in loose stools, whereas magnesium citrate is slightly less absorbable but can increase bowel activity which can be helpful if you tend towards constipation (if you

don't poo at least once a day, this is you). Magnesium is also great if you get PMS (see page 273), PCOS (see page 301), migraines, or have trouble sleeping.

- B vitamins. B1 and B2 are known specifically for their ability to reduce period pain, but it's best to take a vitamin that's a B complex and which contains all the B vitamins as they're all necessary for health and they work together to achieve this.
- Omega-3 Fatty Acids is a powerful anti-inflammatory that can outperform the use of ibuprofen in reducing period pain.
- Curcumin is a molecule found in turmeric and it's another powerful anti-inflammatory that's particularly helpful if you have endometriosis, adenomyosis or heavy periods. Adding turmeric to food isn't enough to make a significant difference as only 3 per cent of it is curcumin, so take a supplement along with a meal as it's best absorbed alongside fat.
- NSAIDs such as ibuprofen work by lowering your production of prostaglandins and are best taken as soon as your period starts (if you use painkillers and they work entirely, that's awesome, but be aware that without any pain you're likely to push on with everything that you need to get done in a day, so remind yourself to slow down – even if you don't feel the pain, your body is struggling somewhat so help it by easing up).
- Heat therapy, the fancy description for a hot bath or water bottle, can improve blood flow and relieve pain, and data from two clinical trials concluded that it can be as effective as treatment with an NSAID.
- Castor oil packs on your lower abdomen can be used to improve flow through the pelvis and reduce period pain. You can find instructions on how to do them on page 83.
- Acupuncture, herbs, and physical therapies such as physiotherapy, reflexology, and the Arvigo Techniques of Maya Abdominal Therapy® (see page 272) can all be a real saviour when it comes to period pain.
- Essential oils can be added to a carrier oil such as almond oil (extra virgin olive oil and coconut oil from your kitchen work beautifully too). As an aromatherapist, I lean towards the following oils as they relieve pain and/or cramps, and/or promote and regularise menstrual flow: black pepper, chamomile, clary sage, fennel, jasmine, juniper, lavender, myrrh, marjoram, peppermint, rose, and rosemary.
- Supplementing with melatonin has been shown to reduce period pain and improve sleep.

- Transcutaneous electrical nerve stimulation (TENS) sounds like it's a form of torture, but it's a small battery-operated pack that has wires that are attached to sticky pads which you apply to your lower abdomen or back. A gentle electrical current then stimulates the affected area which reduces the pain signals going to your spinal cord and brain and encourages the production of pain-relieving endorphins. You're able to control the strength of the current and it usually feels like a tingle. They're a fairly low-cost option and there are lots available to buy secondhand as they're frequently purchased to use as natural pain relief in labour, but if you'd prefer a smaller unit that would be easier to hide under clothing, a TENS device called Livia offers a pricier but more discreet option.
- Orgasms; non-penetrative or penetrative, with your lover or flying solo, it's up to you, but they help by releasing pain-relieving endorphins and oxytocin.
- Keep your womb warm. In Chinese medicine and in many cultures across the world, great emphasis is placed on keeping your feet, abdomen and back warm, and not exposing them to cold or draughts (say goodbye to your crop tops and ballerina slippers), as well as not swimming in cold water whilst menstruating or immediately after a pregnancy loss or birth. I haven't found any scientific research that backs this up, but anecdotally I do find that this advice makes a difference and I think it's worthwhile considering cultural history such as this instead of dismissing them as old wives' tales.
- Cannabidiol (CBD) oil is a product derived from cannabis plants, but it doesn't produce a 'high' or the form of intoxication associated with using weed – that's caused by another cannabinoid known as THC. There's increasing awareness of the potential medical uses of CBD, including using it for pain relief such as period pain by applying it as a cream or oil, or taking it orally in capsule or liquid form.
- Leave your crappy relationship or job. I've had many clients over the years who've found their menstrual cramps disappear entirely when they leave the job they hate or the relationship which isn't working for them.

Endometriosis

Endometriosis is a disease in which tissue that's similar to, but not the same as, the lining of your uterus is found in other places in the body. It can be found on the reproductive organs (uterus, fallopian tubes, ovaries) the utero-sacral ligaments, peritoneum (the membrane that covers your abdomen) or any of the spaces between the bladder, uterus/vagina, and rectum. It can also occur on the bladder, bowels, and in more remote locations such as the diaphragm, lungs, and in rare cases, the eyes and brain.

Every month endometrial tissue goes through the same process as the lining of your womb in that it plumps up, breaks down and then bleeds, except of course the blood and tissue can't exit the body through your vagina like your period does. Instead it causes inflammation that results in an increase in blood supply and congestion which in turn stimulates an immune response, as well as causing adhesions and scarring. In advanced cases, organs that are suspended in the pelvis by ligaments and tissues which are meant to move around to a degree, are bound by scar tissue, and when there's movement – during ovulation, sex, or a bowel movement – it can result in excruciating pain.

Ten per cent of women have endometriosis and symptoms can develop during teen years or later on in life. Symptoms include: chronic pelvic pain, painful periods, painful sex, back pain, infertility, gastro-intestinal symptoms, pain with bowel movements, pain with exercise, bladder pain and urgency/frequency, fatigue, exhaustion, and depression. One person may have a lot of endometriosis but not experience a lot of pain, and another have a minimal amount, but due to the location of the lesion – for example, if it's next to a nerve – may be incapacitated by pain.

It is undoubtedly a condition which can severely impact daily life, work and relationships, and yet one in which physicians do not receive adequate training in diagnosing and treating. Shockingly, and despite its prevalence across all demographics, it takes someone an average of 6–12 years to be diagnosed after presenting with symptoms.

Your healthcare provider might spot things that make them suspect endometriosis from pelvic exams and scans, but it cannot be diagnosed by them. Endo (as it's often referred to as) can only be definitively diagnosed by laparoscopy – keyhole surgery in which a fibre optic instrument is inserted through a small incision in your abdominal wall so that your internal organs and tissues can be viewed. This should ideally be performed by a skilled excision surgeon so that if any endo is removed it is done so in the most appropriate manner.

When it comes to surgical management, there are two options; excision surgery, where the endometrial tissue is cut away, and ablation, where it is burnt away. Generally speaking, excision surgery performed by a highly skilled surgeon is the gold standard. Over the years I've had many clients who've undergone multiple ablation surgeries in which endo is burnt off, but they haven't reduced their symptoms and pain for very long, and commonly caused more scar tissue and problems, so I'm a big believer in one surgery, done well, where possible. That means finding a highly skilled surgeon, finding a way to be treated by them on the NHS (you can request to be referred to a specific surgeon's clinic via the Choose and Book scheme on the NHS) or under your insurance plan (excision surgery is often out of network), travelling to them if they aren't local, and it may require the involvement of more than one surgeon if, for example, you have endo on your bowels or diaphragm which is not within the remit of your gynaecologist to remove. To give you an idea of how tricky this can be, it's estimated that there's only a handful of gynaecologists in the UK who are skilled enough to carry out this surgery, and out of over 400,000 gynaecologists in the USA, only around 150 are. To find a list of skilled excision surgeons and other incredible resources, I highly recommend joining the 'Nancy's Nook Endometriosis Education' group on Facebook and educating yourself about endometriosis and your treatment options (do note that this is an incredible educational resource but not a support group, use the files and search bar!)

Initially, pregnancy can aggravate endo pain but in some cases, pregnancy can lessen the degree to which symptoms are experienced because of the vast increase in production of progesterone, but pregnancy does not 'cure' endometriosis, and neither does hysterectomy. Hysterectomy is only appropriate in a select number of cases because when endometriosis exists outside of the uterus as it frequently does, it's logical that it cannot be cured by removing the uterus. Countless people undergo unnecessary hysterectomies every year because of this outdated understanding and approach to the disease.

Surgery isn't always necessary, and endometriosis can be helped greatly by diet and nutrition, acupuncture and herbs, and physical therapy, and you may find that these methods are enough to manage your symptoms, or you can use them alongside a surgical approach. It doesn't have to be a case of either/or, and it's important that you go down the path that suits you best, which, for a lot of people will involve skilled excision surgery.

Though medication can suppress some symptoms in some people with endo, it does not treat it and only acts as a band-aid. Hormonal birth control doesn't control the growth of endo, and some people will find that their endo progresses while on the pill so even if their symptoms are reduced whilst on it, they're a lot worse once they come off it. Drugs such as Lupron® which suppress the ovaries, essentially instigating a menopausal state, can cause horrendous side effects, can't be used long-term, and again, don't actually treat the endo. The press recently celebrated that the FDA have approved elagolix (brand name, Orlissa™) – the first new endo drug to come on the market for a decade – but Orlissa™ is manufactured by AbbVie, the same pharmaceutical company who hold the patent for Lupron®, which coincidently, after being on the market for a decade, is about to expire and, when it does, generic forms of Lupron® will become available which will be cheaper, thus AbbVie's need to create an updated 'better' drug that they could hold the patent to.

To be clear, hormonal methods may improve symptoms but don't treat the actual endo. Any hormonal treatment to suppress endo may make it harder to find during surgery to remove it and you should speak to your surgeon about their use long before you actually have surgery so that they can advise you when to stop taking them.

You might be wondering how someone ends up with endo, and the truth is that there is no one theory that accounts for all cases. In 1927 Dr. John Sampson came up with a theory that retrograde menstruation – when menstrual flow moves backwards into the pelvis and ovaries – was the cause of endometrial lesions, and despite this being a hugely flawed theory, it remains a prevalent and popular one which continues to cause and complicate management of the disease. Why is it flawed? If you recall, endometrial lesions *resemble* the lining of the womb, but when they're analysed on a microscopic level, they aren't the same. Furthermore, retrograde menstruation occurs in around 90 per cent of menstruators but only 10 per cent have endo, and although it's rare, men can get it too, so clearly retrograde menstruation is not the cause of endometriosis. Other theories include; problems occurring during embryonic development, the migration of stem cells which regenerate the lining of the womb in each menstrual cycle to other areas of the body, and the dysfunction of particular genes. There is certainly a genetic link, if close family members have it then you're more likely to, and one study found endometriosis in 9 per cent of female foetuses, suggesting that it's a disease that individuals are born with which is then triggered by multiple factors later in life such as onset of menstruation, and environmental exposure to chemicals such as dioxins and xenooestrogens (chemicals which mimic oestrogen).

If you have endo, your genes not only over-respond to oestrogen, encouraging more and more endometrial growth, but endo tissue also produces its own oestrogen, so people with endo are really prone to the hormonal imbalance of excess oestrogen. As if that wasn't enough, progesterone receptors are quieted and the inflammation from endo cells results in them being less responsive to progesterone – the hormone that keeps oestrogen in check – which further contributes to overgrowth. This is why administering progesterone as a form of treatment rarely helps, because the progesterone receptors aren't responsive to it.

It can feel like a dismal situation but there are things that can help. Look at the excess oestrogen protocol on page 235, improve your gut and liver function, check out the endometriosis support section in the Resources, and get a top-notch team to support you (naturopath, acupuncturist, physical therapist).

Plan for endometriosis:

- Endometriosis can only be diagnosed by keyhole laparoscopic surgery and if endo is found during the surgery it will be removed, so you really want to have it carried out by someone who is skilled in excision surgery. You can find a list of surgeons in the file section of the 'Nancy's Nook' Facebook group, as well as vast amounts of information on hormonal medications and hysterectomy, and how to prepare for and recover from surgery.
- The suggestions in the painful periods section also apply to the treatment of endo, and it's crucial that you address oestrogen excess and reduce inflammation as endo both creates and is exacerbated by excess oestrogen and inflammation.
- Research suggests that the use of CBD oil may be a particularly helpful strategy for people with endo because of its ability to treat pain as well as the proliferation of the disease.
- Low levels of vitamin D have been linked to endo, and a blood test will show whether you should supplement with vitamin D or not.
- Removing all sources of gluten from your diet can dramatically improve symptoms. One study of women with endo who had not been diagnosed

with celiac disease – a severe allergy to gluten – were put on a gluten-free diet for one year, and 75 per cent of participants reported significant pain relief.

- Stay clear of meat and dairy that's full of hormones; balancing your own hormones is tricky enough without adding in the hormones that are in produce that comes from hormone-laden animals. Opt for grass-fed organic meat and dairy.
- Supplements to consider include; Omega-3 Fatty Acids, curcumin, magnesium, and B vitamin complex.

Adenomyosis

Adenomyosis is a condition of the uterus in which tissue that's normally only found in the lining of the womb (the endometrium), is found in the deeper muscular layer (the myometrium) causing symptoms such as pain and abnormal bleeding. Its symptoms often overlap with those of endo and the two can co-exist, and although it's estimated to affect as many as 20–35 per cent of people with uteruses, it's unclear exactly how prevalent it is as a definitive diagnosis is hard to achieve. Adenomyosis can be suspected from ultrasound or MRI results, but some people who have adeno will have images from these tests that appear normal, so they aren't a reliable way of diagnosing it. A sample of endometrial tissue can be removed during a biopsy to examine it for signs of adenomyosis, but unless the piece of tissue that's removed is from an affected area, it can't be used to confirm it or rule it out, and the procedure itself could cause adenomyosis. The only way to achieve an absolute diagnosis is to perform a hysterectomy and examine the whole of the uterus – not ideal.

The cause of adenomyosis is unclear, but risk factors for it include having uterine surgeries, a termination, or a caesarean birth, as well as being oestrogen dominant, though it's worth pointing out that there are plenty of teens who have never had sex let alone been pregnant who have been found to have adenomyosis, so it's not always caused by surgery or terminations.

Medications which suppress hormones such as the combined birth control pill, Mirena® IUD, high-dose progestins, and other forms of hormone suppressants can be used to relieve some symptoms, but they frequently cause side effects, and some can't be used long-term.

286

Surgical excision, where the area affected is removed, may be suggested in some cases when the disease is clearly defined by ultrasound or MRI, but this is a highly skilled surgery that can lead to severe blood loss, poor outcomes in terms of reduced pain, and although conceiving after this kind of surgery is rare, when pregnancies do occur they are associated with a high rate of pregnancy complications. At present hysterectomy remains the only complete way of resolving adenomyosis, but the dietary, lifestyle, and treatment suggestions in the period pain and endometriosis sections can help to improve symptoms.

No Periods (Amenorrhoea)

Pregnancy, breastfeeding, menopause, and some forms of hormonal birth control can all cause your periods to stop, but if your period has been missing for over three months and none of the above apply to you, it's important to find out what's going on, and if you haven't done a pregnancy test yet, it's always worth doing one to rule it out. There are two types of amenorrhoea; primary amenorrhoea, which is when you've never had a period, and secondary amenorrhoea, which is when you used to have periods but now you don't. It's secondary amenorrhoea that I want to focus on because it's what I see a lot of in my practice. It can be caused by:

- Medications which can interfere with having a regular cycle such as antidepressants, antipsychotics, allergy and blood pressure medications, and of course hormonal birth control.
- Asherman's Syndrome, a condition where scar tissue builds up in the uterus (usually as a result of trauma) which can prevent the normal cyclical build up and shedding of the uterine lining.
- A tumour on the pituitary gland which suppresses your cycle by secreting a hormone called prolactin (these tumours are usually non-cancerous).
- Premature Ovarian Failure, a distressing situation which involves the loss of ovarian function before the age of 40 and instigates premature menopause.
- An overactive or underactive thyroid.
- A condition called hypothalamic amenorrhoea (HA), where the hypothalamus gland in your brain slows or stops the release of Gonadotropin-releasing hormone (GnRH), the hormone which causes

the menstrual cycle to start. HA is common after coming off the birth control pill because while you were on it your hypothalamus stopped communicating with your ovaries and it can take a while for them to get talking again. HA also occurs when there's something off with your diet/exercise/stress levels.

- Polycystic ovarian syndrome (PCOS), a hormonal imbalance which interferes with ovulation and causes long irregular cycles (see page 301 for more details).

I've treated a lot of women whose periods have disappeared; some are waiting for their cycle to return after coming off the pill, and others just haven't had one in a year, or two, or even 10, and in the majority of those that I've treated, the reason for the absence of their period has been because they have hypothalamic amenorrhoea or PCOS. I'm going to be addressing PCOS further on, so let's concentrate on hypothalamic amenorrhoea (HA) for now.

In the absence of a regular cycle, most GPs will recommend that you take the pill in order to have periods, but the problem with this is that you don't have periods on the pill because it prevents you from ovulating, you only have withdrawal bleeds. Withdrawal bleeds happen when your body is subjected to the rapid decline of hormones that comes about when you take the dummy pills in your pack or stop using your patch or NuvaRing®, and while regularly shedding the lining of your womb is important because it reduces your risk of endometrial cancer, it's preferable that you have a real period so that you can receive all the health benefits that come about because of ovulation. Remember, when your periods go MIA what we want is for your hormonal system to start communicating again, so taking the pill and shutting it down again ain't gonna help and it can even prevent recovery from HA.

Survival always trumps reproduction, so if your body determines that this is not a safe or healthy time for you to conceive, your brain tells your ovaries to shut up shop, and you won't ovulate or get your period. This can happen when your stress levels are high for a sustained period of time, or when your body perceives that this is a lean time and therefore not an ideal time to grow a human, because of one of the following scenarios:

- You're not eating enough, or enough of the right types of food; your body needs protein, fat, and carbs in order to make hormones, so if you're on a low-fat/calorie/protein/carb diet, your body's going to struggle to manufacture your reproductive hormones and interprets an inadequate diet as a sign that it's a lean time.

- You skip meals, have an eating disorder, or don't eat frequently enough to match your energy output; you can have an amazingly healthy diet, full of fat and protein, but if you're doing CrossFit or training for a marathon five times a week then you may be doing too much as far as your reproductive health is concerned.

When your periods have stopped it's really important to establish why, especially when it comes to differentiating between HA and PCOS, because with HA you usually need to eat more and exercise less, but with PCOS losing excess weight is a key way of improving symptoms, so you don't want to get them mixed up and inadvertently cause more of a problem by going down the wrong treatment pathway. To get to the bottom of why your periods have stopped, and in order to come up with a suitable treatment plan with any healthcare practitioner you choose to work with, your GP will likely test for the following hormones: thyroid-stimulating hormone (TSH – see box overleaf), prolactin, FSH, LH, testosterone, and a protein called sex hormone binding globulin (SHBG). This initial round of tests is usually enough to suggest why you have amenorrhoea, and further investigations may be carried out to elicit more insight into what's going on. A normal level of TSH can *only* exclude hypothyroidism in the absence of signs and symptoms which indicate a dysfunctional hypothalamic-pituitary-ovarian (HPO) axis, and clearly the absence of periods suggests something has gone awry with the communication of the HPO axis, making more comprehensive thyroid testing necessary (see page 290).

Plan for amenorrhoea:

- Eat more! Especially protein and healthy fat so that you can use them to manufacture hormones. If your current diet excludes or limits carbs, you will need to up your intake of them. I usually recommend that clients with HA eat every 2.5–3 hours, so that they eat three meals a day as well as having healthy snacks that contain protein, that way your body gets the message that food isn't scarce, and you'll have enough energy to have a menstrual cycle, and an increase in body mass index (BMI) is associated with getting your period back.

- Reduce the intensity and frequency at which you exercise and focus on restorative exercise which balances your stress hormones and builds your energy, such as gentle yoga, tai chi, qi gong, swimming, or just going for nice walks. This is a case where less really is more.
- Your focus should be on what you eat and how much you eat, but using supplements such as magnesium, zinc, and a herb called vitex agnus-castus can be supportive too.
- Seed cycling (see page 101) can help to restore optimal hormone levels.
- Use treatments such as acupuncture, herbs and ATMAT® to bring your cycle back.
- Prioritise self-care above all else if you want your period to return.

A Note About Thyroid Testing

Thyroid testing is expensive, and many doctors evaluate thyroid function by only testing for thyroid-stimulating hormone (TSH), the hormone released by your pituitary gland in your brain that's responsible for stimulating your thyroid gland to release thyroid hormone. When thyroid function is optimal, your pituitary and thyroid casually chat back and forth to keep things running as they should, but when thyroid function is sub-optimal, your pituitary gland has to yell at it in order to get it going, and it does this by secreting larger amounts of TSH. That means that a high TSH result indicates that your pituitary gland is working extra hard to compensate for a not-so-great thyroid. If TSH is low, it may be that you're over-producing thyroid hormones and that you have hyperthyroidism. But, what if it's normal? Well, when it comes to testing TSH, what's considered to be 'normal' is controversial.

The normal range for TSH of 0.4–4.5 mU/L is considered by many healthcare professionals to be overly generous, and in light of research suggesting that the upper limit be reduced, there's an emerging consensus that the normal range should be 0.4–2.5 mU/L, particularly when it comes to achieving positive fertility and pregnancy outcomes. When TSH is high it's a sign that your thyroid is underactive (hypothyroidism). But what if your TSH result falls within the reduced range, does that mean your thyroid is doing well? It might, but it might not.

When TSH gets the message to your thyroid that it needs to increase its production of hormones, it produces four different types, helpfully numbered T1, T2, T3, and T4. The main hormone produced by your thyroid is T4, so if your doctor orders a test in addition to TSH, it's likely to be for Free T4 (FT4). Why is it 'free'? The majority of your thyroid hormones are bound up to carrier protein in the blood, but it's the tiny percentage of 'free' thyroid hormones that have an effect in the body, and cause problems, so it makes sense to test the free thyroid hormones, right? High FT4 can indicate an overactive thyroid, and a low level of it indicates an underactive thyroid.

But, if TSH and FT4 are normal, *you can still have hypothyroidism*. In order to be used, T4 must first be converted into Free T3 (FT3), so if your lab work shows that FT3 is low, it could be that your symptoms of hypothyroidism are because you're not converting T4 very well. There's also another inactive form of thyroid hormone called Reverse T3 (RT3) which can attach to the receptors for Free T3 and block it, acting like a brake – a handy mechanism in times of stress or illness when the body wants to slow down your metabolism so that you can use your energy to heal instead of having energy in your muscles for moving and grooving. If Reverse T3 is high, you're probably converting too much T4 to Reverse T3, and not enough to Free T3, and this results in symptoms of hypothyroidism even though TSH and T4 come back as normal.

Okay, what if TSH, FT4, FT3, and RT3 all come back as normal; does that mean you're in the clear? Not entirely. Your labs can all come back as normal, but they can show the presence of thyroid antibodies – a marker and predictor of an autoimmune condition called Hashimoto's hypothyroidism. Testing positive for thyroid antibodies in pregnancy suggests subclinical hypothyroidism and puts you at an increased risk of developing postpartum hypothyroidism.

Hypothyroidism is common in women but is thought to be under-diagnosed, despite it frequently resulting in fertility issues, recurrent miscarriages (because of the increased demand for thyroid hormones in pregnancy), depression, and obesity. It's commonly stated that

1–2 per cent of the population have hypothyroidism, that it is 8–10 times more common in women, and that the likelihood of having it increases with age. But recent large-scale research from Norway suggests that its prevalence rate is higher, with 9 per cent of the women surveyed stating that they had previously received a diagnosis of a thyroid disorder, of which hypothyroidism accounted for 4.8 per cent. And a report from Colorado found that 9.5 per cent of study participants had elevated TSH (>5.1mU/L), a marker of hypothyroidism.

If you have symptoms that suggest thyroid dysfunction such as those listed below then please speak to your GP about comprehensive thyroid testing. If your TSH and T4 results come back as 'normal' and they are unwilling to do further testing that you feel is warranted, then consider seeing another GP or pay for these tests privately if you're able to. Guidance on how to get a diagnosis and work with you doctor can be found at www.thyroiduk.org.uk

Signs of hypothyroidism include:

- Fatigue, particularly upon waking and that may improve over the course of the day
- Weight gain that you can't lose
- High cholesterol
- Feeling cold or having cold hands and feet
- Fluid retention or swollen ankles
- Reduced sweating
- Depression
- Dry rough skin
- Dry hair
- Thin, brittle nails
- Hair loss, especially the outer third of your eyebrows and/or eyelashes
- Low level of sexual desire
- Bowel movements that feel incomplete or occur less than once a day
- Feeling breathless
- Palpitations
- Insomnia
- Tingling in your hands and feet

- Muscle or joint aches, or poor muscle tone (since when was it so hard to open a bottle of wine?)
- Recurrent headaches or migraines
- Dizziness
- Difficulty concentrating, brain feels slow
- Sluggish reflexes
- Bruising easily
- Heavy periods
- Infertility
- Miscarriage

It can be caused by:

- Hashimoto's autoimmune thyroiditis.
- Iodine deficiency.
- A non-cancerous tumour on the pituitary gland which affects its ability to produce TSH (this is a relatively rare cause).
- Thyroid surgery and radiation therapy can diminish or halt production of thyroid hormones.
- Stress and high cortisol levels which inhibit TSH.
- Endocrine disrupting chemicals.
- Goitrogens.
- Vitamin and mineral deficiencies.

Hyperthyroidism can cause weight loss, a rapid or irregular heartbeat, palpitations, feeling nervous or anxious, insomnia, loose stools, shortness of breath, feeling tired and weak, twitching or trembling, sensitivity to heat, and a swelling in your neck caused by a swollen thyroid gland which is called a goitre.

You can support your thyroid by:

- Improving your digestive function. A leaky gut (see page 222) can cause thyroid problems, so cut out problematic foods and have some bone broth to help it heal.
- Considering if you have an intolerance to gluten.

- Eating a nutrient dense diet and chewing your food.
- Getting off your mobile phone – just two hours of use per day can raise TSH and lower T4.
- Practising good sleep hygiene (see page 262) because getting less than 6 hours' sleep is associated with a reduction in TSH and T4.
- Addressing any adrenal imbalance (see page 164) because both too much and too little cortisol can affect thyroid function.
- Avoiding caffeine.
- Avoiding endocrine disruptors in the environment.
- Getting plenty of sunshine.
- Getting your level of vitamin D tested and supplementing if it's low. Vitamin D deficiency is associated with an increase in thyroid antibodies in Hashimoto's patients.
- Exercising can help to restore thyroid function, but overtraining can raise cortisol which, in turn, will negatively impact thyroid hormones.
- On that note, look at how you can reduce sources of stress and take action.

Short and Light Periods

A period which lasts less than two days is considered to be short, though as a period that's short and light can be a sign of deficiency in Chinese medicine, I prefer to work with a more stringent cut off of a period that's less than three days and/or features flow that's light and pinkish in colour rather than red.

'My periods used to be incredibly heavy and full on, sometimes I would flood, but for the last couple of years they've been so much better; really light – hardly there at all – and I only really bleed for a couple of days.' That's what Jess told me when we started working together. It was taking a while for her to conceive so she'd come to me for fertility support, not thinking that her short and light period was a sign that her menstrual cycle was less than optimal. Periods that are short and light are pretty common in my clinic. They indicate a deficiency that can come about after previous heavy blood loss (heavy periods, pregnancy loss, childbirth, surgery), long-term use of the birth control pill, not eating enough nourishing food, and working/ exercising/partying too hard.

Again, it's worth doing a pregnancy test because a period that's suddenly lighter can be an indicator of pregnancy, and it can also be because your previous cycle was one in which you didn't release an egg (an anovulatory cycle) which has the knock-on effect of a period that's a bit off. If you're unsure if you're ovulating or not you can track your BBT throughout your cycle, and you might want to have your oestrogen and iron levels checked as low levels of either can prevent the lining of your uterus from building and plumping up in the way it ought to as you move through your menstrual cycle and cause periods that are lighter and shorter.

If your period has always been on the short side, it's likely that there's nothing wrong, it's simply what's normal for you, though in my practice I do find that there's a tendency for the people who've always had short and light periods and who present as being deficient in Chinese medicine to be long-term vegetarians or vegans. I'm not against vegetarianism or veganism, in fact I was vegetarian for eight years, but there are times when I question how appropriate they are for some of my clients. And yes, I'm prone to deficiency.

Long and/or Heavy Periods

I could get into how much you have to lose in millimetres to be classified as having a heavy period, but I don't think it's all that useful. If you have heavy periods, you likely already know that you do because you:

- Soak through pads and super tampons quickly.
- Have to get up and change them in the night.
- Might have to double up and use tampons and pads or period-wear at the same time.
- May flood.
- Have large clots in your flow.
- Find it hard to leave the house because it's easier to manage your flow if you're at home and near the bathroom.
- Feel really tired from excessive blood loss that's associated with anaemia.

Heavy periods usually have an underlying hormonal imbalance of excess oestrogen and/or low progesterone, which is why they're common in adolescents and during the peri-menopausal years, times in life when you're more likely to have excess oestrogen in relation to progesterone because you ovulate less frequently and therefore don't produce sufficient progesterone. Only 20–45 per cent of adolescents have ovulatory cycles in their first year of having periods, with this figure rising to 75 per cent by 5 years, so it can take a while for things to level out, and in menstruating teens the hormone receptors that detect oestrogen circulating in your blood are also getting used to the presence of oestrogen so they react strongly to it. The oestrogen dominance that's often behind heavy periods is also linked with conditions such as endometriosis, adenomyosis, and fibroids so it's an important factor to address.

People with excessive menstrual bleeding also tend to have an increased rate of prostaglandin production in the lining of their uterus as a period starts. Prostaglandins are a good thing, they help the uterus to contract and expel its lining, but in excess they cause inflammation and pain, which is why menstruators with heavy periods are prone to bad cramps too. It also explains why non-steroidal anti-inflammatory drugs (NSAIDs) and following an anti-inflammatory diet such as the one I've outlined on page 221 can help to reduce excessive flow and relieve period pain. Using NSAIDs such as ibuprofen and mefenamic acid can reduce blood loss by 20–40 per cent.

Heavy periods can also be a sign of hypothyroidism, and a blood clotting disorder called von Willebrand disease, which prevents your blood from clotting and results in heavy periods, accounts for around 20 per cent of cases (if you've always had heavy periods and especially if you have a history of prolonged bleeding after dental work, or heavy blood loss after giving birth or having surgery, ask your GP to test for von Willebrand disease, thrombocytopenia, and platelet function defects as coagulation defects such as these are not as rare as is generally thought and can be treated with medicines which help you to stop bleeding). And some people who use the copper IUD or the Depo-Provera® shot for contraception find that they experience episodes of bleeding that are longer and/or heavier, usually during the first year of use, possibly because of vascular changes to the uterus. Prolonged periods can indicate an anovulatory cycle (I know, those anovulatory cycles can really muck things up) and having a heavy period when you don't usually get them could also be because you were pregnant and are miscarrying.

When you get your period, your body has to strike a balance between keeping your blood liquid enough so that it can flow out and clotting enough so that you don't bleed excessively. It does this by releasing anti-coagulants (proteins that stop the blood from clotting), or if blood loss is heavy, clots will form to limit blood loss and they can be numerous or quite large in size. They can also occur when blood pools in the vagina (if you've been lying down sleeping, for example) or in your uterus (if a condition like adenomyosis interferes with the ability of the uterus to contract, or a growth such as fibroids or polyps which can intrude on the uterine cavity and obstructs flow), so if you feel you're clotting excessively, speak to your GP.

Hormonal birth control such as the pill and the Mirena® IUD are often suggested as ways of treating heavy periods, and although they can reduce blood loss (by up to 90 per cent with the Mirena®), they don't treat the cause of them and won't be helpful if you're keen to avoid hormonal contraception or want to conceive. And some people using hormonal birth control find that their periods are actually heavier and that they experience breakthrough bleeding, in which you bleed outside of the time when you have your withdrawal bleed.

Tranexamic acid, a medication which is taken in pill form during your period, helps your blood to clot and prevents heavy blood loss, but it's controversial as it also increases your risk of developing a blood clot (the sort that can block a blood vessel and end up travelling to your lungs or brain), which is why it's not used in people taking hormonal birth control which has its own risk factor for blood clots.

In cases of severe anaemia and especially if fibroids are present, hormonal medication which is described as a Gonadotropin-releasing hormone analogue (GnRH analogue) may be prescribed. They work by halting the production of sex hormones and suppressing ovulation, resulting in what is essentially a temporary menopausal state.

Endometrial ablation, where the lining of the womb is scraped away or destroyed, results in reduced bleeding 80–90 per cent of the time but comes with a 25–50 per cent chance of developing amenorrhoea (the loss of periods), so it isn't recommended for anyone who plans on having children as it is also associated with an increased risk of miscarriage, haemorrhaging in pregnancy, premature labour, and abnormal placental development. Neither should it be used as a treatment for those who are at an increased risk for endometrial cancer.

Hysterectomy is a very final treatment choice and should only be considered as a last resort. I've had several clients come to me for treatment because they've received a date to have a hysterectomy, but between the treatments they've had and the dietary and lifestyle changes they've made, we've managed to get their bleeding under control. I've also had clients for whom these strategies haven't worked well enough, and that's meant that they've had a hysterectomy knowing that it was absolutely the right choice for them, and they also received crucial support as they worked towards acceptance of their hysterectomy.

If you see your GP they can do a blood test for iron deficiency anaemia, which can come about as a result of heavy blood loss but can also *cause* heavy blood loss, making dietary changes and iron supplementation a great first line treatment option.

Plan for long and/or heavy periods:

- Taking ibuprofen during your period can reduce heavy flow by half, making it a very simple and useful intervention, especially when you're waiting for other interventions to have a preventative effect.
- Supplementing with iron can help to recover from heavy blood loss and prevent further excessive loss.
- Try supplementing with curcumin, the active ingredient in turmeric, as it reduces heavy periods and can also relieve menstrual cramps.
- One study found that taking a herb called shepherd's purse outperforms the NSAID mefenamic acid in reducing blood loss.
- If you have symptoms of excess oestrogen and/or low progesterone, follow my suggestions for them in this section.

Short Cycles

Technically, a short cycle is one which is less than 21 days long, but in my practice, I consider a cycle that's less than 26 days to be short because when a cycle is less than that, it suggests that either the first half of your cycle is short (which is associated with a reduced likelihood of conceiving), or that the second half of your cycle is (linked to problems conceiving and sustaining a pregnancy). Or it can be a bit of both.

In each menstrual cycle, your follicle and egg must grow and mature, and like most things in life, this takes time, energy and nourishment. When you ovulate early, the egg that you release is unlikely to be as fully developed as it could be which is why practitioners often seek to lengthen this phase, especially if you want to conceive.

If you have a short cycle and you don't usually get them, it's probably because a partially matured egg from a previous cycle has escaped the usual process of dying off. Instead, it's had a head start and needs less time to reach maturity, resulting in early ovulation.

It's common in early perimenopause for cycles to shorten by a few days because as ovarian function begins to decline, the brain has to work harder to get your ovaries to release an egg, and it does so by pumping out larger amounts of follicle stimulating hormone (FSH). This results in earlier development of the follicle and therefore earlier ovulation, resulting in a shorter cycle. Short cycles can also be a sign of anovulation, where ovulation hasn't occurred, although it's important to remember that anovulation happens in up to a third of clinically healthy cycles.

If you suspect that the first half of your cycle is normal in length, and that it's the second half that's short, then you may not be producing enough progesterone. Tracking your BBT will help to establish if and when ovulation takes place, and which phase of your cycle is short. You can get a lot of information out of tracking your BBT but might benefit from an experienced practitioner helping you to interpret the data you gather. Hormonal testing on day 3 of your cycle for FSH, LH and oestradiol (E2) can help assess what's going on, but any later than that will produce unreliable results, particularly in the case of short cycles. Testing progesterone in the middle of your luteal phase – which tracking your BBT will help you time correctly – can determine if you're ovulating and if your corpus luteum is producing sufficient progesterone to support the second half of your cycle.

Plan for short cycles:

- I like to work with clients for a decent period of time before they start trying to conceive in order to lengthen their cycle by using acupuncture and my preference is that they have three or more successive optimal length cycles before trying to conceive. Delaying pregnancy plans for this length of time can initially freak some of my clients out, particularly if they feel time is against them in the fertility stakes, but as well as conceiving with ease, I want to ensure that they're in a strong position to sustain a healthy pregnancy and that starts with having healthy mature eggs.

- If your luteal phase is short, support progesterone production (page 159).

Long and Irregular Cycles

A cycle which is longer than 35 days is considered to be long, and it occurs when ovulation is delayed as your luteal phase is fixed at 12–16 days in length, so in long cycles it's always the first phase of your cycle that's too long. They can happen when follicular development is slow, perhaps due to low or decreased sensitivity to FSH, or low levels of oestrogen, which both occur as part of the ageing process.

It's common for long cycles to appear in the teen years as well as during perimenopause. It can take a few years for the menstrual cycle to become regular after first getting a period, and in the absence of other symptoms, isn't something that needs to be investigated or treated. If you're peri-menopausal (the period of time before your periods stop when you experience 'menopausal' symptoms) then you can expect your cycle to go a bit haywire; perhaps having shorter cycles or switching between short and long. Partly this is because your ovaries take a bit more to get going each month, so you pump out more FSH in order to achieve this and this can result in shorter cycles, and you might be ovulating less frequently which can cause both short and long cycles (anovulation is to blame yet again!).

When clients have irregular or long cycles I love recommending BBT tracking because it helps to establish when you ovulate so that you can then calculate when your period will start, and some clients have found that the more comprehensive cycle tracking that we talked about in depth in Section Two has had a regulating effect on their cycles.

If you're having an unusually long cycle, a pregnancy test might reveal the reason why, but if you have consistently long cycles the cause should be investigated as although you could be perimenopausal, 90 per cent of people with oligomenorrhoea (irregular cycles) and amenorrhoea (no periods) go on to be diagnosed with PCOS.

Polycystic Ovarian Syndrome (PCOS)

PCOS is the most common hormonal disorder in ovary owners of reproductive age, affecting up to 15 per cent of us worldwide, though as our knowledge of the syndrome has evolved, its name has been called into question. In the past, the presence of a collection of cysts on the ovaries viewed by ultrasound was enough to receive a diagnosis of PCOS. These cysts are caused when the group of follicles that are put forward for the job of ovulation in each cycle don't end up with a leader – or dominant follicle – and so ovulation isn't achieved. Instead, the underdeveloped follicles form tiny cysts which sit on your ovaries. But polycystic ovaries are very common and are seen on up to 25 per cent of ovary-owners – they're even seen in 14 per cent of people using the contraceptive pill – making the presence or absence of cysts as the sole diagnostic criteria entirely unreliable.

Instead, it's recommended that physicians use the *Rotterdam criteria*, in which two of the following three criteria must be met in order to make a diagnosis; ovarian dysfunction (lack of, or infrequent ovulation which is classified as less than ten periods a year); clinical and/or biochemical signs of excessive amounts of a group of hormones called androgens such as acne and hirsutism (excessive growth of body hair) or high levels of androgens in the blood; and polycystic ovaries. Some experts have criticised the Rotterdam criteria, stating that it can lead to overdiagnosis and misdiagnosis of PCOS. Instead, the Androgen Excess and PCOS Society have recommended that because PCOS is primarily a hyperandrogenic disorder, the definition should be revised to feature hyperandrogenism (hirsutism and/or excess androgens) and ovarian dysfunction (infrequent or absent ovulation and/or polycystic ovaries) so that the Rotterdam criteria would be encompassed, but hyperandrogenism would be required in order to meet the diagnostic criteria.

Androgens

Androgens are a group of hormones (testosterone being the most well-known of them) which have traditionally and incorrectly been referred to as 'male' hormones, but they are important to the health of all sexes. They help us to feel motivated and energised, develop muscle mass and balance body fat, prevent bone loss, stimulate sexual desire, and support fertility. In fact, androgens play a role in over 200 actions in females, and although their levels are much higher in men, in women they're present in higher amounts than oestrogens. But just like all the other hormones, it's a question of balance. High levels of androgens that are common in PCOS can result in the loss of the hair on the scalp, acne, and hirsutism – the growth of hair on specific parts of the body or face, such as the upper lip, chin, forearms, abdomen, and mid-chest.

It's worthwhile getting to know the different androgens, because not only will you be able to understand what your doctor is talking about if you have them tested, but you'll come to understand why treating PCOS as a strictly ovarian issue is short-sighted. Your androgens are:

- Testosterone. Twenty-five per cent of your testosterone comes from your adrenal glands (the ones which sit on top of your kidneys), 25 per cent comes from your ovaries, and 5 per cent is converted from another hormone called androstenedione in your bloodstream. Testosterone is a key hormone when it comes to energy, motivation and sexual desire, as well as developing muscle mass and supporting bone health, so when it's low all of those important facets in life suffer.
- DHEA is mainly produced by your adrenal glands, though around 10 per cent comes from your ovaries and your brain also produces some to protect it from damage caused by high cortisol. It's DHEA which causes you to develop body odour, armpit hair, and pubic hair, and it can be converted into oestrogens in certain parts of the body such as the vagina. From menopause onwards it is the only source of sex hormones for all tissues except the uterus. DHEA is high in the morning and low in the evening (something to consider when you have it tested). Its production peaks in your twenties, and it decreases from the age of 30 and also with the use of some medications such as the birth control pill, metformin, steroids and opioids.
- DHEA-S is made by the adrenals and of all the steroid hormones, DHEA and DHEA-S are the ones which circulate your body in highest numbers though their levels decline with age; in the decade after menopause circulating levels of them are around 70 per cent less than the levels seen in early adult life. DHEA-S is a helpful hormone to test for when

differentiating between PCOS (when it's often high) and hypothalamic amenorrhoea (when it's often low).
- Androstenedione is produced by the ovaries and adrenals (50:50) and it is a precursor hormone that is converted into testosterone and estrone (one of your oestrogen hormones).
- DHT stimulates the production of oil that causes blocked pores and acne which is another indicator of PCOS. Produced by the ovaries and adrenals, as well as circulating levels of DHEA-S.

When we consider that a significant amount of androgens are made by the adrenal glands, it becomes clear that the high levels of androgens which are associated with PCOS are not just an ovarian issue; adrenal function must be assessed and addressed too.

Excess androgens can be caused by high insulin levels, excess body weight, overexercising, and a diet that's low in nutrients. Signs and symptoms include:

- Menstrual cycles that are longer than 35 days
- Acne
- Excess body hair (upper lip, chin, chest, abdomen, and arms)
- Hair loss on the head
- Greasy skin and/or hair
- An increase in body odour
- Unstable blood sugar
- Skin tags
- Infertility
- Reactivity, irritability, and mood swings

You can reduce androgen production by avoiding simple carbohydrates and sugars, losing excess weight, and the following supplements can help: zinc, white peony, liquorice, DIM, reishi mushroom, green tea extract, and saw palmetto.

Low androgens can be caused by the birth control pill and other types of hormonal birth control, low-fat diets, alcohol, lack of exercise, diabetes, hypothyroidism, high prolactin levels, adrenal dysfunction (one quarter of testosterone is made in adrenals so if they aren't functioning correctly then testosterone can be low) and decreased ovarian function (one quarter of testosterone is made in the ovaries, so if there is low ovarian reserve it can result in low testosterone). Signs and symptoms include:

- Low libido
- Painful sex
- Less strong orgasms
- Lower self-confidence
- Lack of lubrication
- Less muscle mass
- Lack of motivation

You can raise your androgens by getting decent sleep, eating a nutrient dense diet, and by weight-training (particularly your legs).

PCOS is a syndrome that people have a genetic predisposition to and it can manifest itself in many ways thanks to its myriad symptoms which include irregular or long menstrual cycles, excess weight gain, resistance to weight loss, sub-fertility, acne, excess hair growth on parts of the body where you probably don't want it such as your chin, arms, chest and abdomen, and hair loss where you do want it – on your head.

Increasingly, researchers and healthcare providers are now describing different types of PCOS in an attempt to group together the varying ways the syndrome expresses itself, and to establish the best course of action when it comes to treating it. Receiving a PCOS diagnosis is upsetting; not only are the symptoms unpleasant, but it's linked to diminished fertility, insulin resistance, type 2 diabetes, gestational diabetes, and cardiovascular disease as well as depression and diminished confidence. The great news is that it is *highly responsive* to simple diet and lifestyle interventions, and by taking charge of your health you will be able to significantly reduce your symptoms, improve your cycle, your fertility, your skin, and your overall health.

Now for your chance to take a guess at how conventional medicine 'treats' PCOS … any takers? Yep, you guessed correctly; the all-singing, all-dancing birth control pill! While the correct intention is there – 'let's regulate your cycle' – the pill cannot regulate your cycle because it works by *preventing* ovulation, and with PCOS, you really want to be ovulating because it's ovulation that will lead to menstruation, and it's important for your reproductive health that the lining of your womb is shed regularly. Although the pill can achieve this by giving you withdrawal bleeds, it can also impair insulin resistance after just three months of taking it which people with PCOS already have an issue with, contribute to weight gain (in most cases of PCOS, weight loss is the goal because a 5 per cent reduction in body weight can result in a significant improvement in symptoms), and the oral contraceptives most commonly used to manage PCOS are the ones with the highest risks for developing blood clots (if you've got PCOS you're already at an increased risk for getting them).

When you stop taking the birth control pill it can sometimes take a few months or a couple of years for you to start ovulating again and during this time, cysts can appear on your ovaries as eggs try to ovulate but don't quite make it and accumulate on the surface instead. When you come off some birth control pills you can also experience a short-term surge in androgens which can cause what's described as post-pill PCOS.

Metformin is a medication which can lower blood sugar levels and it's often prescribed to treat the insulin resistance associated with PCOS, in which your body's cells don't respond properly to the hormone insulin and can cause type 2 diabetes. But it frequently brings with it the unpleasant side effects of nausea and vomiting, diarrhoea, bloating and abdominal discomfort, so using other interventions such as exercise, diet and supplements to improve insulin resistance is preferable.

It's common and normal for teens to have polycystic ovaries (because you produce a lot of follicles when you're younger), irregular cycles (remember that it can take 2–5 years for you to have ovulatory cycles and for your cycle to become regular after you first start menstruating), high levels of LH and androgens, as well as experiencing insulin resistance. It's therefore recommended that teens should meet *all three* of the Rotterdam criteria in order to receive a diagnosis of PCOS. In the absence of very clear signs and symptoms of PCOS, it's wise to hold off on diagnosing it until your twenties because of the impact it can have on body confidence and unnecessary use of the pill.

It's important to have lab testing to differentiate between PCOS and hypothalamic amenorrhoea (HA), as with a diagnosis of PCOS you may be told to restrict your intake of calories and if what you actually have is HA, then you'll really need those calories to start menstruating again.

PCOS is not just an ovarian issue: your adrenal glands produce roughly the same amount of testosterone and androstenedione as the ovaries, as well producing the majority of DHEA, and all of DHEA-S, so adrenal function should be assessed and ways to limit and manage stress be brought in. Around half of your testosterone is made in your body fat, which is why losing excess body weight can result in the improvement of signs of excess androgens such as acne and hirsutism. Thirty to seventy-five per cent of people with PCOS are obese but not everyone with PCOS is overweight, in fact some people with it can have a thin stature and are described as having 'lean PCOS'.

Investigations used to confirm PCOS and rule out other conditions which present with similar signs and symptoms include:

- Fasting insulin or a glucose tolerance test.
- Haemoglobin A1c, which looks at your average blood sugar over the past 2–3 months.
- FSH, LH and oestradiol, preferably on day 3 of your period (admittedly this can be tricky if you only have two periods a year, in which case a random day is fine).
- Progesterone (preferably mid-luteal phase, again, timing this can be tricky).
- 17-hydroxyprogesterone, a hormone that can indicate a glandular disorder that can result in insufficient cortisol production and excess androgen production.
- Prolactin, a hormone that can suppress the menstrual cycle.
- Testosterone, sex hormone binding globulin (SHBG), androstenedione and DHEA-S.
- Full thyroid panel (TSH, T3, T4, thyroid antibodies, and reverse T3). In my experience GPs tend not to order a full thyroid panel but it's important with PCOS because an underlying thyroid issue can interfere with all your hard work to improve your symptoms.
- Diurnal cortisol.
- Fasting lipids, to test your cholesterol and other fats in your blood.
- Serum vitamin D. Up to 85 per cent of people with PCOS are deficient in vitamin D, which is associated with obesity, metabolic and hormonal imbalances, so testing for it and supplementing with it if necessary is wise.
- Transvaginal (internal) ultrasound to assess the ovaries for cysts.

Plan for PCOS:

- I can't emphasise the value of working one-on-one with a qualified naturopath enough. They can help you to figure out what the best diet and exercise plan is *for you*. Different things work for different people and that's especially true when it comes to PCOS and the variety of ways it can manifest.
- Generally speaking, an anti-inflammatory diet is highly beneficial (see page 220). It's really important to strike a balance between weight loss (*if* you are overweight), managing insulin secretion, and stabilising your blood sugar, all of which can be tricky, so a naturopath is the best person to help you do this.
- Address stress because it can result in high cortisol and elevated androgens, and PCOS can be an adrenal gland issue.
- Improve gut and liver function.
- Exercise; strength training can improve insulin sensitivity by 24 per cent, HIIT, yoga, pilates. Lots of cardio to try and lose weight can result in a stress response which can cause further hormonal dysregulation, so slow and steady might be more appropriate.
- Abdominal castor oil packs.
- Supplements to consider: Inositol, d-chiro-inositol, berberine, N-Acetyl-Cysteine (NAC), Omega-3 Fatty Acids, chromium, green tea (EGCG) or drink several cups a day, magnesium, B vitamins, vitamin D, zinc, white peony, liquorice, Vitex agnus-castus, Dong quai, melatonin, reishi mushroom, probiotics … the list goes on and on. There are a lot of ways to improve PCOS through diet and supplements, and although having so many options might feel overwhelming to you, it's actually really good because it means that there are specific ways to support the symptoms that you get. But it does mean that hunting down a naturopath who loves to work with PCOS is your best way of finding which ones are most appropriate for you.

Ovarian Cysts

Functional ovarian cysts are cysts which are perfectly normal. They form when either a developing follicle fills with fluid, or when the corpus luteum that forms after ovulation fills with fluid or blood (a blood-filled cyst is called a haemorrhagic cyst). Both these types can grow to 6cm across, but many don't cause symptoms, and most resolve themselves without treatment within a few menstrual cycles. In my experience this is rarely fully explained to clients, resulting in a lot of unnecessary tears and sleepless nights.

When cysts do cause symptoms, these include: pelvic pain or discomfort, sudden severe pain if a cyst bursts or if it develops a stalk which it twists on and stops the cyst's blood supply, and pain if the cyst is large enough to impinge on nearby organs and structures like your bladder or rectum, difficulty emptying your bowels, pain during penetrative sex, a frequent need to urinate, changes to your cycle or period, and feeling full and bloated.

They're diagnosed by ultrasound or MRI, often quite matter-of-factly when other conditions are being investigated, and a watch and wait approach is most common and most disappear of their own accord. If they don't and they're sizeable and/or causing symptoms, then non-invasive keyhole laparoscopic surgery may be suggested. Sometimes traditional surgery is required.

Dermoid cysts (sometimes called ovarian teratomas) tend to be quite large – up to, and occasionally beyond, 15cm across. They develop from germ cells which go on to form eggs, and because eggs have the potential to form a multitude of tissue types and structures, they can contain hair, fat, and parts of teeth or bone. This kind of cyst accounts for up to 20 per cent of non-cancerous ovarian growths, they don't usually produce any symptoms and are often discovered incidentally and are usually removed by surgery.

Cyst-adenomas develop from cells that cover the outer part of the ovary and there are two main types; serous cyst-adenomas which are usually small, and mucinous cyst-adenomas which can grow very large (up to 30cm across) and exert pressure on other organs such as the bladder and bowel, resulting in digestive issues like constipation and pain, and a frequent need to urinate.

Cysts are diagnosed by ultrasound which is usually repeated a few months later to determine if it's resolved itself. Your GP may suggest testing your blood for a protein called CA125 as an elevated level of it is a marker for ovarian cancer (around 5 per cent of ovarian cysts are cancerous). If you get recurrent functional cysts, ask your doctor to test your thyroid as thyroid dysfunction can be the root cause of them. You don't have to do anything to treat cysts as they usually take care of themselves, but ATMAT® and castor oil packs can help and are supportive of overall reproductive function, so in my book they're always worth doing.

Fibroids

Uterine fibroids are abnormal growths of muscle tissue that form in, or on, the walls of the uterus. Most grow in the uterine wall and are referred to as *intramural*. If they project into the uterine cavity they're called *submucosal* and if this type is attached to the lining of the uterus by a stalk, then they are referred to as *pedunculated*. When they grow outwards from the uterus and into other places in the pelvis they are described as *subserous.*

They're the most common non-cancerous tumour during the reproductive years and occur in 77 per cent of people with a uterus at some point in their lifetime. They're the single most common reason for someone to have a hysterectomy, though up to 50 per cent of people with them don't have any symptoms and won't know that they have them until they have an ultrasound scan during pregnancy.

Problems that they can cause include heavy and/or painful periods, dysfunctional uterine bleeding between periods, iron deficiency anaemia, pelvic pain, needing to wee frequently if the fibroid presses against the bladder, or constipation if it imposes itself against the colon or rectum. Depending on their size, number and location, they can also cause fertility challenges and complications in pregnancy. Fibroids are associated with hormonal imbalances such as excess oestrogen, and as such they can shrink after menopause when hormone production diminishes. They're more common in people whose family members have them, and in those with an African ancestry.

Unless it's particularly large or causing problems, a watch and wait approach is usually adopted. You won't be surprised to hear that medications used to treat the symptoms of fibroids include hormonal birth control and hormonal suppressants such as GnRH agonists which induce a menopausal state, but they are typically only used prior to surgery, as although GnRH agonists can result in up to a 50 per cent reduction in the size of the fibroid, within a few months of not taking it, they grow back to their former size.

Medical management includes non-invasive procedures which cut off the blood supply to the fibroid, such as uterine artery embolisation, in which a tiny tube called a catheter is inserted into an artery in your leg, and guided through the arteries that supply the uterus with blood until the artery that supplies the fibroid is reached, at which point some very small particles of plastic are injected via the catheter to deprive the fibroid of blood.

Surgery can also be performed to remove problematic fibroids; a myomectomy is minimally invasive and involves the removal of the fibroid through either keyhole laparoscopic surgery to the abdomen, or abdominal surgery if the fibroid(s) is quite large, but in severe cases a hysterectomy may be suggested.

Acupuncture can be used to reduce the size of fibroids, and Chinese herbs have a good track record of treating fibroids but they must be prescribed by someone who's qualified to ensure that they're used safely. There's also a lot that you can do to help yourself, including:

- Follow my excess oestrogen protocol on page 235.
- Eat a diet that's low in red meat and high in green vegetables.
- Get plenty of Omega-3 Fatty Acids in your diet by eating fatty fish or by supplementing with fish oil, or algae if you don't consume fish.
- Reduce alcohol intake as there's a strong association between consumption of booze and fibroids.
- Use castor oil packs, ATMAT®, acupuncture, and Chinese herbs to improve flow through the pelvis and reduce the size of the fibroids.

I hope that this chapter has helped you to identify any issues that you might have and given you some ideas of what you can do to improve your symptoms. Many conditions can be improved or resolved entirely with the suggestions I've provided, but do seek out help if you need it. You can find a list of my suggestions for further reading, as well as where to find a qualified practitioner, in the Resources section.

EPILOGUE

When I set out to write this book, my sole aim was to help you to feel better in yourself; to help you to understand your body and what it gets up to during your menstruating years. After helping women with menstrual and reproductive health issues in my treatment room for over a decade, I know that most of us have not grown up with the knowledge of our bodies that we ought to, and how powerful that information can be.

I also wanted to reassure you about what's normal, and to highlight the importance of seeking out medical help – in whatever way you deem as appropriate – when things go awry. And according to a 2018 report by Public Health England, the majority of us do experience reproductive health symptoms. Their research found that 80 per cent of women have experienced at least one reproductive health symptom in the last year, and half of the participants reported menstrual issues, with this figure rising to three quarters of women in the 16 to 24 year old age group. But despite such a high prevalence of reproductive health issues, less than half of women with symptoms sought out medical help and this figure was unrelated to the severity of their symptoms. Please, please, please, if you have any concern about your reproductive or hormonal health, speak to your GP and/or a qualified alternative health practitioner who is experienced in treating issues like the ones in this book. It is not your lot in life to put up with pain and suffering and you have a right to reproductive healthcare which improves your symptoms and your quality of life.

Beyond the necessity of receiving appropriate treatment, it's important that we report the problems we have because when we do, medical statistics become more accurate and representative of our experiences, and funding for medical research into reproductive conditions is more likely. In addition to this, when we inform healthcare practitioners about positive and negative outcomes, including reporting side effects, then there is the potential for efficacy and safety rates to improve.

Whatever you choose to do with the information in this book, I hope that it has helped you to become more aware of your body and that you're feeling the benefits of tracking your cycle. If you haven't started tracking yet, the cycle dial on page 313 is a quick and easy way to get started and may well end up changing your life, just as it did mine. You can download a blank dial for free from my website (*see* Resources).

When I was racked with horrific pain every month, I lived in fear of my period. I loved who I was in my Spring and Summer and felt right at home there, but my relationship with my Winter was rocky at best. Tracking my cycle made me realise that the first two days of my period were the only ones where I actually stopped and took care of myself, and that was only because I had no choice but to hide in bed with a pack of ibuprofen and a hot water bottle. Sure, I could've continued popping painkillers like nobody's business, but that would have meant ignoring my body. Instead, I chose to listen. I listened to my body's needs throughout the whole of my cycle and worked my way through the pain with the support of a Chinese medicine practitioner and a nutritionist. And I'm glad that I did because although I didn't know it at the time, something in me was being born; an awareness of myself and my place in the world, both of which ultimately led to the creation of this book.

Where will *Period Power* take you?

APPENDIX

Below is an example of a dial I completed to track my own cycle. You can download a blank dial from my website (*see* Resources).

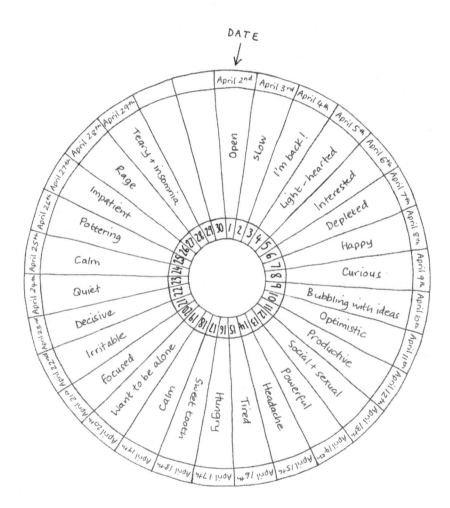

GLOSSARY

Amenorrhoea The absence of periods during the reproductive years.

Androgens A group of hormones traditionally referred to as 'male', but which people of all genders have. Testosterone is an example of an androgen hormone.

Anovulatory cycle A menstrual cycle in which ovulation did not take place, and therefore no progesterone was produced by the corpus luteum.

Basal body temperature (BBT) The lowest body temperature reached during rest. It is taken immediately after waking in the morning and because temperatures are higher after ovulation and throughout the second half of the cycle, it can be used to identify when ovulation has taken place.

Bisphenol A (BPA) An endocrine disruptor which mimics oestrogen. It's present in lots of goods, from water bottles and food containers to the thermal paper receipts are printed on, and it can cause breast cancer and other illnesses and abnormalities.

Corpus luteum Following ovulation, the follicle which contained the egg for that month collapses and forms the corpus luteum, a temporary gland which produces and secretes progesterone in the second half of your cycle.

Cortisol A hormone that's produced by the adrenal glands which regulates a large number of processes in the body, including blood sugar levels and the immune response. It's also released in response to stress.

Endocrine disruptors Chemicals in food, pesticides, personal care products, plastics, and solvents which interfere with how the endocrine system functions.

Endocrine system The hormone producing glands in your body, such as your pituitary, hypothalamus, thyroid, adrenals, and ovaries.

Endometrium The inner lining of the uterus. In each menstrual cycle it plumps up in preparation for potential implantation of a fertilised egg and is shed during menstruation if conception doesn't take place.

Fertility awareness method (FAM) Fertility awareness is a way to identify fertile and non-fertile times in the menstrual cycle, including the use of BBT charting and can be used to avoid or achieve pregnancy.

Follicle A fluid-filled sac that contains an immature egg. During ovulation a mature egg is released from its follicle, the follicle then collapses and forms the corpus luteum.

Follicle stimulating hormone (FSH) A hormone produced by your pituitary gland which stimulates the follicles in your ovaries, instructing them to grow and mature.

Follicular phase The first half of the menstrual cycle, beginning when a period starts and ending at ovulation, in which ovarian follicles grow and mature until one releases an egg at ovulation. During this phase the lining of the uterus thickens in preparation for implantation of a fertilised egg.

Gonadotropin-releasing hormone (GnRH) A hormone released by the hypothalamus gland which stimulates the pituitary gland to release FSH and LH.

Hirsutism Excess hair growth on the face and body, often caused by excess androgens.

Hyperthyroidism When the thyroid gland is overactive and produces too much thyroid hormones.

Hypothalamic amenorrhoea (HA) When periods stop because the hypothalamus gland stops or slows production of GnRH.

Hypothyroidism When the thyroid gland is underactive and doesn't produce enough thyroid hormones.

Hysterectomy The surgical removal of the uterus. When the ovaries and cervix are also removed it is referred to as a total hysterectomy, but when the ovaries and cervix are not removed, it is called a partial hysterectomy.

Luteal phase The second half of your cycle – from ovulation to the start of your period – which is typically 12–16 days in length.

Luteinising hormone (LH) A hormone produced by the pituitary gland. The acute rise of LH towards the end of the first half of the cycle triggers ovulation and the development of the corpus luteum.

Menarche The first period you ever have.

Menopause The end of your menstruating years, officially reached one year after your last period.

Menstrual cycle Starts on the first day of your period and ends when your next period begins.

Menstruation Your period.

Microbiome The community of microorganisms that populate your body, or a specific part of the body – such as the gut and vagina – and which carry out lots of body processes, including manufacturing hormones.

Oestrogen The umbrella term for the three forms of oestrogen; oestradiol, oestrone, and oestriol. Oestrogen is responsible for the development and regulation of the female reproductive system, but it's also present in males.

Oestrogen detoxification The ways that you metabolise (process) oestrogen.

Ovulation Occurs when an ovarian follicle releases a mature egg.

Perimenopause The period of time when hormonal changes occur prior to your periods stopping which can result in symptoms such as hot flushes and insomnia.

Postpartum The period of time which begins after giving birth and never ends.

Pregnenolone A hormone made by the adrenal glands which is the precursor to several other hormones, such as cortisol, oestrogen, progesterone, and testosterone.

Premenstruum The week or two preceding menstruation.

Premenstrual dysphoric disorder (PMDD) A very severe form of PMS that causes mental and physical distress in the premenstruum and which is relieved within a few days of a period starting.

Premenstrual syndrome (PMS) The physical and emotional symptoms that can occur in the premenstruum.

Progesterone The hormone made by the ovary after ovulation which is necessary in order to sustain a pregnancy.

Progestin A synthetic hormone which is similar to but not the same as progesterone.

Sex hormone binding globulin (SHBG) A protein that's made by your liver which binds to excess hormones, such as oestrogen and testosterone.

Testosterone A hormone known as an androgen. It's produced in small amounts by the adrenal glands and the ovaries in females and is found in larger amounts in males.

Vagina The internal tube which connects your vulva to your cervix (neck of the uterus).

Vulva Your external genitals, including your clitoris and labia. In other words, all the bits you can see.

Withdrawal bleed The monthly bleeding produced when someone using hormonal birth control such as the pill experiences a drop (or withdrawal) of hormones when they take the placebo pills in their pack, causing their endometrium to shed.

RESOURCES

You can download a free cycle charting kit at maisiehill.com/chartmycycle

Further reading

A Blessing Not a Curse, Jane Bennett.

Come As You Are, Dr. Emily Nagoski.

Doing Harm: The Truth About How Bad Medicine and Lazy Science Leave Women Dismissed, Misdiagnosed, and Sick, Maya Dusenbery.

Healing PCOS, Amy Medling.

Hormonal: How Hormones Drive Desire, Shape Relationships, and Make Us Wiser, Dr. Martie Haselton.

Inferior: How Science Got Women Wrong – and the New Research That's Rewriting the Story, Angela Saini.

Killing the Black Body: Race, Reproduction, and the Meaning of Liberty, Dorothy Roberts.

Medical Bondage: Race, Gender, and the Origins of American Gynaecology, Deirdre Benia Cooper Owens.

Sweetening the Pill, Holly Grigg-Spall.

Taking Charge of Your Fertility, Toni Weschler.

The Period Repair Manual, Lara Briden.

The Pill: Are You Sure it's for You? Jane Bennett and Alexandra Pope.

Why I'm No Longer Talking to White People About Race, Reni Eddo-Lodge.

Wild Power, Alexandra Pope and Sjanie Hugo-Wurlitzer.

Your No Guilt Pregnancy Plan: A revolutionary guide to pregnancy, birth and the weeks that follow, Rebecca Schiller.

Your Silence Will Not Protect You: Essays and Poems, Audre Lorde.

8 Steps to Reverse Your PCOS, Dr. Fiona McCulloch.

Websites

Bleedingwhiletrans.com to learn more about transgender periods.

CoppaFeel.org are a breast cancer awareness charity who promote early detection of breast cancer by encouraging women and men to regularly check their breasts and chest.

Daysy.me is a fertility tracker that uses the fertility awareness method to tell you when you're fertile or not.

Endowhat.com an educational and empowering documentary about endometriosis.

Eveappeal.org.uk is a UK charity who raise awareness and fund research into gynaecological research.

Fpa.org.uk is a sexual health charity that provide information on contraception, STIs and pregnancy choices.

healinghistamine.com has lots of information and tools to heal histamine intolerance.

helloclue.com is a free period tracker.

iapmd.org the International Association for Premenstrual Disorders.

justisse.ca for fertility awareness education and natural birth control.

kindara.com is a free fertility charting app.

laylafsaad.com

menstrual-matters.com

menstruationresearch.org

modernwomen.bigcartel.com for Sarah Gottessdiener's Many Moons Lunar Planner.

Nancy's Nook Endometriosis Education and Discussion Group: facebook.com/groups/418136991574617

Nicolejardim.com for programs to fix your period.

Ourbodiesourselves.org for education about reproductive health and medical care.

pcosdiva.com learn about the latest news, research, and diets/meal plans for PCOS.

pms.org.uk National Association for Premenstrual Syndrome

rachelcargle.com for her lecture on Unpacking White Feminism.

sibocenter.com and sibosos.com for information on small intestinal bacterial overgrowth, including how to test and treat it.

sweeteningthepill.com

5thvitalsign.com

Where to find a practitioner

Arvigo Techniques of Maya Abdominal Therapy: arvigotherapy.com

Association of community and multibed acupuncture clinics: acmac.net

Association of Naturopathic Practitioners: theanp.co.uk

British Acupuncture Council: acupuncture.org.uk

National Certification Commission for Acupuncture and Oriental Medicine: nccaom.org

The American Association of Naturopathic Physicians: naturopathic.org

Women's health physiotherapists: pelvicphysiotherapy.com/list-of-therapists

Medical and wellness tests

American Gut Project is an opportunity to test your gut microbiome whilst contributing to medical research: humanfoodproject.com/americangut

Atlas Biomed offer DNA and microbiome testing: atlasbiomed.com

British Gut Project is a collaboration between the TwinsUK team at King's College London and The American Gut Project to understand the bacterial diversity of the British Gut, and is a way to discover the health of your microbiome whilst contributing to medical research: britishgut.org

DUTCH test: https://dutchtest.com/

Lifecode Gx offer genetic testing that includes information about oestrogen pathways, histamine, detoxification and methylation: lifecodegx.com

Oura is a wellness ring and app that shows how your body responds to your lifestyle by analysing your sleep, activity levels, daily rhythms and the physiological responses in your body: ouraring.com

uBiome offer microbiome testing as a health and wellness tool, as well as tests which must be ordered with your doctor, including the SmartJane screening test for vaginal flora, HPV and STIs: ubiome.com

Supplement brands
BioCare
Designs for Health
Nutri Advanced
Pure Encapsulations
Thorne Research
Seeking Health
Cytoplan
Terranova
Viridian

Menstrual Supplies
Fluxundies.com
Gladrags.com
Holysponge.net
lunapads.com
Modibodi.com
Myfreda.com
Natracare.com
Ohne.co
Pyramindseven.com
Sustainnatural.com
thecupeffect.org
wearedame.co
Wuka.co.uk

Sex and relationships
Babeland.com is a women-friendly sex shop and website.
Dameproducts.com for sex toys.
Drannacabeca.com/products/julva for Dr. Anna Cabeca's DHEA vaginal cream.

Ohnut.co is an intimate wearable that allows users to customise penetration depth and reduce pain.

Sustainnatural.com for vagina-friendly lubricant and condoms.

thehavelockclinic.com are a team of highly specialised doctors and psychologists who treat sexual problems in their clinics and over Skype, as well as through their excellent online therapy workshops which you can attend anonymously.

Sh-womenstore.com is a female-focused pleasure and sex shop.

Yesyesyes.org for natural, pure and certified organic intimate lubricants, moisturisers and washes.

Food, kitchen and home

beeswrap.com the natural alternative to plastic wrap for food storage.

Coombefarmorganic.co.uk for grass fed organic meat.

ewg.org/foodnews for the Environmental Working Group's guide to pesticides in produce, and their Dirty Dozen and Clean Fifteen lists (updated annually).

Eversfieldorganic.co.uk for 100 per cent grass fed organic meat.

Glass containers are available from Ikea.

Lodgemfg.com make cast iron cookware.

ntrs.nasa.gov/archive/nasa/casi.ntrs.nasa.gov/19930073077.pdf for the NASA clean air study and a list of houseplants which improve indoor air quality.

Riverford.co.uk for 100 per cent organic and seasonal produce, delivered to your door from their farm.

seafoodwatch.org for the Monterey Bay Aquarium –

Theberkey.com for water filters and purification.

Thekitchn.com for instructions on how to make homemade kefir and kombucha.

Skincare and cosmetics

Acure.com for natural, organic, and vegan skin, hair and beauty products.

Beautycounter.com for safe and effective skin care and cosmetics that are EWG verified.

Cocokind.com for superfood-based skincare and make-up.

ewg.org/skindeep for the Environmental Working Group's (EWG) guide to choosing safer personal care products.

greenpeople.co.uk for natural and organic skincare.

iliabeauty.com for make-up that's effective and safe.

Livinglibations. Neem enameliser paste to replace toothpaste.

Naturaldeoco.com make effective natural deodorants.

Paiskincare.com for certified organic skincare that's suitable for sensitive skin.

Skinandtoniclondon.com

Weleda.co.uk for 100 per cent natural, organic herbal medicine and body care products.

W3llpeople.com for toxin-free cosmetics that are EWG verified.

REFERENCES

Information about the reproductive system and the menstrual cycle has been drawn from the following texts:

Fritz, M.A. and Speroff, L. (eds.) (2011) *Clinical Gynaecologic Endocrinology and Infertility*. 8th ed. Philadelphia: Lippincott Williams and Wilkins.

Johnson, M.H. (2018) *Essential Reproduction*. 8th ed. Hoboken, NJ: Wiley.

Leung, P.C.K. and Adashi, E.Y. (eds.) (2004) *The Ovary*. 2nd ed. San Diego: Elsevier.

Nicolle, L. and Woodriff Beirne, A. (eds.) (2010) *Biochemical Imbalances in Disease*. London: Singing Dragon.

Chapter 1

'couldn't identify the vulva on a medical diagram': https://inews.co.uk/news/health/female-anatomy-identify-vagina-vulva-eve-appeal/

'1 in 5 women attending a sexual health clinic had adhesions': Aerts, L. *et al* (2017) The prevalence of clitoral adhesions in women presenting to the sexual medicine practice, *The Journal of Sexual Medicine*, 14(4), p. e110.

'the clitoris changes in volume over the course of a menstrual cycle': Battaglia, C. *et al* (2008) Menstrual cycle-related morphometric and vascular modifications of the clitoris, *The Journal of Sexual Medicine*, 5(12), pp. 2853–2861.

'decrease in size when you use hormonal birth control': Battaglia, C. *et al* (2011) Sexual behavior and oral contraception: A pilot study, *The Journal of Sexual Medicine*, 9(2), pp. 550–557.

'all forty women experienced a decrease in clitoral volume': Battaglia, C. *et al* (2014) Clitoral vascularization and sexual behavior in young patients treated with drospirenone-ethinyl estradiol or contraceptive vagina ring: A prospective, randomized, pilot study, *The Journal of Sexual Medicine*, 11(2), pp. 471–480.

'18 per cent of women orgasm through penetration alone': Herbenick, D. *et al* (2017) Women's experiences with genital touching, sexual pleasure, and orgasm: Results from a U.S. probability sample of women ages 18 to 94, *Journal of Sex and Marital Therapy*, 44(2), pp. 201–212.

'eight erections per night': Fisher, C. *et al* (1983) Patterns of female sexual arousal during sleep and waking: Vaginal thermoconductive studies, *Archives of Sexual Behaviour*, 12(2), pp. 97–122.

'as young as nine years old seeking them out': Mackenzie, J. (2017) *Vagina surgery 'sought by girls as young as nine'*. [Online]. Available from: https://www.bbc.co.uk/news/health-40410459 [Accessed 3 March 2018].

'lack of a healthy vaginal microbiome can result in': Aslan, E. and Bechelaghem, N. (2018) To 'douche' or not to 'douche': hygiene habits may have detrimental effects on vaginal microbiota, *Journal of Obstetrics and Gynaecology*, 38(5), pp. 678–681.

'Although cervical screening undoubtedly has its benefits and saves lives, there are downsides': Kyrgiou, M. *et al* (2016) Adverse obstetric outcomes after local treatment for cervical preinvasive and early invasive disease according to cone depth: systematic review and meta-analysis, *The British Medical Journal*, p. 354.

'Smoking cigarettes and cannabis negatively impacts on the motility of your fallopian tubes': Talbot, P. and Riveles, K. (2005) Smoking and reproduction: the oviduct as a target of cigarette smoke, *Reproductive Biology and Endocrinology*, 3(52).

'increases your risk of ectopic pregnancy': Bouyer, J. *et al* (2003) Risk factors for ectopic pregnancy: a comprehensive analysis based on a large case-control, population-based study in France, *American Journal of Epidemiology*, 157(3), pp. 185–194.

Chapter 2

'as little as 12.4 per cent of us actually have': Vollman, R. F. (1977) *The Menstrual Cycle*, New York; Knopf, pp. 51–52.

'She makes your features appear more symmetrical': Scutt, D. and Manning, J.T. (1996) Symmetry and ovulation in women, *Human Reproduction*, 11(11), pp. 2477–2480.

'only 13 per cent of women trying to conceive': Hampton, K. and Mazza, D. (2009) Should spontaneous or timed intercourse guide couples trying to conceive?, *Human Reproduction*, 24(12), pp. 3236–3237.

'We don't sync up with each other': Clue (2017) *Do menstrual cycles sync? Unlikely, finds Clue data.* [Online]. Available from:https://helloclue.com/articles/cycle-a-z/do-menstrual-cycles-sync-unlikely-finds-clue-data [Accessed 4 February 2018].

'One study found that sperm can be present in pre-ejaculate fluid which dribbles out prior to the main event': Kovavisarach, E., Lorthanawanich, S. and Muangsamran, P. (2016) Presence of sperm in pre-ejaculatory fluid of healthy males, *Journal of the Medical Association of Thailand*, 99 Supplement 2, pp. 38–41.

'though other small studies found no sperm in some pre-ejaculate': Zukerman, Z., Weiss, D.B. and Orvieto, R. (2003) Does preejaculatory penile secretion originating from Cowper's gland contain sperm? *Journal of Assisted Reproduction and Genetics*, 20(4), pp. 157–159. And: Politch, J.A., Mayer, K.H. and Anderson, D.J. (2016) HIV-1 is undetectable in pre-ejaculatory secretions from HIV-1-infected men on suppressive HAART, *AIDS*, 30(12), pp. 1899–1903.

'and the failure rate of using the withdrawal method is 4–18.4 per cent which is similar to the 2–17.4 per cent achieved with condoms': Fritz, M.A. and Speroff, L. (eds.) (2011, p. 1134) *Clinical Gynecologic Endocrinology and Infertility*. 8th ed. Philadelphia: Lippincott Williams and Wilkins.

'at ovulation 4.8 per cent of menstruators will experience spotting': Dasharathy, S.S. *et al* (2012) Menstrual bleeding patterns among regularly menstruating women, *American Journal of Epidemiology*, 175(6), pp. 536–545.

'Ovulation largely happens in the morning in spring and in the evening during autumn and winter': Testart, J., Frydman, R. and Roger, M. (1982) Seasonal influence of diurnal rhythms in the onset of the plasma luteinizing hormone surge in women, *Journal of Clinical Endocrinology and Metabolism*, 55(2), pp. 374–377.

'Younger women tend to ovulate from alternating ovaries, whereas women over the age of 30 are more likely to ovulate from the same ovary': Fukuda, M. *et al* (2001) Characteristics of human ovulation in natural cycles correlated with age and achievement of pregnancy, *Human Reproduction*, 16(12), pp. 2501–2507.

'the remaining fallopian tube picking up the egg from the ovary': Ross, J.A. *et al* (2013) Ovum transmigration after salpingectomy for ectopic pregnancy, *Human Reproduction*, 28(4), pp. 937–941.

Chapter 3

'poor hygiene and freezing temperatures have resulted in death': Bowman, V. (2018) Woman in Nepal dies after being exiled to outdoor hut during her period, *The Guardian*, 12 January 2018. [Online]. Available from: https://www.theguardian.com/global-development/2018/jan/12/woman-nepal-dies-exiled-outdoor-hut-period-menstruation [Accessed 27 March 2018].

'an online survey conducted by YouGov found that 30 per cent of women have taken time off work': YouGov (2017) *82% of women say their employers make no accommodations for period pain*. [Online]. Available from: https://today.yougov.com/topics/lifestyle/articles-reports/2017/08/23/82-women-say-their-employers-make-no-accommodation [Accessed 3 June 2018].

'number of menstrual products per packet goes down': Reference for Business [no date] *Company Profile, Information, Business Description, History, Background Information on Tambrands Inc*. [Online]. Available from: https://www.referenceforbusiness.com/history2/43/Tambrands-Inc.html [Accessed 7 July 2018].

'Plan UK reports that one in 10 girls': Plan International UK (2017) *Plan International UK's research into period poverty and stigma*. [Online]. Available from: https://plan-uk.org/media-centre/plan-international-uks-research-on-period-poverty-and-stigma [Accessed 17 January 2018].

'a report by the charity WaterAid and UNICEF found that more than a third of girls in South Asia': WaterAid (2018) *Menstrual hygiene management in schools in South Asia.* [Online]. Available from: https://washmatters.wateraid.org/publications/menstrual-hygiene-management-in-schools-south-asia [Accessed 2 August 2018].

'*When a girl misses school because of her period, cumulatively that puts her behind her male classmates by 145 days. And that's the mitigated setback if she opts to stay in school, which most do not*': Markle, M. (2017) 'Periods affect potential', *Time*, [Online]. Available from: http://time.com/4694568/meghan-markle-period-stigma/ [Accessed 2 April 2018].

'*Period poverty is not just financial poverty – sometimes it's poverty of knowledge, confidence, sustainability, or access and schools can address this right now.*': Quint, C. (2018) *Period Positive.* [Online]. Available from: https://periodpositive.wordpress.com/news/ [Accessed 6 July 2018].

'70 per cent of girls aren't allowed…almost two-thirds worry about leaking in class': Plan International UK (2018) *Locked Out.* [Online]. Available from: https://plan-uk.org/act-for-girls/girls-rights-in-the-uk/break-the-barriers-our-menstrual-manifesto/locked-out [Accessed 5 June 2018].

'One in three women worldwide don't have access to a safe place to go to the toilet': Unilever [no date] We can't wait, a report on sanitation and hygiene for women and girls. [Online]. Available from: https://www.unilever.com/Images/we-can-t-wait-a-report-on-sanitation-and-hygiene-for-women-and-girls-november-2013_tcm244-425178_1_en.pdf [Accessed 6 June 2018].

'up to 70 per cent of menstruators who get migraines': Cleveland Clinic (2014) Hormone headaches and menstrual migraines. [Online]. Available from: https://my.clevelandclinic.org/health/diseases/8260-hormone-headaches-and-menstrual-migraines [Accessed 5 December 2017].

'when a girl's first period is acknowledged positively or celebrated': Schooler, D. *et al* (2005) Cycles of shame: menstrual shame, body shame, and sexual decision-making, *Journal of Sex Research*, 42(4), pp. 324–334.

'have been found to have a deficiency in magnesium': Mauskop, A., Altura, B.T. and Altura, B.M. (2002) Serum ionized magnesium levels and serum ionized calcium/ionized magnesium ratios in women with menstrual migraine, *Headache*, 42(4), pp. 242–248.

'related to blood loss and low levels of iron': Calhoun, A.H. and Gill, N. (2017) Presenting a new, non-hormonally mediated cyclic headache in women: end-menstrual migraine, *Headache*, 57(1), pp. 17–20.

'endorphins are produced even in the absence of severe pain': Laatikainen, T. *et al* (1985) Plasma B-endorphin and the menstrual cycle, *Fertility and Sterility*, 44(2), pp. 206–209.

Chapter 4

'features take on a more symmetrical appearance': Scutt, D. and Manning, J.T. (1996) Symmetry and ovulation in women, *Human Reproduction*, 11(11), pp. 2477–2480.

'As oestrogen increases, your memory and mental agility will improve': Sherwin, B.B. (1994) Estrogen and cognitive functioning in women: Lessons we have learned, *Behavioural Neuroscience*, 126(1), pp. 123–127.

'high levels of oestrogen can make you more prone to injury': Yim, J., Petrofsky, J. and Lee, H. (2018) Correlation between mechanical properties of the ankle muscles and postural sway during the menstrual cycle, *The Tohoku Journal of Experimental Medicine*, 244(3), pp. 201–207.

Chapter 5

'we do walk more around ovulation': Fessler, D.M.T. (2003) No time to eat: An adaptationist account of periovulatory behavioural changes, *The Quarterly Review of Biology*, 78(1), pp. 3–21.

'features become softer and more symmetrical': Scutt, D. and Manning, J.T. (1996) Symmetry and ovulation in women, *Human Reproduction*, 11(11), pp. 2477–2480.

'around 85 per cent of women don't experience spontaneous desire…30 per cent of us rarely or never experience spontaneous desire for sex': Nagoski, E. (2014) I drew this graph about sexual desire…I think it might change your life. 16 June. *The Dirty Normal*. [Online]. Available from: https://www.thedirtynormal.com/post/2014/06/16/i-drew-this-graph-about-sexual-desire-and-i-think-it-might-change-your-life/ [Accessed 22 June 2018].

'pill users have four times the amount of SHBG': Panzer, C. *et al* (2006) Impact of oral contraceptives on sex hormone-binding globulin and androgen levels: a retrospective study in women with sexual dysfunction, *The Journal of Sexual Medicine*, 3(1), pp. 104–113.

'still hadn't returned to the baseline level': Panzer, C. *et al* (2006) Impact of oral contraceptives on sex hormone-binding globulin and androgen levels: a retrospective study in women with sexual dysfunction, *The Journal of Sexual Medicine*, 3(1), pp. 104–113.

'singletons experience a heightening of desire at ovulation more than people in long-term relationships': Caruso, S. *et al* (2014) Do hormones influence women's sex? Sexual activity over the menstrual cycle, *The Journal of Sexual Medicine*, 11(1), pp. 211–221.

'75 per cent of us will experience at some point': The American College of Obstetricians and Gynecologists (2017) *When sex is painful*. [Online]. Available from: https://www.acog.org/-/media/For-Patients/faq020.pdf [Accessed 20 September 2018].

'87 per cent of participants with IC experienced pain': Peters, K.M. *et al* (2007) Prevalence of pelvic floor dysfunction in patients with interstitial cystitis, *Urology*, 70(1), pp. 16–18.

'resulted in a 47 per cent improvement in IC symptoms': Weinstock, L.B., Klutke, C.G. and Lin, H.C. (2008) Small intestinal bacterial overgrowth in patients with interstitial cystitis and gastrointestinal symptoms, *Digestive Diseases and Sciences*, 53(5), pp. 1246–1251.

'occurs in around a third of all clinically normal menstrual cycles': Prior, J.C. *et al* (2015) Ovulation Prevalence in Women with Spontaneous Normal-Length Menstrual Cycles – A Population-Based Cohort from HUNT3, Norway, *PLoS One*, 10(8).

'Not eating enough calories': De Souza M.J. *et al* (2007) Severity of energy-related menstrual disturbances increases in proportion to indices of energy conservation in exercising women, *Fertility and* Sterility, 9788(4), pp. 971–975.

'and carbs': Chavarro, J.E. *et al* (2009) A prospective study of dietary carbohydrate quantity and quality in relation to risk of ovulatory infertility, *European Journal of Clinical Nutrition*, 63(1), pp. 78–86.

'drinking caffeinated soft drinks': Chavarro, J.E. *et al* (2009) Caffeinated and alcoholic beverage intake in relation to ovulatory disorder infertility, *Epidemiology*, 20(3), pp. 374–381.

'can suppress your appetite': Leeners, B. *et al* (2017) Ovarian hormones and obesity, *Human Reproduction Update*, 23(3), pp. 300–321.

'decreased appetite before ovulation often coincides with a peak in sexual desire': Roney, J.R. and Simmons, Z.L. (2017) Ovarian hormone fluctuations predict within-cycle shifts in women's food intake, *Hormones and Behavior*, 90, pp. 8–14.

'binge drinking is known to increase oestrogen levels': Reichmann, M.E. *et al* (1993) Effects of alcohol consumption on plasma and urinary hormone concentrations in premenopausal women, *Journal of the National Cancer Institute*, 85(9), pp. 722–727.

'sometimes testosterone and LH too': Schliep, K.C. *et al* (2015) Alcohol intake, reproductive hormones, and menstrual cycle function: a prospective cohort study, *The American Journal of Clinical Nutrition*, 102(4), pp. 933–942.

'alcohol is a depressant': Royal College of Psychiatrists (2018) *Alcohol and depression*. [Online]. Available from: https://www.rcpsych.ac.uk/healthadvice/problemsanddisorders/alcoholdepression.aspx [Accessed 2 October 2018].

'falling asleep and staying asleep': Moline, M.L., Broch, L. and Zak, R. (2004) Sleep in women across the life cycle from adulthood through menopause, *The Medical Clinics of North America*, 88, pp. 705–736.

'Summer is when you're likely to hit your PBs': Sung, E. *et al* (2014) Effects of follicular versus luteal phase-based strength training in young women, *SpringerPlus*, 3, p. 668.

'(ACL) is 4–8 times more likely to be injured now': Herzberg, S. D. *et al* (2017) The effect of menstrual cycle and contraceptives on ACL injuries and laxity: A systematic review and meta-analysis, *Orthopaedic Journal of Sports Medicine*, 5(7).

'report feeling more satisfied in their relationships': Aron, A. *et al* (2000) Couples' shared participation in novel and arousing activities and experienced relationship quality, *Journal of Personality and Social Psychology*, 78, pp. 273–284.

'couples to feel emotionally attuned': Stel, M. and Vonk, R. (2010) Mimicry in social interaction: benefits for mimickers, mimickees, and their interaction. *British Journal of Psychology*, 101(2), pp. 311–323.

Chapter 6

'your gut instinct – is astonishingly accurate 90 per cent of the time': Tsetsos, K., Chater, N. and Usher, M. (2012) Salience driven value integration explains decision biases and preference reversal, *PNAS*, 109(24), pp. 9659–9664.

'more likely to interpret other people's expressions negatively': Conway, C. *et al* (2007) Salience of emotional displays of danger and contagion in faces is enhanced when progesterone levels are raised, *Hormones and Behavior*, 51(2), pp. 202–206.

'*the lack of understanding or support, rejection, and pathologization commonly found in heterosexual women's accounts*': Ussher, J. and Perz, J. (2008) Empathy, egalitarianism and emotion work in the relational negotiation of PMS: the experience of women in lesbian relationships, *Feminism and Psychology*, 18(1), pp. 87–111.

'As oestrogen declines, so does serotonin, causing dip in mood and an increase in appetite': Dye, L. and Blundell, J.E. (1997) Menstrual cycle and appetite control: implications for weight regulation. *Human Reproduction*, 12(6) pp. 1142–1151.

'a higher intake of alcohol is associated with an increase in oestrogen': Muti, P. *et al* (1998) Alcohol consumption and total estradiol in premenopausal women, *Cancer Epidemiology, Biomarkers and Prevention*, 7(3) pp. 189–203.

'Alcohol intake is associated with an increase in premenstrual anxiety and mood changes, and smoking is associated with menstrual cramps and back pain': Gold, E. *et al* (2007) Diet and lifestyle factors associated with premenstrual symptoms in a racially diverse community sample: study of women's health across the nation (SWAN), *Journal of Women's Health*, 16(5).

'a review of 27 studies concluded that it reduces REM sleep': Ebrahim, I.O. *et al* (2013) Alcohol and sleep: effects on normal sleep, *Alcoholism, Clinical and Experimental Research*, 37(4), pp. 539–549.

'caffeine elimination is slowed in the late luteal phase': Lane, J.D. *et al* (1992) Menstrual cycle effects on caffeine elimination in the human female, *European Journal of Clinical Pharmacology*, 43(5) pp. 543–546.

'Trouble falling and/or staying asleep increases your production of the stress hormone cortisol': Vgontzas, A.N. *et al* (1998) Chronic insomnia and activity of the stress system: a preliminary system, *Journal of Psychosomatic Research*, 45(1) pp.21–31, and Vgontzas, A.N. *et al* (2001) Chronic insomnia is associated with nyctohemeral activation of the hypothalamic-pituitary-adrenal axis: clinical implications, *Journal of Clinical Endocrinology Metabolism*, 86(8) pp. 3787–3794.

'one night of interrupted sleep can mess up your blood sugar': Van den Berg, R. *et al* (2016) A single night of sleep curtailment increases plasma acylcarnitines: Novel insights in the relationship between sleep and insulin resistance, *Archives of Biochemistry and Biophysics*, Jan 1: pp. 145–151.

'sleep deprivation in the second half of your cycle increases premenstrual mood disturbances': Jehan, S. *et al* (2016) Sleep and premenstrual syndrome, *Journal of Sleep Medicine and Disorders*, 3(5).

'regular aerobic exercise greatly reduces the symptoms of PMS': Samadi, Z., Taghian, F. and Valiani, M. (2013) The effects of 8 weeks of regular aerobic exercise on the symptoms of premenstrual syndrome in non-athlete girls, *Iranian Journal of Nursing and Midwifery Research*, 18(1) pp.14–19, and Ghanbari, Z., Manshavi, F.D. and Jafarabadi, M. (2008) The effect of three months regular aerobic exercise on premenstrual syndrome, *Journal of Family and Reproductive Health*, 2(4), pp. 167–171.

'race-based discrimination and poor health outcomes that education and income do not offer protection from': Martin, N. and Montagne, R. (2017) Nothing protects black women from dying in pregnancy and childbirth, *ProPublica*. [Online]. Available from: https://www.propublica.org/article/nothing-protects-black-women-from-dying-in-pregnancy-and-childbirth [Accessed 7 July 2018].

'Black couples are twice as likely as white couples to be infertile': Chandra, A., Copen, C.E. and Stephen, E.H. (2013) Infertility and impaired fecundity in the United States, 1982–2010: Data from the National Survey of Family Growth, *National Health Statistics Reports; no. 67*. Hyattsville, MD: National Center for Health Statistics.

'Black women are more likely than white women to have unnecessary surgeries such as hysterectomies': Bower, J.K. *et al* (2009) Black-white differences in hysterectomy prevalence: The CARDIA study, *American Journal of Public Health*, 99(2), pp. 300–307.

'black women are *five* times more likely to die in the childbirth year than white women': MBRRACE-UK (2018) *Saving Lives, Improving Mothers' Care: Lessons learned to inform maternity care from the UK and Ireland Confidential Enquiries into Maternal Deaths and Morbidity 2014–16*, Oxford: National Perinatal Epidemiology Unit, University of Oxford.

'black women are twice as likely to have a stillbirth': Gray, R. *et al* (2009) Towards an understanding of variations in infant mortality rates between different ethnic groups in England and Wales, in: *Inequalities in Infant Mortality Project Briefing Paper 3*, Oxford: National Perinatal Epidemiology Unit.

'Pain is undertreated in black women': Hoffman, K.M. *et al* (2016) Racial bias in pain assessment and treatment recommendations about biological differences between blacks and whites, *PNAS*, 113(16), pp. 4296–4301.

References

'incorrectly diagnosed with pelvic inflammatory disease': Chatman, D.L. (1976) Endo-metriosis and the black woman, *The Journal of Reproductive Medicine*, 16(6), pp. 303–306.

'a belief that is unbelievably still rampant today': Hoffman, K.M. *et al* (2016) *Ibid.*

'black people receiving less pain relief than white people': Staton, L.J. *et al* (2007) When race matters: disagreement in pain perception between patients and their physicians in primary care, *Journal of the National Medical Association*, 99(5), pp. 532–538.

'analysed data from the medical records of over 900,000 children': Goyal, M.K. *et al* (2015) Racial disparities in pain management of children with appendicitis in emergency departments, *JAMA Pediatrics*, 169(11), pp. 996–1002.

'a third of Puerto Rican women being robbed of their reproductive rights': PBS [no date]. *The Puerto Rico Pill Trials*. [Online]. Available from: https://www.pbs.org/wgbh/americanexperience/features/pill-puerto-rico-pill-trials/ [Accessed 21 June 2018].

'*1978 FDA audit of a Depo-Provera trial at Emory University in Atlanta discovered the reckless disregard for the health of the 4,700 black subjects*': Roberts, D. (1997) *Killing the Black Body*. Vintage Books.

'the loss of their jobs if they did not consent': Kaufman, C.E. (2000) Reproductive control in apartheid South Africa, *Population Studies*, 54(1), pp. 105–114.

'gardening and reading both lead to decreases in cortisol': Van Den Berg, A.E. and Custers, M.H. (2011) Gardening promotes neuroendocrine and affective restoration from stress, *Journal of Health Psychology*, 16(1), pp. 3–11.

Chapter 7

'In the first two years of having periods, around half of cycles are ones where ovulation takes place': Borsos, A. *et al* (1988) Ovarian function after the menarche and hormonal contraception, *International Journal of Gynaecology and Obstetrics*, 27(2), pp. 249–253.

'75 per cent by five years, and over the following few years 80 per cent of cycles are ovulatory': Metcalf, M.G. *et al* (1983) Incidence of ovulation in the years after menarche, *Journal of Endocrinology*, 97(2), pp. 213–219.

'21 to 45 days is considered typical': World Health Organization multicenter study on menstrual and ovulatory patterns in adolescent girls. II. Longitudinal study of menstrual patterns in the early postmenarcheal period, duration of bleeding episodes and menstrual cycles. World Health Organization Task Force on Adolescent Reproductive Health, *Journal of Adolescent Health Care*, 7(4), pp. 236–244.

'can lead to low bone density in your twenties': Nose-Ogura, S. *et al* (2018) Low bone density in elite female athletes with a history of secondary amenorrhea in their teens, *Clinical Journal of Sport Medicine*.

'lost an average of 4 per cent of their spinal bone': Prior, J.C. *et al* (1994) Amenorrhea and anovulation: Risk factors for osteoporosis that precede menopause, in: Lorrain J.,

Plouffe L., Ravnikar V.A., Speroff L. and Watts N.B. (eds) *Comprehensive Management of Menopause. Clinical Perspectives in Obstetrics and Gynecology*. New York: Springer, pp. 79–96.

'one million women in Denmark': Skovlund, C.W. *et al* (2016) Association of hormonal contraception with depression, *JAMA Psychiatry*, 73(11), pp. 1154–1162.

'linked to inflammatory bowel disease': Khalili, H. *et al* (2013) Oral contraceptives, reproductive factors and risk of inflammatory bowel disease, *Gut*, 62(8), pp. 1153–1159.

'levels of SHBG still remained high': Panzer, C. *et al* (2006) Impact of oral contraceptives on sex hormone-binding globulin and androgen levels: a retrospective study in women with sexual dysfunction, *The Journal of Sexual Medicine*, 3(1), pp. 104–113.

'One study of 22 healthy women': Battaglia, C. *et al* (2011) Sexual behaviour and oral contraception: a pilot study, *The Journal of Sexual Medicine*, 9(2), pp. 550–557.

'it can also suppress ovulation in up to 85 per cent of cycles': Kailasam, C. and Cahill, D. (2008) Review of the safety, efficacy and patient acceptability of the levonorgestrel-releasing intrauterine system, *Patient Preference and Adherence*, 2, pp. 293–302.

'so far trials have been abandoned because of the unwanted side effects participants experienced': Behre, H.M. *et al* (2016) Efficacy and safety of an injectable combination hormonal contraceptive for men, *The Journal of Clinical Endocrinology and Metabolism*, 101(12), pp. 4779–4788, and, Mathew, V. and Bantwal, G. (2012) Male contraception, *Indian Journal of Endocrinology and Metabolism*, 16(6), pp. 910–917.

'an association between long-term pill use (5–10 years) and a thin uterine lining': Talukdar, N. *et al* (2012) Effect of long-term combined oral contraceptive pill use on endometrial thickness, *Obstetrics and Gynaecology*, 120 (2 Pt 1), pp. 348–354.

'the pill has a negative impact on ovarian volume and AMH': Birch Peterson, K. *et al* (2015) Ovarian reserve assessment in users of oral contraception seeking fertility advice on their reproductive lifespan, *Human reproduction*, 30(10), pp. 2364–2375.

'reduces your ability to absorb key vitamins and minerals': Palmery, M. *et al* (2013) Oral contraceptives and changes in nutritional requirements, *European Review for Medical and Pharmacological Sciences*, 17(13), pp. 1804–1813.

'in the absence of breast/chestfeeding you can ovulate as early as three weeks after giving birth': Jackson, E. and Glasier, A. (2011) Return of ovulation and menses in postpartum nonlactating women: A systematic review, *Obstetrics and Gynecology*, 117(3), pp. 657–662.

'1 in 18 new mothers develop it': Stagnaro-Green, A. (2012) Approach to the patient with postpartum thyroiditis, *The Journal of Clinical Endocrinology and Metabolism*, 97(2), pp. 334–342.

'43 per cent of cases present with only hypothyroidism': Stagnaro-Green, A. (2012) *Ibid.*

'women who develop postpartum thyroiditis have a 25–30 per cent chance of developing hypothyroidism within the following 5–10 years': Keely, E.J. (2011) Postpartum thyroiditis: An autoimmune thyroid disorder which predicts future thyroid health, *Obstetric Medicine*, 4(1), pp. 7–11.

'test positive for thyroid antibodies in the third trimester of pregnancy, 80 per cent will go on to develop postpartum thyroiditis': Prummel, M.F., and Wiersinga, W.M (2005) Thyroid peroxidase autoantibodies in euthyroid subjects, *Best Practice and Research: Clinical Endocrinology and Metababolism*,19, pp.1–15.

'Hysterectomy increases your long-term risk of vaginal prolapse and urinary incontinence': Forsgren, C. *et al* (2012) Vaginal hysterectomy and risk of pelvic organ prolapse and stress urinary incontinence surgery, *International Urogynecology Journal*, 23(1), pp. 43–48.

'Up to 45 per cent of the thyroid glands of women over sixty shows signs of hypothyroidism': Felicetta, J.V. (1987) Thyroid changes with aging: significance and management, *Geriatrics*, 42(1), pp. 86–92.

'up to 20 per cent of women over sixty have subclinical hypothyroidism': Surks, M.I. *et al* (2004) Subclinical thyroid disease: a scientific review and guidelines for diagnosis and management, *JAMA*, 291(2), pp. 228–238.

'83 per cent of women experience no mood changes…likelihood of having depression does increase in perimenopause': Cohen L.S. *et al* (2006) Risk for new onset of depression during the menopausal transition: the Harvard study of moods and cycles, *Arch Gen Psychiatry*, 63(4), pp. 385–390.

'Before I started testosterone, I had a moderate 3–5-day cycle that came with few side effects. But after 3–4 months on hormones, my period became extremely irregular, lasted up to two weeks, and caused the worse cramps I've ever experienced in my life. This continued for the six months I was on testosterone and hasn't slowed down since I had to stop hormones due to financial and insurance issues.': Bliss, C. (2018) What trans and non-binary menstruators should know about periods, *Seventeen*, 1 June 2018. [Online]. Available from: https://www.seventeen.com/health/a20963434/trans-and-non-binary-periods/ [Accessed 20 June 2018].

'The fact that an organ in your body has the ability to shed its lining every once in a while does not determine who you are as a person, or how the world should recognise you ... Your period does not define who you are.' Bliss, C. (2018) *Ibid.*

Chapter 8

'small amounts of pulses on a daily basis': Winham, D.M. and Hutchins, A.M. (2011) Perceptions of flatulence from bean consumption among adults in 3 feeding studies, *Nutrition Journal*, 10:128.

'12-year study of over 70,000 women conducted by Harvard found that consuming dairy does not reduce fracture risk': Feskanich, D. *et al* (1997) Milk, dietary calcium, and bone fractures in women: a 12-year study, *American Journal of Public Health*, 87(6), pp. 992–997.

'Low-fat and fat-free milk...reducing ovarian function': Chavarro, J.E. *et al* (2007) A prospective study of dairy foods intake and anovulatory infertility, *Human Reproduction*, 22(5), pp. 1340–1347.

'One study found that supplementing with melatonin can improve quality of sleep and period pain': Keshavarzi, F. *et al* (2018) Both melatonin and meloxicam improved sleep and pain in females with primary dysmenorrhoea – results from a double-blind cross-over intervention pilot study, *Archives of Women's Mental Health*, 21(6), pp. 601–609.

'Exposure to blue light in the evening and at night': Chang, A-M. *et al* (2015) Evening use of light-emitting eReaders negatively affects sleep, circadian timing, and next-morning alertness, *Proceedings of the National Academy of Sciences of the United States of America*, 112(4), pp. 1232–1237.

'Mobile device use is also associated with a decline in production of thyroid hormones': Mortavazi, S. *et al* (2009) Alterations in TSH and thyroid hormones following mobile phone use, *Oman Medical Journal*, 24(4), pp. 274–278.

'Turn your phone off for portions of the day (71 per cent of Britons never do this)... (a third of Britons check their phones right before going to bed)': Wakefield, J. (2018) Phone and internet use: number of mobile calls drops for first time, *BBC*, 2 August 2018. [Online]. Available from: https://www.bbc.co.uk/news/technology-45033302 [Accessed 21 August 2018].

'people with Hashimoto's test positive for gluten specific inflammatory antibodies ... test positive for the inflammatory antibodies linked to celiac disease': Jiskra, J. *et al* (2003) IgA and IgG antigliadin, IgA anti-tissue transglutaminase and antiendomysial antibodies in patients with autoimmune thyroid diseases and their relationship to thyroidal replacement therapy, *Physiological Research*, 52(1), pp. 79–88.

'that one study found that using products without phthalates, parabens and phenol': Harley, K.G. *et al* (2016) Reducing phthalate, paraben, and phenol exposure from personal care products in adolescent girls: findings from the HERMOSA intervention study, *Environmental Health Perspectives*, 124(10), pp. 1600–1607.

Chapter 9

'only 12.4 per cent of cycles are 28 days long': Vollman, R. F. (1977) *The Menstrual Cycle*, New York; Knopf, pp. 51–52.

'research shows that hospital staff take women's pain less seriously': Hoffmann, D.E. and Tarzian, A.J. (2001) The girl who cried pain: A bias against women in the treatment of pain, *The Journal of Law, Medicine and Ethics*, 29(1), pp. 13–27.

'a 2014 study investigating the incidence of depressive symptoms premenstrually': Prasad, A. *et al* (2014) Depressive symptoms and their relationship with endogenous reproductive hormones and sporadic anovulation in premenopausal women, *Annals of Epidemiology*, 24(12), pp. 920–924.

'failed to provide clear evidence in support of the existence of a specific premenstrual negative mood syndrome in the general population': Romans, S.R. *et al* (2012) Mood and the menstrual cycle: A review of prospective data studies, *Gender Medicine*, 9(5), pp. 361–384.

'PMDD is believed to be a genetic disorder…variation in their oestrogen receptor': Huo, L. *et al* (2007) Risk for premenstrual dysphoric disorder is associated with genetic variation in ESR1, the estrogen receptor alpha gene, *Biological Psychiatry*, 62(8), pp. 925–933.

'more likely to be sensitive to the effects of oestrogen and progesterone': Dubet, N. *et al* (2016) The ESC/E(Z) complex, an intrinsic cellular molecular pathway differentially responsive to ovarian steroids in premenstrual dysphoric disorder, *Molecular Psychiatry*, 22(18), pp. 1172–1184.

'As many as 84 per cent of us have primary dysmenorrhoea': Grandi, G. *et al* (2012) Prevalence of menstrual pain in young women: what is dysmenorrhoea?, *Journal of Pain Research*, 5, pp. 169–174.

'hot bath can be just as effective': Akin, M. *et al* (2004) Continuous, low-level, topical heat wrap therapy as compared to acetaminophen for primary dysmenorrhoea, *Journal of Reproductive Medicine*, 49(9), pp. 739–745.

'exercise throughout your cycle is associated with an improvement': Dehnavi, Z.M., Jafarnejad, F. and Kamali, Z. (2018) The effect of aerobic exercise on primary dysmenorrhoea: a clinical trial study, *Journal of Education and Health Promotion*, 7(3).

'Omega-3 Fatty Acids is a powerful anti-inflammatory that can outperform the use of ibuprofen in reducing period pain': Zafari, M., Behmanesh, F., and Mohammadi, A.A. (2011) Comparison of the effect of Omega-3 Fatty Acids and ibuprofen on treatment of severe pain in primary dysmenorrhoea, *Caspian Journal of Internal Medicine*, 2(3), pp. 279–282.

'data from two clinical trials concluded that it can be as effective as treatment with an NSAID': Wang, S.F., Lee, J.P. and Hwa, H.L. (2009) Effect of transcutaneous electrical nerve stimulation on primary dysmenorrhoea, *Neuromodulation*, 12 (4), pp. 302–309, and Kannan, P. and Claydon, L.S. (2014) Some physiotherapy treatments may relieve menstrual pain in women with primary dysmenorrhoea: a systematic review, *Journal of Physiotherapy*, 60(1), pp. 13–21.

'Supplementing with melatonin has been shown to reduce period pain and improve sleep': Keshavarzi, F. *et al* (2018) Both melatonin and meloxicam improved sleep and pain in females with primary dysmenorrhoea – results from a double-blind cross-over intervention pilot study, *Archives of Women's Mental Health*, 21(6), pp. 601–609.

'excision surgery performed by a highly skilled surgeon is the gold standard': Pundir, J. *et al* (2017) Laparoscopic excision versus ablation for endometriosis-associated pain: an updated systematic review and meta-analysis, *Journal of Minimally Invasive Gynecology*, 24(5), pp. 747–756.

'retrograde menstruation occurs in around 90 per cent of menstruators': Halme, J. *et al* (1984) Retrograde menstruation in healthy women and in patients with endometriosis, *Obstetrics and Gynaecology*, 64(2), pp. 151–154.

'endometriosis in 9 per cent of female foetuses': Signorile, P.G. *et al* (2009) Ectopic endometrium in human foetuses is a common event and sustains the theory of müllerianosis in the pathogenesis of endometriosis, a disease that predisposes to cancer, *Journal of Experimental and Clinical Cancer Research*, 28(1), p. 49.

'CBD oil may be a particularly helpful strategy': Bouaziz, J. *et al* (2017) The clinical significance of endocannabinoids in endometriosis pain management, *Cannabis and cannabinoid research*, 2(1), pp. 72–80.

'Low levels of vitamin D have been linked to endo': Ciavattini, A. *et al* (2017) Ovarian endometriosis and vitamin D serum levels, *Gynaecology Endocrinology*, 33(2), pp. 164–167.

'gluten-free diet for one year': Marziali, M. *et al* (2012) Gluten-free diet: a new strategy for management of painful endometriosis related symptoms? *Minerva Chirurgica*, 67(6), pp. 499–504.

'can even prevent recovery from HA': Falsetti, L. *et al* (2002) Long-term follow-up of functional hypothalamic amenorrhea and prognostic factors, *Journal of Clinical Endocrinology Metabolism*, 87(2), pp. 500–505.

'an increase in body mass index (BMI) is associated with getting your period back': Falsetti, L. *et al* (2002) Long-term follow-up of functional hypothalamic amenorrhea and prognostic factors, *Journal of Clinical Endocrinology Metabolism*, 87(2), pp. 500–505.

'an emerging consensus that the normal range should be': The Practice Committee of the American Society for Reproductive Medicine (2012) Evaluation and treatment of recurrent pregnancy loss: a committee opinion, *Fertility and Sterility*, 99(1), pp. 103–111.

'research from Norway suggests that its prevalence rate is higher': Asvold, B.O., Vatten, L.J. and Bjøro, T. (2013) Changes in the prevalence of hypothyroidism: the HUNT study in Norway, *European Journal of Endocrinology*, 169(5), pp. 613–620.

'report from Colorado found that': Canaris, G.J. *et al* (2000) The Colorado thyroid disease prevalence study, *Archives of Internal Medicine*, 160(4), pp. 526–534.

'two hours of use per day can raise TSH and lower T4': Mortavazi, S. *et al* (2009) Alterations in TSH and thyroid hormones following mobile phone use, *Oman Medical Journal*, 24(4), pp. 274–278.

References

'getting less than 6 hours' sleep is associated with a reduction in TSH and T4': Kessler, L. *et al* (2010) Changes in serum TSH and free T4 during human sleep restriction, *Sleep*, 33(8), pp. 1115–1118.

'Vitamin D deficiency is associated with an increase in thyroid antibodies': Unal, A.D. *et al* (2014) Vitamin D deficiency is related to thyroid antibodies in autoimmune thyroiditis, *Central European Journal of Immunology*, 39(4), pp. 493–497.

'Only 20–45 per cent of adolescents have ovulatory cycles in their first year of having periods': Borsos, A. *et al* (1988) *Ibid.*

'with this figure rising to 75 per cent by 5 years': Metcalf, M.G. *et al* (1983) *Ibid.*

'Using NSAIDs such as ibuprofen and mefenamic acid can reduce blood loss': Lethaby, A., Augood, C. and Duckitt, K. (2000) Nonsteroidal anti-inflammatory drugs for heavy menstrual bleeding, *The Cochrane Database of Systematic Reviews*, 2.

'von Willebrand disease … accounts for around 20 per cent of cases': Edlund, M. *et al* (1996) On the value of menorrhagia as a predictor for coagulation disorders, *American Journal of Hematology*, 53 (4), pp. 234–238. Kadir, R.A. *et al* (1998) Frequency of inherited bleeding disorders in women with menorrhagia, *Lancet*, 351(9101), pp. 485–489.

'some people who use the copper IUD': Hubacher, D., Chen, P.L. and Park, S. (2009) Side effects from the copper IUD: do they decrease over time?, *Contraception*, 79(5), pp. 356–362.

'or the Depo-Provera® shot for contraception find that they experience episodes of bleeding': Jacobstein, R. and Polis, C.B. (2014) Progestin-only contraception: injectables and implants, *Best Practice and Research. Clinical Obstetrics and Gynaecology*, 28(6), pp. 795–806.

'can reduce blood loss (by up to 90 per cent with the Mirena®)': *BMJ* (2004) 328:1199.

'Endometrial ablation, where the lining of the womb is scraped away or destroyed, results in reduced bleeding 80–90 per cent of the time…but comes with a 25–50 per cent chance of developing amenorrhoea (the loss of periods)': Royal Devon and Exeter NHS Foundation Trust (2017) *Endometrial Ablation.* [Online]. Available from: https://www.rdehospital.nhs.uk/documents/patient-information-leaflets/gynaecology/patient-information-leaflet-endometrial-ablation.pdf [Accessed 21 June 2018].

'also associated with an increased risk of miscarriage': Kohn, J.R. *et al* (2017) Pregnancy after endometrial ablation: a systematic review, *BJOG*, 125(1), pp. 43–53.

'Supplementing with iron can help to recover from heavy blood loss and prevent further excessive loss': Taymor, M.L., Sturgis, S.H. and Yahia, C. (1964) The etiological role of chronic iron deficiency in production of menorrhagia, *JAMA*, 187, pp. 323–327.

'a herb called shepherd's purse outperforms the NSAID mefenamic acid in reducing blood loss': Naafe, M. *et al* (2018) Effect of hydroalcoholic extracts of capsella bursa-pastoris on heavy menstrual bleeding: A randomized clinical trial, *Journal of Alternative and Complementary Medicine*, 24(7), pp. 694–700.

'the first half of your cycle is short (which is associated with a reduced likelihood of conceiving)': Small, C.M. *et al* (2006) menstrual cycle characteristics: associations with fertility and spontaneous abortion, *Epidemiology*, 17(1), pp. 52–60.

'linked to problems conceiving and sustaining a pregnancy': Mesen, T.B. and Young, S.L. (2015) Progesterone and the luteal phase, a requisite to reproduction, *Obstetrics and Gynecology Clinics of North America*, 42(1), pp. 135–151.

'90 per cent of people with oligomenorrhoea (irregular cycles) and amenorrhoea (no periods) go on to be diagnosed with PCOS': Allahbadia, G. and Merchant, R. (2011) Polycystic ovary syndrome and impact on health, *Middle East Fertility Society Journal*, 16(1), pp. 19–37.

'affecting up to 15 per cent of us worldwide': Ding, T. *et al* (2017) The prevalence of polycystic ovary syndrome in reproductive-aged women of different ethnicity: a systematic review and meta-analysis, *Oncotarget*, 8(56), pp. 96351–96358.

'polycystic ovaries are very common and are seen on up to 25 per cent of ovary-owners': Polson, D.W. *et al* (1988) Polycystic ovaries – a common finding in normal women, *Lancet*, 1(8590), pp. 870–872.

'it can also impair insulin resistance after just three months of taking it': Adeniji, A.A. *et al* (2016) Metabolic effects of a commonly used combined hormonal oral contraceptive in women with and without polycystic ovary syndrome, *Journal of Women's Health*, 25(6), pp. 638–645.

'strength training can improve insulin sensitivity by 24 per cent': Van Der Heijden, G.J. *et al* (2010) Strength exercise improves muscle mass and hepatic insulin sensitivity in obese youth, *Medicine and Science in Sports and Exercise*, 42(11), pp. 1973–1980.

'more common in people whose family members have them, and in those with an African ancestry': Templeman, S.F. *et al* (2009) Risk factors for surgical removed fibroids in a large cohort of teachers, *Fertility and Sterility*, 92(4), pp. 1436–1446.

'strong association between consumption of booze and fibroids': Templeman, S.F. *et al* (2009) Risk factors for surgical removed fibroids in a large cohort of teachers, *Fertility and Sterility*, 92(4), pp. 1436–1446.

Epilogue

'a 2018 report by Public Health England': Public Health England (2018) *What do women say? Reproductive health is a public health issue*: London.

ACKNOWLEDGEMENTS

Thank you to everybody at Bloomsbury: to my editor, Charlotte Croft, when we met I knew that you understood the importance of *Period Power* and that you would be as dedicated to it as I am. I'm incredibly thankful to you and Holly Jarrald for your enthusiasm and hard work, for asking *all* the questions that needed to be asked, and for not making me cut the forty thousand extra words that ended up in this book. Thank you to Katherine Macpherson and Lizzy Ewer for getting it out there in the world, to Helen Crawford-White for the perfect cover, and to Jasmine Parker for bringing my words to life with your beautiful illustrations.

Thank you to Julia Silk, my fabulous agent, it was you who told me that I had something, who pushed me to crack on when I was in the depths of motherhood and had no idea how to answer your emails let alone write a book, and you who held my hand in so many ways over the past year – and put a glass of wine in it too.

I am indebted to Alexandra Pope and Sjanie Hugo Wurlitzer for introducing me to the inner seasons of the cycle, for allowing me to use them in this book, and for your part in changing my own experience of my cycle, thank you.

My heartfelt thanks go to Jane Bennett, Layla Saad, Mars Lord, Holly Grigg-Spall, Sarah Gottesdiener, Catarina, Sandra, Natalie, Cass Bliss, and Kenny Jones for allowing me to use your words – this book is better for them. Thank you to my clients who've allowed me to use their stories anonymously. Thank you to Dr. Carrie Jones for agreeing to proofread the book and for helping me to sort out the niggles. Thank you to Ash Ambirge for coining 'The Cycle Strategy', and to Jen Sincero for your goat story.

Thank you to my friends and teachers who have inspired, challenged and educated me: Christine Hall, Hilary Lewin, Rosita Arvigo, Diane Macdonald, Nicole Jardim, Jessica Drummond, Giusi Pezzotta, Jani White, Martin Benwell, Kim Wager, Ian Appleyard, Nicola Goodall, Kicki Hansard, Naomi Absalom, and Michaela Christmann. Thank you to Reina James for your wisdom and gentle guidance, for helping me to know myself and my place in the world. Lisa Lister, for telling me that the world needs my medicine – the words that kept me going through it all. Thank you, Jason Stein, for repeatedly telling me to write, and to everyone in the Heart Crew for holding me as I figured it all out. Pippa Wright and Brigid Moss, your early interest and encouragement was what initiated this whole process, thank you. To Sophie Heawood for quoting me. And to my junior school teacher, Mrs Thompson, who told me that I could write and that I should.

Thank you to Amy Redmond and Anna Jones, my most fervent supporters, for your belief in me and this work and your eagerness to shout about it. Thank you to every single woman who has shared their experiences with me, whether it's been in my treatment room, the labour ward, on one of my workshops, or on a bus, thank you for that privilege.

To my friends: Holly Barringer, Ainslie McLennan, Charlotte Frische, Sharmin and Fergus Jackson, Anna Batchelor, Samantha Holmes, Andy Allen, and Nikole Lowe. Thank you to the women of Margate for all your encouragement, particularly Gemma Pearson, Catherine Dawson, Anna Fewster, Cynthia Lawrence John, Jenefer Odell, and Rosie Ray. To everyone in The Rabbit Hole, thank you for giving me a place to rage and celebrate, and for all your support as I negotiated work and motherhood. Rebecca Schiller, thank you for showing me that it could be done, for telling me I needed an agent, introducing me to Julia, and for doula-ing me through the deadlines. Thank you to Boe and Henry at Mar Mar, your coffee and croissants fuelled this book and your stunning plants aided the process too. Thank you to Richard and Craig for being such awesome neighbours, for all the moments of peace you gave me, and for feigning interest in vaginas. Thank you to Paula Toogood and everyone at Space for Play for taking such good care of Nelson, this book would not have been possible without you.

Natalie and Christos Georgas, thank you for your generosity and support. Nat, you picked me up when I was collapsing and always knew how to get me going again, you have saved me on an almost daily basis and I am eternally grateful for your friendship.

Octavia Bright, like a sea goddess sent to help me, you arrived in Margate as I started writing and left as I came to the end. When I found myself in turbulent waters, you were there to either smooth them or get me to dig deeper. I hope that as you read this book you'll feel the marks of our conversations. Thank you.

Thank you, Mum, for your love and belief in me – everything in this book came from you. Sam, there aren't enough words to describe what you mean to me, I'm proud to call you my brother and my friend and I'm grateful for all the ways in which you have helped me and for how you continue to inspire me. Thank you to my son Nelson, your arrival in the world made me want to be better, and so much of this book was written in my head on the many, many occasions when I was up feeding you in the night. And finally, thank you to Paul, for your love and belief in me, for being my safe place, for all the things you've done so that I could achieve my dream, for letting me go to do it and for still being there when it was done. You are my favourite human.

INDEX

acne   174, 183, 223, 238, 245, 248
acupuncture   65, 105, 107, 160, 173, 262, 280, 290, 310
adenomyosis   83, 286–7
adrenal dysfunction   164–6, 200–1
adrenal glands   30, 160, 260–1, 294, 302, 303, 306, 307
adrenaline   30, 160–1
aerobic exercise   132, 151
ageing   42, 160, 300, 302
   see also menopause; perimenopause; post-menopause
alcohol   107, 125, 131, 141, 149–50, 257, 310
amenorrhoea   104–6, 183–4, 206, 243, 249, 262, 287–8, 297, 300
'amplification' strategy   118
ampulla   24
anaemia   97, 295, 297, 298
anaerobic exercise   102–3
androgens   301–4, 306, 307
androstenedione   302, 303, 306
anger   152–8
anovulation   129, 170, 171–2, 202, 296, 299, 300
anti-depressants   116–17, 125, 130, 220, 276
antibiotics   41, 129, 227, 229–30, 255
anxiety   28, 63, 103, 116, 117, 149, 208, 220, 223, 238, 248, 263
   see also premenstrual dysphoric disorder (PMDD); premenstrual syndrome (PMS)
appetite   45, 47, 112, 130, 149
apps, phone   54, 212
Arvigo Techniques of Maya Abdominal Therapy (ATMAT)   23, 160, 191, 204–5, 272, 280, 290, 308, 310
Asherman's syndrome   287
atresia   25, 202
autoimmune paleo protocol   221–2
Autumn phase (luteal phase) see luteal phase (Autumn)

bacteria, healthy see gut health; microbiome; vaginal microbiome
bacterial vaginosis (BV)   40–1
Bartholin's glands   17
basal body temperature (BBT)   33–4, 35, 45, 63, 83, 128, 160, 172, 191, 295, 299, 300
bioidentical hormones   65, 207–8
birth control pills, hormonal   2, 15, 35, 45, 123–4, 156, 158, 159, 173–4, 176–84, 278, 284, 286, 288, 297, 304–5, 309
birth, giving   21–2, 194, 227–8
Bisphenol A (BPA)   170, 204, 266
Black, Indigenous and People of Colour (BIPOC)   154–8, 182–3
Blackwell, Dr Anona   41
bladder   23, 127–8, 230, 282
   weakness   89, 204
bleeding, abnormal uterine   204–5
Bliss, Cass   210–11, 212
blood sugar levels   45, 130, 149, 150, 161, 166, 198, 201, 242, 243–4, 252, 254, 258, 262, 305, 307
blue light   163, 166, 263–4
bone density   28, 174, 178, 180, 254
bowel movements   32, 131, 239–40, 278
   see also constipation
brain fog   145, 201, 206, 220
breakfast, what to eat for   242–3
breast cancer   108, 170, 179, 232
breastfeeding/chestfeeding   19, 125, 196, 228
Burke, Tarana   157

caesarean births   41, 83, 227–8, 286
caffeine   150, 163, 166
cancer   44, 108, 170, 177, 179–80, 232, 288, 308
Candida albicans   40
cannabidiol oil (CBD)   281, 285
carbohydrates   252
castor oil packs, abdominal   83–5, 307, 310

Index

Index

Sjogren's syndrome   19
Skene's glands   17
skin conditions   88, 174, 183, 220, 223, 238, 245, 248, 301, 302, 306
sleep   44, 47, 131, 141, 150, 159, 162, 163, 164, 177, 202, 219, 221, 229, 259–63, 294
small intestine bacterial overgrowth (SIBO)   128, 230–2
smoking   24, 41, 201, 279
Soft Cups   81
solvents   267
sperm   21, 24, 37, 178, 188
spotting   32, 38, 129, 192, 204, 270
Spring phase (follicular phase) see follicular phase (Spring)
Steinem, Gloria   8
stress   30, 124, 127, 160–7, 208, 229, 260–1, 294, 307
   see also anger; cortisol; premenstrual dysphoric disorder (PMDD); premenstrual syndrome (PMS)
sugars   253–4, 303
Summer phase (follicular phase) see follicular phase (Summer)
supplements, dietary   105, 107, 116, 160, 173, 174, 221, 249, 277, 279–80, 286, 290, 298, 303, 307, 310
surfactants   266–7
surgical menopause   205–6
sympto-thermal method   34–5

tampons   6, 7, 42, 87–8, 90, 211
teenage periods   169–77, 179, 295–6, 305
temperature changes   8, 33–4, 35, 45, 63, 83, 128, 160, 172, 191, 295, 299, 300
TENS devices   281
terminations   41, 83, 286
testosterone   25, 28, 43, 95, 111, 115, 120, 123–4, 131, 180, 204, 209–10, 211, 237, 245, 289, 302, 304, 306
thrush   40
thyroid function   289, 290–1, 308
thyroid glands   30, 34, 180, 198–200, 206–7, 258, 287
thyroid hormone binding globulin (THBG)   180

thyroid hormones - TSH, T3 and T4 264
thyroid-stimulating hormone (TSH)   289, 290–1
tiredness/fatigue   58, 63, 68, 96, 97, 125, 131, 149, 199, 201, 214, 220–1, 238, 244, 252, 255, 282, 292, 293, 295
   see also energy levels; resting and menstruation; sleep
tone policing   154–5
trans fats   249
transgender people   209–12
transition days   58–60, 93–4, 111–12, 135–6
trichomoniasis 'trich'   41
Trump, Donald   6

urethra   13, 17
urinary tract infections   229–30
uterine cycle   30
uterus (womb)   11, 13, 19, 20, 21, 22–3, 30, 45, 205, 286, 287, 309

vaginal dryness   16, 19, 42, 106, 196
vaginal microbiome   20, 40–1, 87, 268–9
vaginal opening   17–18
vaginal ring, contraceptive   15
vaginal wall   17
vaginas   13, 19–20
vaginismus   127
veganism/vegetarianism   257–8, 295
vegetables   245–6
vitamin D   285, 294
von Willebrand disease   296
vulva   13
vulvodynia   90, 127, 222
vulval vestibule   17

water   252
   see also dehydration/hydration
weight, body   161, 200, 206, 220, 229, 244–5, 255, 289, 303, 306, 307
Winter phase (menstruation) see periods/menstruation (Winter)
womb (uterus) see uterus (womb)
womb lining   22–3, 24, 36, 45
   see also endometrium
work and periods   74–5, 114–15, 118–20